# Toward a Science of Clinical Psychology: Laboratory Evaluations and Interventions

# Toward a Science of Clinical Psychology: Laboratory Evaluations and Interventions

Luciano L'Abate
Editor

**Nova Science Publishers, Inc.**
*New York*

For permission to use material from this book please contact us:
Telephone 631-231-7269; Fax 631-231-8175
Web Site: http://www.novapublishers.com



**LIBRARY OF CONGRESS CATALOGING-IN-PUBLICATION DATA**

Toward a science of clinical psychology : laboratory evaluations and interventions / Luciano L'Abate, editor.
p. ; cm.
Includes bibliographical references and index.
ISBN 978-1-60456-062-6
1. Clinical psychology--Standards. 2. Diagnosis, Laboratory. I. L'Abate, Luciano, 1928-
[DNLM: 1. Psychology, Clinical--standards. 2. Evidence-Based Medicine. 3. Mental Disorders--diagnosis. 4. Mental Disorders--therapy. WM 105 T737 2007]
RC467.T69 2007
616.89--dc22 2007046667

*Published by Nova Science Publishers, Inc. ✢ New York*

*To future clinical psychologists who, in dealing with complex human relationships, may learn to practice more as compassionate scientists than as impressionable artists*

# CONTENTS

# FOREWORD

This edited volume by Dr. Luciano L'Abate is a major contribution to the literature addressing the link between clinical research and clinical practice. When we currently think of clinical evidence, we tend to think in terms of randomized clinical trials — a methodology that seeks to determine if a therapeutic approach works. These trials have certainly been important in answering questions about if a treatment works and, to some extent, for whom it works. However, these designs provide much less information about the theoretical mechanisms of treatment — why or how an intervention works. The aim of this volume is to present various types of methodologies that pair clinical research and practice.

This emphasis on gathering evidence to support our clinical practice has been part of clinical psychology for over 50 years. It was following the conference held in 1949 at the University of Colorado in Boulder, in the United States of America, that there was endorsement of a training model outlining that clinical psychologists should be trained as research scientists. As well as the skills necessary for clinical practice, obtaining a research degree, namely the Ph.D, was considered essential to prepare psychologists for dual career roles – as both practitioners that can evaluate research, and as active scientists that can carry out research and contribute to the literature. This model has been termed the scientist-practitioner model.

A few years later, a "single case" research model, conceptualizing good clinical practice as applied science became prominent in the United Kingdom. Through the manipulation of hypothesized variables and carefully monitoring their effects on baseline measures of a problem, the practitioner could ascertain the effectiveness of an intervention. Echoing the early writings by Wundt, clinical practice was considered analogous to conducting an experiment in which there was a single subject, and there was an immediate need to ensure that assessments were individually tailored.

By the time of the next major American conference on training, this time in Vail, Colorado, the assumption that there was insufficient firm knowledge to allow practitioners to generate evidence-based solutions to practical problems was disputed. The Vail model emphasized professional training, endorsed the newly emerging qualification, the Doctor of Psychology (PsyD), and suggested that there is no need to train practitioners in methodologies for conducting science, and conceptualized training as preparing professionals to be consumers of science.

This historical context has resulted in two ways in which practitioners can use evidence for practice. One way entails the systematic gathering of data to document client progress, and to be able to adjust treatment plans according to data on client change. The other way is to base one's practice on procedures and principles that have been shown to be effective in other settings and in the hands of other practitioners. The two ways are not incompatible, but in recent years there has been a particular emphasis on the second strategy: the implementation of validated procedures, and there is now a division between research and practice.

The distance between research and practice is also apparent when one examines the methods sections of published studies of psychotherapy. Only a minority of published studies outline methodologies are representative of the fluid and intricate nature of clinical practice. There has been an attempt to label research as either "effectiveness" (methods reflective of clinical practice) or "efficacy" (tightly controlled methods), but the reality is that most studies exist on the continuum between these two extremes. In the application of evidence, the practitioner must go beyond the narrow confines of 'efficacious' systematic treatment selection, and draw upon theory in order to develop a clear understanding of the patient and to be able to construct a realistic treatment plan. Clearly, there is need for a stronger relationship between underlying philosophy and theory, clinical research, and clinical practice.

Through his own work with patients, research, and writing, Dr. L'Abate has been able to appreciate the obstacles and complexities in pairing research and practice. Instead of yielding to these challenges, Dr. L'Abate has edited this volume to utilize the laboratory method as a framework for making clinical psychology accountable for its practices, facilitating the refinement and development of low-cost procedures in evaluation and intervention. Specifically, the objectives were to bridge the distance between research and practice, with the expressed intent of developing new methods to address the growing number of mental health concerns influencing the population, and provide some clarity to the increasingly complex literature on assessment and treatment. The integration of theory, clinical experience, research throughout this book models the joining of these aspects of clinical science. Dr. L'Abate, and the contributors to this volume share an optimistic view that the practitioners and their managers can use standard, uniformly replicable methods and practices.

It has been a privilege to have this opportunity to read and comment on a volume with such ambitious objectives. It has also been an honor to collaborate with Dr. L'Abate on various projects surrounding the utilization of between-session (homework) tasks to enhance patient progress towards their therapeutic goals. Thus, it also gives me great pleasure to see our work placed within the broader context of current developments in clinical psychology. I join with Dr. L'Abate and his contributors in calling for a greater connection between theory, research, and practice – as we facilitate the evolving science of clinical psychology.

Nikolaos Kazantzis, Ph.D.

# PREFACE

The aim of this edited work is to put under one cover various types of laboratory practices that pair clinical practice with research using standard operating procedures (SOPs) in evaluations and in interventions. Again and again in most clinical psychology texts research and practice are treated separately, even though the laboratory method, practiced years ago in neuro-psychology by Ralph Reitan and by a few neuro-psychologists, is now practiced in quite a few settings, as, for instance, in many college and university centers. In spite of its use in various settings around the world, there is no way of knowing who is using this method unless attention to it is brought about by an integrating text such as this one.

The Internet has changed the way psychological evaluations and interventions are going to be delivered in the not too distant future. The chaotic nature of evaluations and interventions in face-to-face practices (thousands of tests and 400+ different psychotherapies?) will become even more chaotic when practiced online. It is important, therefore, to rely more and more on standardized, uniform practices, SOPs that will assure that those practices go hand in hand with research. Rather than research and practice going along two separate tracks, as it has happened in the past and it is still happening in the present, the laboratory method (LM) would allow for both practice and research to go along the same track, a monorail, so to speak, hand in hand rather then separately, as practiced by this writer years ago.

## PLAN OF THE BOOK

In the introductory Chapter 1, L'Abate expands on what characteristics compose the LM and why it is important to include standard, uniformly replicable procedures in evaluation and interventions, possibly in the hands of professionals as well as of middle-level semi-professionals and paraprofessionals, equipment, computers and the Internet. There are at least three reasons why the LM is needed in clinical practices: (1) bridge the considerable gap existing between practitioners and researchers, and (2) deal with the multitude of growing mental health problems facing our Nation, and (3) introduce some systematic order in a bewildering array of tests and interventions in clinical psychology.

Section I includes two contributions about the LM in the evaluation and treatment of children and their families. In Chapter 2 Eleonora Maino reviews the main assessments methods for children with disabilities – used in Italy and abroad with a focus on the assessment and diagnostic procedures carried out by the Rehabilitation Center at "La Nostra Famiglia" in Northern Italy. This Rehabilitation Center is a facility for children and adolescents (age range: 0-18 years) with organic pathologies (genetic diseases, rare syndromes, mental retardation, neuromotor pathologies, head injury and child brain tumors) or with psychopathology. This chapter describes the different assessment protocols used in the Rehabilitation Center and the multidisciplinary work of practitioners with different backgrounds and skills which allow to obtain an accurate picture of the abilities and deficits of the children and their families for timely and cost-effective rehabilitation planning.

In Chapter 3 Andrea M. Chronis and Tana L. Clarke introduce an integrated treatment for depressed mothers of children with ADHD developing and evaluating an integrated cognitive-behavioral intervention for depressed mothers of children with ADHD. They summarize a number of pilot studies that show that this topic is important to pursue, namely because: (1) maternal depression predicts the developmental course of conduct problems in children with ADHD and (2) because maternal depression predicts suboptimal treatment outcomes for children with ADHD. This intervention involves skills training--behavioral parenting skills and cognitive-behavioral skills to manage depression.

Section II is devoted to the LM in prevention using psycho-social-educational skills training programs.

In Chapter 4 Douglas W. Nangle, Erika Carpenter Rich, Elizabeth J. Shepherd, and Jessica Fales look at the evolution of a social-skills intervention for at-risk preschoolers in an applied setting because the preschool period is an opportune time for social-skills intervention. Children's social knowledge is still emerging and peer status has not yet crystallized. Nonetheless, intervention research has focused more on elementary-aged children and relatively few studies have targeted preschoolers. After a literature review, this chapter describes the research team's ongoing collaborative relationship with a large community agency coordinating more than 20 Head Start classrooms in Eastern Maine. A series of intervention studies will be presented along with a discussion of the challenges posed by the applied setting and future directions.

In Chapter 5, Raymond G. Miltenberger focuses on teaching safety skills to children from the viewpoint of important issues in training and generalization. Safety skills are a specific type of social skill that involves behavioral skills training and strategies for promoting generalization of those skills.

In Chapter 6, Pamela Orpinas, Katherine Raczynski, and Arthur (Andy) Horne review the use social skills training to reduce bullying and aggression in schools. A number of social skills training programs have been developed to address the problem of bullying and aggression in schools. These programs have demonstrate varying degrees of impact and effectiveness. This chapter provides a brief overview of the extent of the problem of aggression in schools, followed by a review of prevention programs that have been developed. The final portion of the chapter addresses the difficulty of implementing manualized approaches to reducing aggression and bullying provide recommendations for steps and procedures for more effective program implementation.

In Chapter 7, Douglas C. Smith tackles the topic of social emotional literacy (SEL) which encompasses not only social skills training in the traditional sense but other aspects of social and emotional competence such as anger management, impulse control, interpersonal problem solving, etc. The SEL framework might provide a nice umbrella for a section focusing on children and adolescents with some of the topics listed being. There are a number of empirically validated SEL programs that tend to be school-based that are comprehensive in the sense that they often include family interventions as well. Typically, these programs target children and youth from primary through secondary grade levels. This chapter provides an overview of school-based approaches to social skills development and review a sample of SEL interventions that have empirical support.

Section III is devoted to the LM in psychotherapy through manualized and structured treatments.

In Chapter 8, William C. Sanderson, Simon Rego, and Katherine Muller review the history and development of manualized treatments in psychotherapy: (1) historically, the late Gerald Klerman, MD, who was at NIMH at the time, is credited with moving psychotherapy research in this direction), (2) a broad overview about the science generated from the use of manuals in psychotherapy research because a literature review would be too extensive; and (3) the use of manuals in clinical practice and clinician's feelings about evidence-based manuals and their relevance to clinical practice.

In Chapter 9, T. Mark Harwood and Larry E. Beutler inspect the varieties of research-based practice. The proponents of common factors treatment models have generally neglected to appreciate the complexity of psychotherapy process and have tended to employ simplistic statistical models in their research. These authors present research findings that illustrate the complexity of the psychotherapy process (e.g., ATIs) and demonstrate how these treatment elements interact in various ways with patient attributes. Additionally, this chapter discusses the development and application of a manualized and flexible patient-treatment matching model and a computer-driven system of patient-treatment matching.

In Chapter 10, Michael Lambert and Jason Whipple use outcome measurement and research based on algorithms to improve clinical practice. Of course, it is hard to put this research in a category because it includes both evaluation and intervention. Participants fill out a pre-therapy measure as well as at every subsequent session. These authors have empirically derived algorithms that are applied during the process of psychotherapy with a feedback of this information to therapists and patients. Participants are also asked to take an additional measure if they are not making adequate therapeutic progress. These measures are used as part of decision making about the failing case. Outcome studies show fairly dramatic improvements in participant treatment response. Thus, this approach involves both interventions in the form of feedback and reliance on evaluations.

In Chapter 11 Terry McClanahan showcases his cognitive treatment of chronic pain. The assessment consists of a standardized clinical interview, along with the Beck Depression Inventory, BAI, and Pain Outcomes Questionnaire, The treatment is a 9 week group format and is very much manualized with a participant workbook. The nine sessions cover: (1) biopsychosocial model of chronic pain, (2) sleep hygiene & neurophysiology, (3) medications, addiction v. dependence, (4) 3 ps of chronic pain (pacing, prioritizing, planning), (5, 6, & 7) cognitive behavioral therapy and chronic pain, (8) communication skills, (9) treatment review and treatment planning. There is also a booster session at 4 week post- treatment. Outcome data indicate that the program produces significant changes in the attitudes and behaviors of participants.

In Chapter 12 Mary McMurran reviews her extensive research about treatments for people with personality difficulties. This chapter includes: Stop & Think!, a social problem solving therapy for people with personality disorder/difficulties, and 2. COVAID, Control of Violence for Angry Impulsive Drinkers. Stop & Think is better evaluated, but there is still work to do on the manuals; COVAID manuals are in good shape, but the evaluation data are limited.

In Chapter 13, Roland A. Carlstedt summarises the results of integrative evidence-based clinical psychology. A field-tested protocol incorporates psychophysiological monitoring and outcome measures. In addition, qEEG normative databases are used to guide treatment of certain disorders (ADD) as well chart the course of psychopharmacological interventions by routinely monitoring all psychotherapy sessions using heart rate variability analyses and monitoring devices in-the-field to help anxiety/phobia participants. In the context of addiction/weight loss and depression exercise is also used as an adjunct treatment.

Section IV is devoted to miscellaneous laboratory methods that could not be classified otherwise.

In Chapter 14, Anthony Chambers and Jay Lebow consider common and unique factors in assessing African American couples. They discuss how assessing African American couples shows both similar and different factors than those found in assessing Caucasian couples. This topic has emerged as being of greatest interest given its crucial importance in the world of couple/family therapy.

In Chapter 15, Patrick W. Corrigan, Jennifer Rafacz, and Abigail Wassel review evidence-based treatments in psychiatric rehabilitation. Consensus of interdisciplinary panels has identified seven interventions as evidence-based that include: (1) strategic administration of psychoactive medications; (2) assertive community treatment that helps people live independently in their communities; (3) supported employment and education to help people achieve vocational goals; (4) Supported Education (SEd), (5) family therapies that teach better management skills for all relevant people in the family; (6) integrated treatment for people with dual disabilities (psychiatric and substance induced); and (7) illness management and recovery (largely cognitive strategies that help the person manage disability-related symptoms). Current research is determining whether other treatments meet evidence-based criteria. These criteria include consumer operated services and faith-based initiatives. Important in this stage of development is identifying strategies that facilitate the dissemination and subsequent use of these treatments.

In Chapter 16 Max M. North, Sarah North, and Chad B. Burwick review the evolution of Virtual Reality Therapy (VRT). Their chapter covers the historical development and recent research for various applications of VRT to phobias and related anxieties. In Chapter 17. Piero De Giacomo, Andrea De Giacomo, Francesco Margari, Rita Marcellis, and Wanda Santamato review the use of methodology online psychotherapy with functional and dysfunctional populations. In Chapter 18, Mario Cusinato and Walter Colesso administered a laboratory task to evaluate the validity of a likeness model derived from relational competence theory. Results supported applications of this task to functional and dysfunctional participants for therapeutic purposes

In Section V the conclusive Chapter 19, L'Abate discusses the implications of the LM involving: (1) working at a distance from participants through a hierarchy of personnel and instrumentation; (2) using various types of distance writing and the nonverbal medium, (3) evaluated through objective test batteries or interventions; and (4) administered by middle-level semi-professionals or para-professionals, or through mechanical devices, such as computers and the Internet. He suggests a sieves or stages model of psychotherapy that includes recent advances in distance writing, homework assignments, and low-cost approaches to promote physical and mental health.

Appendix A includes a proposal for a graduate degree for structured interventions online that includes a two-year curriculum for a certificate or master degree program.

## Intended Audiences for this Book

There are at least three major audiences that hopefully could profit by reading this book: (1) our primary audience would include clinical psychologists in private or independent practice who would like to bridge the existing gap between clinical psychology as a profession and clinical psychology as a science; (2) academic clinical psychologists who might tend to view clinical psychology more as a science rather than as a profession; and (3) the students in graduate clinical psychology programs who are looking at reconciling diverse, conflicting, and often times confusing ideologies and value systems existing among their academic teachers and their clinical supervisors. It would be delightful, of course, if other mental health professionals in related disciplines were to consult the contents of this volume to improve their own practices.

Luciano L'Abate<br>
*Atlanta, GA*<br>
*July 21$^{th}$, 2007*

In: Toward a Science of Clinical Psychology
Editor: Luciano L'Abate, pp. 1-34
ISBN: 978-1-60456-062-6


*Chapter I*

# WHAT IS THE LABORATORY METHOD IN CLINICAL PSYCHOLOGY?

***Luciano L'Abate***

## ABSTRACT

The aim of this edited volume is to gather under one cover various types of laboratory practices that pair clinical practice with research using standard operating procedures (SOPs) in evaluations and interventions. The laboratory method (LM) in clinical psychology, therefore, means the use of SOPs in both evaluation and interventions. Standard means uniformity in operations that are replicable in both evaluations and interventions. Uniformity of operations assures replicability, which is a desideratum of any science. Without replicability there is no assurance that any operation (evaluation or intervention) can be repeated within the same professional, among professionals, and among curative (clinics, hospitals) or punitive (prisons) or even private practice settings. Without replicability we will never know whether our evaluations and interventions are valid and reliable. Without replicability the profession of clinical psychology will not able to account for its practices. As Lilienfeld, Fowler, Lohr, and Lynn (2005) commented on this issue: "....the field of clinical psychology has for too long neglected a problem that now has come home to roost: the burgeoning industry of pseudoscientific and unscientific psychotherapies" (p. 187)."Kendall (2006) in his introduction to a whole issue dedicated to the present status and future of clinical psychology commented: "...clinical psychology is nevertheless struggling with the inherence differences between our science side and our professional side" (p. 203).

## CHARACTERISTICS OF THE LABORATORY METHOD

There are at least four characteristics that describe the LM in clinical psychology. The LM is: (1) systematic; (2) replicable; (3) progressive; and (4) requiring a hierarchy of personnel or instruments. Of course, these characteristics are not free from controversies which, although important, would take this chapter away from its primary focus (Gelso, 1985; Heppner & Anderson, 1985; Howard, 1985a, 1985b, 1985c; Keeney & Morris, 1985; Kiesler, 1994; Stricker, 1992).

## The Laboratory Method is Systematic

A method means a thought-out combination of various tasks or a sequence or series of steps that follow some kind of rational or empirical system. This combination or sequence is used to develop ways and means to duplicate whatever is performed by practitioners and by participants. Sometimes the combination or sequence is performed by semi- or non-professionals using specialized instruments under the supervision of a professional. Evaluations, for instance, consist of a combination of various tests, while interventions are structured according to a sequence or series of predetermined steps or tasks. These tasks are usually prescribed in writing rather than verbally (exercises, homework assignments, handouts, worksheets, practice exercises, protocols, workbooks, etc.) making them replicable, as in the case of many psychosocial skills training programs, as well as in some cases in psychotherapy with manuals for specific clinical conditions. Some thought and some evidence has been given beforehand to provide the very best possible evaluation and treatment for whatever target (population, syndrome, condition, disorder or symptom) needs to be changed for the better. Standardization of evaluations and of interventions might link clinical practice with research in ways that are not possible otherwise.

## The Laboratory Method is Replicable

Replicability is the cornerstone of the scientific method (Hayes, Follette, Dawes, & Grady, 1995). Most standard, objective, self-report, paper-and-pencil psychological tests are by definition replicable because they are printed and require writing on the part of participants or examiners. However, the psychotherapeutic community tends to avoid the use of objective tests in evaluation and tends to use the very subjective, talk-based (tb) interview instead, go figure! Without this quality of replicability, there may exist artistic and religious beliefs and practices that could produce some healing in some people. However, these beliefs or practices based on personal beliefs and intuitive gimmicks will not produce progress in the practice and science of clinical psychology. When practices are based on faith, and on a host of uncontrolled placebo effects that are difficult to identify, these effects lead to a chaotic state of affairs in both evaluations and interventions. The fact that most tests are structured to require writing, either on the part of participants or on the part of examiners, for instance, will determine how responses will be evaluated and converted into single scores, profiles, and recommendations for treatment. However, there is no way of knowing whether the recommended treatment follows from the original evaluation as long as interventions are based on face-to-face (f2f) talk, as in many preventive and psychotherapeutic practices (L'Abate, 2006, 2007d).

Dealing with interventions, either in health promotion, illness prevention, treatment, or rehabilitation, requires replicability in items, instructions, questions, tasks, exercises, or homework assignments that can be replicated only when the required tasks are reproducible in writing. Progress in science, business, government, medicine, or law is not based on the spoken word. It is based on the written word. Skyscrapers are not built on the basis of words. They are based a blueprints that are the outcome of architectural design and engineering calculations. This is why, for instance, enrichment programs for couples and families were originally written *verbatim* to assure replicability of operations (L'Abate & Weinstein, 1987; L'Abate & Young, 1987). This replicability is now present in manuals, that, however, are still based, at least in part, on the spoken word of both professionals and participants (LeCroy, 1994; Van Hasselt & Hersen, 1996), essentially maintaining and propagating the status quo in psychotherapy (L'Abate, 2005). As long as talk remains the major or only vehicle of communication and healing, it will be difficult if not impossible to replicate operations and obtain valid and reliable results. Replicability is assured only by research grants to few worthy academics but will not be available to the clinical, practicing profession of clinical psychology at large. Hence, the existing gap between clinicians/ practitioners and academics/ researchers would grow even wider, as mentioned below.

Without replicability there is no accountability because when operations are not standard and replicable there is no way of knowing what factor or combination of factors is responsible for whatever results one may obtain, either in evaluations or in interventions.

## The Laboratory Method is Progressively Cumulative

Because of its systematic replicability that allows *accumulation of information*, the LM can assure progress and advancement in how more people who need help will be reached and helped in the future. As mentioned above and in previous writings (L'Abate, 2003c, 2004c; 2005, 2006a, 2007a; 2007b, 2007d), and repeatedly here, as long as talk remains the major if only vehicle of communication and healing, there will not be progress in clinical psychological and psychotherapeutic practices. As long as clinical, psychological practices are viewed as an art or a religion strictly on faith and considered as "private," progress will be very slow and difficult. There is no progress if clinical practices are left solely to whims and wills of individual practitioners. Consequently, there will not be accumulation of information and of knowledge, since this information is kept strictly within the individual practitioner's mind and experience and nowhere else. Furthermore, if such information is not evaluated externally by others, how is one to know whether it is valid and reliable? Without accumulation of knowledge progress is not going to occur and, if it does, it will be slow and arduous. It will remain "private" and "independent" from external examination. Therefore, this process would not contribute to the accumulation of knowledge available to improve both professional practices and help participants.

## The Laboratory Method uses a Hierarchy of Intermediary Personnel and Instruments

Laboratory evaluations and interventions imply that different levels of education and training will be necessary to assure that these levels perform different operations to obtain maximum cost-effectiveness and objectivity in producing results. Why should doctorate level professionals spend time to perform repetitive tasks that can and should performed by personnel with baccalaureate or master degrees? This point will be elaborated later in this chapter. The criterion of cost-effectiveness in clinical procedures suggests a functional division of labor expanded even further in Chapter 19 of this volume. Laboratory procedures can be administered by paraprofessional, technical-level intermediaries with a college degree and personal qualities (warmth, regard, and empathy), who are directed and supervised by a full-fledged clinical psychologist at the doctorate+ level. Hence, in this hierarchy, professionals work at a distance from participants, often times without ever seeing them face-to-face (f2f) but through a structure that is already present in medical and legal professions. Some para-professionals acting as intermediaries between participants and supervising professionals, however, have been replaced by computers, the Internet, and standard equipment, as shown in various chapters of this volume.

A hierarchy of intermediary personnel does not apply only to the human realm. Clinical psychologists are relying more and more on other modalities of intervention, such as computers, equipments, instruments, and mechanical devises to perform services once administered by psychologists themselves. A prime example of mechanical intermediaries, among others, can be found in Virtual Reality Therapy (Chapter 16 this volume), where treatment is performed by an instrument rather than by the professional. Another example can be found in distance writing performed away from the therapist's presence, as discussed in Chapter 19 this volume. Even more preposterously, the beginning of treatment could start with a dictionary (L'Abate, 2007a, 2007c, 2007d).

## WHY THE LABORATORY METHOD (LM)?

The LM aims to bridge the considerably wide gap that exists between clinicians/practitioners versus academic researchers, as acknowledged in a variety of sources, a few among many (Lilienfeld, Fowler, Lohr, & Lynn, 2005; Persons, 1995) and especially in psychotherapy (Elliott & Bradley, 1994; Stiles, 1994). First, the LM is one way to cope with the chaotic state of affairs in psychological evaluations, especially in the number of existing tests, which is grown to uncontrollable extremes. There are more tests than there are conditions to evaluate not only for individuals but also for couples and for families, as discussed below. Second, the LM is one way to systematize and evaluate the incredible number of structured interventions and unstructured psychotherapies available on the market. According to some sources, there are at least 400 types of psychotherapies existing on the market place of psychotherapy (Bergin & Garfield, 1994).The foregoing estimate does not consider and count the possibility that there are as many psychotherapies as there are psychotherapists, as long as talk is the norm for psychological interventions. Third, therapists practicing privately on their own are non-replicable events in ways that make those events impossible to apply to other settings. This privacy or independence makes it impossible to duplicate and replicate whatever is said or done by practitioners in the secrecy of their offices. Variability within and among psychotherapists makes it impossible to replicate methods of treatment from one psychotherapist to another. Consequently, it is practically impossible to identify and eliminate opportunistic charlatans from responsible professionals.

Even manuals do not assure replicability because the means of communication between therapists and participants remains still based on f2f personal contact and on talk between professionals and participants (LeCroy, 1994; Van Hasselt & Hersen, 1996). Manuals still leave the responsibility for change solely on the shoulders of professionals, thus avoiding and minimizing interactive involvement of participants in the process of change. Furthermore, since the major medium of communication between professionals and participants includes only talk, their communications need to be recorded, transcribed, and coded. As already noted, this process is expensive and available only to researchers who receive grant moneys to evaluate process and outcome. Consequently, as long as manuals use talk as the only medium of communication between participants and professionals, nothing will change in the field of psychotherapy and the status quo in that field of endeavor will prevail (L'Abate, 2005).

Furthermore, current mental health practices based on f2f tb interventions between professionals and participants are not sufficient to deal with the increasingly serious disturbances from childhood to seniority facing our country (and other nations). For example, the following statistics, provided by the National Institute of Drug Abuse, indicate that of the 21.1 million people who needed but did not receive treatment in 2004, an estimated 1.2 million (5.8 percent) reported that they felt they needed treatment for their alcohol or drug use problem. Of the 1.2 million persons who felt they needed treatment, 441,000 (35.8 percent) reported that they made an effort but were unable to get treatment, and 792,000 (64.2 percent) reported making no effort to get treatment. Among people who needed but did not receive treatment and felt they needed treatment for a substance abuuse problem, the most often reported reasons for not receiving treatment were not ready to stop using (40.0 percent) and cost or insurance barriers (34.5 percent). *However, among the people who made an effort but were unable to get treatment, 42.5 percent reported cost or insurance barriers, and only 25.3 percent reported that they were not ready to stop using* (underlying mine). These results are based on 2003 and 2004 combined data.

The number of persons needing treatment for an illicit drug use problem in 2004 (8.1 million) was higher than the number needing treatment in 2003 (7.3 million); similarly, the number of persons receiving treatment for drug use at a specialty facility was higher in 2004 (1.4 million) than in 2003 (1.1 million). These 2004 estimates were similar to the corresponding estimates in 2002 (7.7 million needing treatment, 1.4 million receiving treatment). Of the 21.1 million people who needed but did not receive treatment in 2004, an estimated 1.2 million (5.8 percent) reported that they felt they needed treatment for their alcohol or drug use problem. Of the 1.2 million persons who felt they needed treatment, 441,000 (35.8 percent) reported that they made an effort but were unable to get treatment, and 792,000 (64.2 percent) reported making no effort to get treatment .(underlying mine). 6.6 million people needed but did not receive treatment for an illicit drug use problem in 2004 (underlying mine). Of these, 598,000 (9.0 percent) felt they needed treatment. This number increased from 362,000 in 2002 and from 426,000 in 2003. Of the 598,000 persons who felt they needed treatment in 2004,194,000 (32.4 percent) reported that they made an effort but were unable to get treatment, and 404,000 (67.6 percent) reported making no effort to get treatment.

These staggering statistics, plus the reports of the Surgeon General (US Publish Health Servicce, 1999) and the President's New Freedom Commission on Mental Health (2003), indicate the need for the creation of middle-level specialists who will be able to deal with functional or semi-functional populations to decrease the burden put on existing mental health facilities by many overwhelming dysfunctionalities and ever increasing mental health needs (Appendix A). Among those who do need professional f2f talk and/or medication, there are those who might not need either of those (expensive) interventions, but who could use interventions directed toward promoting healthier solutions to their concerns thus decreasing the intensity of problems that, left unattended, may exacerbate into full-blown disorders (L'Abate, 2007a).

According to both reports cited above, promotion of physical and mental health, as well as prevention and treatment of mental health illnesses, have not even been attempted for a variety of reasons. One reason includes the creation of specialties trained to deal effectively with both promotion and prevention. These specialties could assist existing mental health professions to deal with as many functional and semi-functional populations who avoid existing mental health facilities but who could profit by working on their problems online in the privacy of their homes (Appendix A).

If costs are an issue in the delivery of mental health services, any responsible and validated innovation that would reduce costs should be relevant. In this case, the curriculum presented in Appendix A would allow specialists graduating from this program to help deliver low-cost online interventions that could be added to existing, more expensive, traditional f2f tb interventions, either on their own or in addition to those traditional practices (L'Abate, 1992).

Given the staggering numbers of conditions needing help, there is no way that the f2f tb paradigm used in the past century will remain relevant to clinical and research practices in this century. Computers are fast becoming the third avenue of delivery for mental health services after medication and psychotherapy (Bracy, 1992; Bradley, Welch, & Skilbeck, 1993). The question to answer is *whether* computers can fulfill some functions until now preserved by f2f tb psychotherapy and, if they do, *how* can they be utilized in the prevention and treatment of mental disorders. Software for such delivery has already been created to deal with individual, marital, and family problems (L'Abate, 1992, 2004a, 2004c, 2007c). An additional nuanced discussion of the LM on the Internet is available in Chapter 19 of this volume.

## THE BACKGROUND OF THE LABORATORY METHOD

An excellent but outdated standard treatise about clinical psychology (Walker, 1983) does not mention the LM, neither does a more recent treatise (Hersen, Kazdin, & Bellack, 1991). Except for a plea by Kihlstrom and Kihlstrom (1998) and a more recent mention of the LM "in medicine" by Kihlstrom (2002), this writer knows only of six secondary references about clinical psychology as a science (Hayes, Barlow, & Nelson-Gray, 1999; Hayes,

Follette, Dawes, & Grady, 1995; Lilienfeld, Lohr, & Lynn, 2004; McFall, 1996; Routh & DeRubeis, 1998; Treat, Bootzin, & Baker, 2007).

Hayes, Barlow, and Nelson-Grey (1999) were essentially concerned with the same goal of this volume, the combination of practice and research. In spite of this goal, however, their major concern was research methodology. They did advocate but did not suggest any specific means by which practice can be linked with research. The edited volume by Hayes, Follette, Dawes, and Grady (1995) serves as the background for this chapter and for the whole volume. All contributors, some of which are cited throughout this chapter, were critical of current practices in clinical psychology that were not replicable and, therefore, questionable. Most views expressed in that work echo what this writer argued more than 40 years ago (L'Abate, 1964, 1968a, 1968b). Lilienfeld, Fowler, Lohr and Lynn (2005), repeating what Lilienfeld, Lynn and Lohr (2003) reviewed earlier, are essentially critical of assessment tools based on the projective hypothesis, like the Rorschach, and of questionable treatments like Eye Movement Desensitization and Reprocessing (EMDR). McFall (1996) published a manifesto for a science of clinical psychology that should be considered the predecessor of this book. Unfortunately, few clinical psychologists followed his suggestions to compare psychotherapy results between clinical and research centers. Even in Routh and DeRubeis' work (1998), with the exception of Kihlstrom and Kihlstrom's chapter already mentioned, most chapters were devoted to research on the causes and risks factors in psychopathology, new assessment instruments in psychotherapy, and outcome research about psychotherapy for various disorders (anxiety, depression, etc.). Again, no specific suggestions were given on how to combine practice with research. In other words, the aims and contents of at least three major references do not overlap with contents of this volume.

More recently, Kihlstrom's replied to this writer's query about the seeming failure of the LM in clinical psychology (John F. Kihlstrom, personal communication, February 2, 2005): "I don't know why laboratory assessments aren't more popular than they are. They were clearly what David Shakow and others thought we should be headed toward, and my training at Penn under Julius Wishner (who, you remember, proposed laboratory measurements of "psychological efficiency") was oriented toward that goal as well. Of course, it's also true that experimental psychopathology, which presumably would provide the scientific basis for such laboratory tests, has fallen on hard times. Everybody seems to be much more interested in biology these days. Another factor might be the science-practice split. Many clinicians might think that they don't have anything to learn from scientists, and, as I have argued elsewhere , altogether too many scientists don't care what goes on in the clinic. And then there is sheer organizational inertia (or is that just a fancy name for sheer laziness?). As long as DSM is organized around signs and symptoms, nobody's going to take the trouble to devise laboratory tests."

A volume in honor of Richard McFall (Treat, Bootzin, & Baker, 2007) includes contributions to: (1) the history and epistemology of psychological clinical science; (2) applications of clinical science to topics of applied significance; (3) model integrative research programs; and (4) future directions for research, applications and training. Among various chapters, only one by G. T. Wilson on manual-based treatment and beyond overlaps with the topics considered in the present volume.

## Clinical Psychology as a Laboratory Science

It is now over forty years since an attempt was made to reconcile clinical practice with research through the LM (L'Abate, 1964, 1968a,b,c, 1971, 1973a). Many changes and tremendous growth have taken place in the profession, expanding from a psychodiagnostic specialty, usually ancillary to psychiatry, to an independent involvement in private practice and especially psychotherapy (L'Abate & De Giacomo, 2003). This section, therefore, summarizes forty years of expansions for the LM from individual psychodiagnosis to recent Internet applications through programmed writing (L'Abate, 1992, 1996, 2007c). This latter approach minimizes f2f talk and relies mainly on cost-effective, mass-produced, and easily replicable operations that can serve as data bases for research purposes. Hence, the LM allows responsible clinicians to operate at the same time also as researchers, bridging the considerable gap that exists between the two fields.

### Psychodiagnostics

The first psychodiagnostic laboratory for children was founded in 1964 in St. Louis Children Hospital. That laboratory is still in existence and has mushroomed into twelve doctorate level clinical psychologists (Russell Hoffmann, III, personal communication, April 18, 2006). However, the LM is no longer practiced, presumably because there is no interest in research. At that time, the budget allowed for one full-time secretary, a part-time graduate student (to administer the Rorschach & Wechsler Intelligence Scales), and part-time, non-paid volunteers (to administer simple tests like the DAP, Bender-Gestalt, and Peabody Intelligence Test, among others. Complete test batteries were administered to all children and assembled on the basis of age (six months to 3 years, 3 to 6 years, 7 to 12 years, etc.) to evaluate at least three different aspects of a child's functioning that were of interest to referring physicians, that is, pediatricians, psychiatrists, and neurologists: (1) intellectual level, (2) emotional make-up, and (3) possible neurological impairment. This approach, reduced the cost of a psychological evaluation, estimated at the time at about \$120.00, down to \$34.00 per child, without reducing the quality of the evaluation or using shortcuts in the evaluation.

After my move to Atlanta and the Department of Psychiatry at the Emory University School of Medicine (1964), in addition to a laboratory in that Department, two additional psychodiagnostic laboratories were founded, one in the Department of Pediatrics and another at Aidmore Children Hospital. With my move to Georgia State University (1965), the laboratory from the Psychiatry Department was transferred to the Psychology Department of GSU. In this fashion, I was able to evaluate an average of ten children a week in one day of my time, a task that would have taken about a week of my time were I to test each child f2f personally (L'Abate, 1969).

If I could be allowed one admittedly self-serving anecdotal testimonial to this approach, it was given by a retired pediatrician who had referred children to the GSU laboratory 20+ years earlier. At a social function with a group made up by a child psychiatrist and another psychologist, without knowing the identity of this writer who was present, he was asked about psychological testing for children. He replied that he valued it a great deal and that he had seen quite a few reports by many Atlanta clinical child psychologists, but that he only believed and valued reports given by "that fellow at GSU with an Eyetalian name. They were the most complete psychological reports I have ever read." When he was informed of my identity he was quite surprised. When additionally I appraised him that very likely I had only shaken the children's hands but not seen them otherwise, even though I had supervised the test administration (by graduate students) and I did write the report, his dismissive reply was: "I don't believe it."

An attempt to differentiate test reports written on the basis of personal contact with and test evaluation by me versus psychological test reports written without the professional test administration of the child (except to meet and greet the child and writing the final report) and administered by a technician failed completely. A diplomate level judge could not distinguish above chance between the two types of reports.

## Playtherapy

From psychodiagnostics, the LM was expanded to an automated playroom that allowed to monitor everything the child did in a two rooms, one for aggression and the other for construction (L'Abate, 1968d, 1971, 1973a). Results from this application were reported (L'Abate, 1979) and have been summarized in an unpublished paper (L'Abate, 2003b). A doctoral dissertation related the dialogue between children and therapists to objective results derived from standard pre-and post-psychodiagnostic evaluations.

Finding that accepting children in play therapy stigmatized them as "identified patients," and that this acceptance would consequently diminish the family's involvement in therapeutic process, with the advent of family therapy in the early 70s, both play therapy rooms were converted into family therapy rooms. With the advent of virtual reality, however, it is now possible to reconstruct a playroom that would contain both aggressive and constructive toys and games at various developmental levels (L'Abate, 2003b).

## Enrichment Programs

To train graduate students to deal with multi-relational systems, as in couple and family therapy, instructions were written down to follow verbatim in dealing with either mock couples and families through role playing or with volunteer couples and families who did not need therapy but who could use "booster shots" in the form of "enrichment" (L'Abate & Weinstein, 1987; L'Abate & Young, 1987). This approach allowed to reach and help around 300 couple and families using graduate students as intermediaries, with a very small number of drop-outs, training quite a few graduate students to deal with multi-relational systems rather than with individuals (L'Abate & Jessee, 1981). Various dissertations stemmed from this approach (L'Abate & De Giacomo, 2003).

### Programmed Writing and Self-help Mental Health Workbooks

By relying more and more on the written medium at a distance from the professional rather than f2f talk, using systematically written homework assignments (L'Abate, 1986, 1990, 1992, 1996, 2001, 2002, 2003a, 2003c, 2004a, 2004c, 2007c;L'Abate & De Giacomo, 2003), I was able to expand clinical practice beyond the confines of the professional office and indicate how it is possible to help troubled people (individuals, couples, and families) through the infinite possibilities of the Internet. Workbooks or protocols were developed for non-clinical respondents (primary prevention) or for at-risk participants conceived as secondary prevention because of their targeted nature. They can be administered solely by themselves in primary prevention or in conjunction with crisis interventions, psychotherapy, and medication (tertiary prevention). A meta-analysis of mental health workbooks versus physical health workbooks produced a medium effect size of 0.44 for workbooks and a low effect size of 0.25 for physical health workbooks (Smyth & L'Abate, 2001).

## The Laboratory Method in Evaluation

Historically, psychological tests were developed to fulfill two basic scientific requirements, and that is: to understand and to predict, but not to control or to prescribe (Butcher, 2006). Control, in the form of interventions or psychotherapy, remained uniquely separate from understanding and predicting, with almost no connection between these processes. Therefore, the major issue with psychological tests lies in their being completely separated from interventions, that is: they were constructed to evaluate not to treat. Hence, there is almost no connection between psychological evaluations and treatments. Even if there were a connection, such a connection cannot be demonstrated as long as treatment occurs verbally. This is why I developed self-report, paper-and-pencil tests that were directly connected to written homework assignments, protocols or workbooks, such as, among many others, the Self-Other Profile Chart for individuals, couples, and families, and the Problems-in-Relationships Test for couples, Negotiation and Planned Parenting for parents. These prescriptive instruments are prime examples of connecting evaluation with treatment, as long as treatment is based on writing rather than on talk (L'Abate, 1990, 1992, 2006, 2007d; McMahan & L'Abate, 2001).

There is no way of counting and estimating how many tests, inventories, questionnaires, or rating sheets exist currently on the psychological marketplace . Nor would such estimate make a difference to the thesis that it is impossible to evaluate anybody with one single test or rating scale for intelligence, personality, work performance, or psychiatric diagnosis (Maruish, 1999; Sajatovic & Ramirez, 2001; Sperry, 2004; Touliatos, Perlmutter, & Straus, 1990; Woody, 1980). Practitioners who do use multi-dimensional tests like the Minnesota Multiphasic Personality Inventory-2 (MMPI-2), for instance, apparently do also use projective techniques, like the Rorschach inkblots, supposedly to acquire a more in-depth understanding of people's problems and personalities. A single test, inventory or questionnaire, in and by itself, is not sufficient to set a baseline to evaluate treatment and is not sufficient to even capture the multifaceted aspects of personalities and whatever other qualities make up that personality, including intelligence level. Nor will a single test be sufficient to develop a treatment plan. A professional cannot, will not, and should not make recommendations about a person's life based on a single test, no matter how valid and reliable that test may be.

Hence, even multi-dimensional tests such as the Wechsler Intelligence Scale or the MMPI-2 need to be administered together with other intelligence and personality tests to reach a moderate understanding of an individual, besides the intelligence level as an established base. How are we going to find "What Works for Whom?" (Roth & Fonagy, 1996) unless we determine what assets and liabilities are present in individuals, couples, or families? How can we even dream of helping people without a clear understanding of their problems and, even more importantly, without a clear view or plan of how to help them?

Again and again, research and practice are treated separately in most texts, even though the LM, pioneered years ago in neuro-psychology by Ralph Reitan and a few neuro-psychologists, as discussed in Chapter 19 of this volume, is now practiced in quite a few settings. In spite of its use in various settings around the world, there is no way of knowing who is using this method unless attention to it is brought about by an integrating text, as provided by this volume.

## The Notion of Battery in Psychological Evaluations

The notion of a battery derives from the military practice to shoot at a moving target from different vantage points with different weapons to triangle and assure enveloping and hitting that target one way or another. By the same token, a battery of psychological tests attempts to evaluate a variety of dimensions that are relevant and that compose the particular nature of the target being evaluated (Hunsley & Mash, 2007). Using the compilation of a wide range of tests, usually called a "test battery" implies some systematic thought about the reasons for assembling such a series based on the: (1) nature of the target population (i.e., learning disabled, acting out rebellion, etc.), target disorder or syndrome (i.e., schizophrenia), or target symptom (i.e., anxiety); (2) age of target population (i.e., children, single adults, senior citizens); (3) composition of target population, (i.e., singles, couples, families, etc.), (4) special considerations, such as comorbidity, ethnic diversity, socio-economic status, or gender, and, last but not least (5) costs involved in the administration, scoring, and interpretation of test results (L'Abate, 1973b, 1994b, 2004b). Should tests consist of only paper-and-pencil self-reports or should they be administered by professional, semi-professional, or technical personnel? For instance, the greater the involvement of doctorate-level professional personnel the higher the costs of administration will be. Would test results be scored manually or by computer? How about interpretation of test results? Would it be computer-driven or given by a professional? Answers to these questions determine the costs of a test battery, including length of administration and time needed to assemble one (Cone, 1995;Hunsley & Mash, 2007).

## Professional versus Technical Skills

The differentiation between professional and technical skills has not yet occurred in most clinical practices, in spite of its being stressed in previous writings (L'Abate, 1992, 1994a, 2001, 2002, 2003a). By technical is meant any ability that requires evidence of interpersonal skills (courtesy, empathy, personal regard, sensitivity) plus skills to follow written instructions in a manual, as in the case of most psychological tests. A bachelor degree level of education may be necessary to administer and score most psychological tests, including projective techniques, provided written instructions are followed to the letter. Professional skills, on the other hand, require knowledge of statistics, test construction, and psychometric properties of any test instrument. That knowledge involves a doctorate level of education plus extensive supervised clinical experience, as well knowledge of psychopathology, and in specialties like neuro-psychology knowledge of cerebral functions..

Given this differentiation, for instance, it may take one hour to administer a standard intelligence test and ten to fifteen minutes to score it. In some cases, this process has been taken over by computers. It will take a few minutes of either computer or professional time to interpret test results. However, the meaning of results from one test needs to be integrated with results from other tests. This process does indeed require a professional level of knowledge relevant to the target being examined as well as the professional context within which the evaluation is taking place (L'Abate, 1994a, p. 212). For instance, writing a report about the meaning and interpretation of results requires a level of knowledge above and beyond just statistics, test-construction, etc. It requires knowledge of psychopathology, some basic understanding of neurological and cerebral functions, and other contextual factors that are relevant to whoever is referring a case for evaluation. Consequently, professionals would direct, supervise, and support middle-level and sub-professionals in the administration and scoring of psychological tests. Ultimately, the professional is responsible for whatever the outcome will be: the final psychological report (L'Abate, 2007a).

One important issue relating to psychological testing refers to differentiating among various levels of above-average to superior personality functioning. No matter what the level of functioning may be, there are not yet tests devised to differentiate among levels of above average to superior functioning, as far as I know. Most psychological tests have been developed and validated to evaluate levels and types of psychopathology and dysfunctionality. The importance of this differentiation is related to identifying and specifying which individuals, couples or families need what kind of help. Given the nature of the referral, what strengths are present to decide whether to use primary, secondary, or tertiary prevention approaches? (Barrera & Sandler, 2006). Since there are no tests that, to my knowledge, can produce such a discrimination, it will be necessary to rely on actual self-reports about individual and relational positively constructive activities that would determine the level of functioning and the type of intervention necessary to satisfy the reason for referral . One way to evaluate higher-than-average functioning is to rely on what positive and pleasant individual and relational activities participants engage inside and outside their homes. Are participants assuming leadership positions outside of home and work? Are they passive recipients of other people's initiatives? These questions have been answered conceptually (L'Abate, 2005) but need to be evaluated empirically (L'Abate, 2007d).

Table 1.1 includes a list of positive individual, dyadic, and multi-relational activities that should help to differentiate among below-average, average, and above-average levels of activities according to four dimensions of frequency, duration, intensity, and satisfaction. Even though it has not been validated, it may become a starting point in differentiating which participants are at risk, who are in need, and who are in crisis.

Given this differentiation, for instance, it would be possible to narrow-down which participants are *at risk* but functional enough to require universal low-cost approaches with additional possibly generic home-work assignments (L'Abate, 2007c), which participants are *in need* of specific activities and homework targeted to their specific needs, and which participants are *in crisis*, not able to perform most positive activities requiring f2f tb crisis intervention and psychotherapy.

**Table 1. Constructive Patterns: Checklist of Behaviors Necessary to Discriminate Levels of Functioning in Individuals, Couples, and Families.**

Instructions:

Circle the number that best represents how often, how long, how strong, and how satisfying behaviors listed below are from 1 to 5. If an activity is not included in this list, there are two available spaces where such an activity can be added. Write the name of that added activity and rate it accordingly. To rate the following activities you need to understand these definitions: Frequency means how often a behavior occurs, ranging from not at all (1) to very often (5). Duration means how long a behavior lasts, ranging from very short (1) to very long (5). Intensity means how strong a behavior is, ranging from very weak (1) to very strong (5).

Satisfaction means how much pleasure a behavior gives you, ranging from very little pleasure (1) to a great deal of pleasure (5).

| Individuals: | Frequency | Duration | Intensity | Satisfaction |
|---|---|---|---|---|
| Nutrition: Diet, food intake, vitamins, supplements, herbs | 1 2 3 4 5 | 1 2 3 4 5 | 1 2 3 4 5 | 1 2 3 4 5 |
| Physical Activities: | | | | |
| Exercise, sports, hunting, games | 1 2 3 4 5 | 1 2 3 4 5 | 1 2 3 4 5 | 1 2 3 4 5 |
| Pleasant and pleasurable activities | | | | |
| Hobbies, collecting, gardening and similar activities | 1 2 3 4 5 | 1 2 3 4 5 | 1 2 3 4 5 | 1 2 3 4 5 |
| Reading: | | | | |
| Preferred books, magazines, newspapers | 1 2 3 4 5 | 1 2 3 4 5 | 1 2 3 4 5 | 1 2 3 4 5 |
| Television: | | | | |
| How much time spent, programs watched, reliance on tapes, disks, etc | 1 2 3 4 5 | 1 2 3 4 5 | 1 2 3 4 5 | 1 2 3 4 5 |
| Computer and Internet Use: | | | | |
| Enrichment: education extra-home, school/work interests | 1 2 3 4 5 | 1 2 3 4 5 | 1 2 3 4 5 | 1 2 3 4 5 |
| Entertainment: | 1 2 3 4 5 | 1 2 3 4 5 | 1 2 3 4 5 | 1 2 3 4 5 |
| Friendships: | | | | |
| Nature of friends and frequency of meetings | 1 2 3 4 5 | 1 2 3 4 5 | 1 2 3 4 5 | 1 2 3 4 5 |

**Table 1. (Continued)**

| Individuals: | Frequency | Duration | Intensity | Satisfaction |
|---|---|---|---|---|
| Correspondence: | | | | |
| Writing versus computer-driven e-mails, etc. | 1 2 3 4 5 | 1 2 3 4 5 | 1 2 3 4 5 | 1 2 3 4 5 |
| Use of Car: Strictly for work and shopping purposes, joy riding/vacations | 1 2 3 4 5 | 1 2 3 4 5 | 1 2 3 4 5 | 1 2 3 4 5 |
| Use of alcohol, smoking, wine | 1 2 3 4 5 | 1 2 3 4 5 | 1 2 3 4 5 | 1 2 3 4 5 |
| Computer & Internet use | 1 2 3 4 5 | 1 2 3 4 5 | 1 2 3 4 5 | 1 2 3 4 5 |
| Volunteering: Where, when, for how long? | 1 2 3 4 5 | 1 2 3 4 5 | 1 2 3 4 5 | 1 2 3 4 5 |
| Pets or animal companions… | 1 2 3 4 5 | 1 2 3 4 5 | 1 2 3 4 5 | 1 2 3 4 5 |
| Collecting (what?________________) | 1 2 3 4 5 | 1 2 3 4 5 | 1 2 3 4 5 | 1 2 3 4 5 |
| Other ____________ | 1 2 3 4 5 | 1 2 3 4 5 | 1 2 3 4 5 | 1 2 3 4 5 |
| Other ____________ | 1 2 3 4 5 | 1 2 3 4 5 | 1 2 3 4 5 | 1 2 3 4 5 |
| Couples and Families: | | | | |
| Affection (touching, hugging, holding, huddling, kissing, cuddling) | 1 2 3 4 5 | 1 2 3 4 5 | 1 2 3 4 5 | 1 2 3 4 5 |
| Attending movies, plays, concerts, symphonies, or operas | 1 2 3 4 5 | 1 2 3 4 5 | 1 2 3 4 5 | 1 2 3 4 5 |
| Camping and hiking | 1 2 3 4 5 | 1 2 3 4 5 | 1 2 3 4 5 | 1 2 3 4 5 |
| Celebrations (birthdays, special occasions, promotions, etc.) | 1 2 3 4 5 | 1 2 3 4 5 | 1 2 3 4 5 | 1 2 3 4 5 |
| Cooking together | 1 2 3 4 5 | 1 2 3 4 5 | 1 2 3 4 5 | 1 2 3 4 5 |
| Eating together | 1 2 3 4 5 | 1 2 3 4 5 | 1 2 3 4 5 | 1 2 3 4 5 |
| Entertainment (parties, reunions, etc.) | 1 2 3 4 5 | 1 2 3 4 5 | 1 2 3 4 5 | 1 2 3 4 5 |
| Playing cards or board games | 1 2 3 4 5 | 1 2 3 4 5 | 1 2 3 4 5 | 1 2 3 4 5 |
| Sex, sexuality, and sensuality | 1 2 3 4 5 | 1 2 3 4 5 | 1 2 3 4 5 | 1 2 3 4 5 |
| Shopping together | 1 2 3 4 5 | 1 2 3 4 5 | 1 2 3 4 5 | 1 2 3 4 5 |
| Vacations | 1 2 3 4 5 | 1 2 3 4 5 | 1 2 3 4 5 | 1 2 3 4 5 |
| Watching at home together vs. apart: movies, CD-rom, TV | 1 2 3 4 5 | 1 2 3 4 5 | 1 2 3 4 5 | 1 2 3 4 5 |
| Other ____________ | 1 2 3 4 5 | 1 2 3 4 5 | 1 2 3 4 5 | 1 2 3 4 5 |
| Other ____________ | 1 2 3 4 5 | 1 2 3 4 5 | 1 2 3 4 5 | 1 2 3 4 5 |

Feel free to add any comments that may relate to the activities listed in this form by adding more information about these activities. For instance, giving more information about activities that needed to be specified above but there may have not been much space to allow more information

## Using Middle-Level Semi- or Para-professionals in Evaluations (and Interventions)

Given the differentiation between technical and professional skills, not only in evaluation but also in interventions, a great many functions can be allocated and delegated to semi-or para-professionals with evidenced responsible and responsive technical and interpersonal skills (see Chapter 19 this volume). Objections to this thesis, for instance, have consisted of assigning to doctorate level professionals the mystique of possessing unique skills that cannot be found at the technical level. Observations of an examinee;s extra-test behaviors, for instance, consist of participant's or examinee's comments or reactions above and beyond the performance requested by the test itself. The attribution of specific, mystical observational skills to doctorate level professionals does not seem to be supported by any evidence known to me. Any sensitive, responsible, and well trained technician can report all these observations as well as any professional.

## THE LABORATORY METHOD IN PSYCHOTHERAPY: PRACTICING CLINICAL PSYCHOLOGY IN THE 21ST CENTURY

The major choice that practicing psychological professionals (promoters, preventers, psychotherapists, and rehabilitators) need to make nowadays is whether to continue working according to models from the past century or whether to accept, assimilate, and apply models necessary to practice in this century. If they choose to practice in this century, clinicians will need to give up at least seven major models (biases, dogmas, or myths) that determined clinical practices in the past century. The major if not the only vehicle of communication and healing in the past century has been psychotherapy, that is, a more or less prolonged, f2f tb relationship between participants and professionals, usually based on fees or on public funds. Consequently, this section will highlight the dangerous influence of professional biases that hamper, detour, and delay progress in the field of psychotherapy, as the major form of psychological intervention. This field has been subjected to many undeserving and unwarranted criticisms that deny its relevance for promoting mental health and prevent illness in countless participants. These attacks have been more frequent and perhaps more acerbic over the last few years (Albee, 2000; Dineen, 1996; Sykes, 1992; Watters & Ofshe, 1999). There is not need to rehash them here. They have been considered and summarized in greater detail elsewhere (L'Abate, 2002).

A more recent criticism (Keen, 2000) has been directed toward the field's inability to distinguish superficial and trivial from serious, relevant problems. Consequently, everybody is treated with the same panaceas. No distinction in treatments is made to deal with trivial rather than with really serious clinical problems. Keen's (2000) possibly justified criticism, however, like many others critics of psychotherapy, fails to give a realistic solution. If not a solution, at least a practical and relevant suggestion should be given for corrective approaches to differentiate superficial from serious problems. If there is no baseline evaluation, for instance, except for a subjective and usually unreliable tb interview, how is it possible to determine which treatment to follow? How are therapists going to separate the trivial from the troublesome? How can we distinguish superficial from serious problems without an objective and thorough evaluation? Using a rating scale about frequency, rate, duration, and intensity of these activities like the one proposed here (Table 1.1) could be one way to differentiate objectively among different levels of functionality.

Furthermore, if treatment is based on talk, how is it possible to document what happened or went on in the privacy of a professional's office, except perhaps for self-serving therapist's notes? For instance, if pre-post-treatment evaluations were adopted as SOPs, as done routinely in some fields of medicine, the distinction between serious versus superficial problems could be addressed more objectively than heretofore. Furthermore, one could argue that the presence of a professional should be made contingent on completing an evaluation and even written homework assignments, minimizing personal contacts and talk between participants and professionals only to critical and severe psychological conditions and after participants have shown their willingness to work for change on their own rather than relying solely on the therapist's shoulders (L'Abate, 2006, 2007d).

The major issue here, of course, lies in defining what does constitute "progress" in psychotherapy? If we are not clear, concerned, and competent to address this issue, the status quo will continue to prevail and nothing is going to change. Consequently, *progress in psychotherapy means helping more people in need of help per unit of professional time in more cost-effective ways than it is possible through f2f and talk alone*. Progress would mean using cost-effective, mass-oriented ways of helping people who want professional help by distinguishing among: (1) who is *at risk* (primary prevention); (2) who is *in need* (secondary prevention); and (3) who is *in crisis* (tertiary prevention) (L'Abate, 1990, 2007a). Unless we make this crucial distinction, we shall continue to practice psychotherapy pall-mall, using the same reactive approach for everybody without any distinction of severity, type, and content of dysfunctionalities.No specificity in treatment means that everybody is treated the same way without regard to age, gender, education, socio-economic status, and referral question. Everybody, regardless of complaint, is treated with the same personal gimmicks, games, and gambits dear to the hearts, whims and wills of many psychotherapists. Without any distinction about type and level of dysfunctionality everybody is treated the same: reactively. Participants say something and the therapist reacts to what has been said. If we cannot distinguish what is relevant from what is irrelevant, as Keen wants us to do, then we are destined to continue operating in the same way, no change will take place, no progress will occur, and the status quo will prevail (L'Abate, 1997, 1999a, 1999b).

A second issue that is relevant to the lack of progress in psychotherapy lies in the profession's inability to define what characteristics constitute a competent therapist (Teyber & McClure, 2000). Fortunately, this shortcoming is being resolved through examination of the variables that define therapeutic effectiveness. Huppert, Bufka, Barlow, et al. (2001, p. 747) started by looking at the outcome of the interaction between treatment and therapist characteristics. They found that therapists significantly differed in the magnitude of change among caseloads. Effect sizes for therapist impact on outcome measures varied from 0% to 18%, suggesting that this impact varies from nil to something that is too unreliable to base a whole method of treatment. Furthermore, as suggested earlier, therapists are too variable within themselves to allow the possibly erroneous human equation to deal with serious and severe human problems.

In spite of these positive developments, certain professional biases are still exerting a powerful influence on how psychotherapy is still practiced at the present time. As already noted, there are at least seven major models or biases in the field of psychotherapy. Here one is tempted to use the term "dogmas" but biases denote the presence of followers of dogmas. One would estimate that many psychotherapists, regardless of professional identity and ideological orientation, subscribe in one way or another, and to a degree or another, to at least one if not all of the following interconnected biases. Calling these models "dogmas" in this case is equivalent to implying that they are based on magic, superstitions, and unexplainable beliefs present through personal faith and impressions beyond any objective reality. In fact, for some therapists, in my opinion, psychotherapy is like a religion. You either believe in it or you do not. Any attack or criticism is ignored and the status quo prevails against any attack. Of course, no matter how many criticisms are leveled against it, as cited above, there is no question that the field of psychotherapy has flourished and is still flourishing, considering the many texts and training programs that in many cases are at the source of these cults, oops!! dogmas. Some books and training programs are responsible for preserving and promoting practices based on dogmas as accepted facts.

## Models from the Last Century

Seven models have dominated the clinical practice of psychotherapy in the last century: (1) f2f talk; (2) personal presence of professionals; (3) therapeutic alliance; (4) subjective impressions; (5) anti-empirical stance; (6) practices without theory, and (7) successes without failures.

### *Face-to-face Talk*

There are shortcomings in the f2f talk-based (tb) paradigm. This paradigm is so ingrained in our traditional mental health practices that to question it tantamount to heresy. The magic of the spoken word is stressed at the expense of the other two media: written and non-verbal. Because of its over-reliance on talk, there is an inability to provide a record of process and progress in the course of intervention. Only the subjective and likely biased recollections of the therapist furnish such a record (L'Abate, 1997, 1999a, 1999b).

Since scant information about the process of note taking could be found. in the extant literature , in a pilot survey I obtained answers to a structured questionnaire about the note-taking process in psychotherapy from a sample of 56 from 100 participants drawn from the National Register of Health Service Providers in Psychology. They gave demographic information about themselves and about their use and functions of notes and record-keeping in psychotherapy. Most answers indicated the importance of note-taking and record-keeping as an integral part of the psychotherapy process. The results of this survey raise the possibility of computer analyses of these notes in their relationship to specific outcomes in psychotherapy. If psychotherapy is to become more of a science, it might need to relate the process of note-taking and record-keeping to specific psychopathologies and to the therapist-participant relationships as assessed by these notes. Managed care companies, to be sure, do require written treatment plans, but these plans are useless, since there is no one to check whether they were followed, except for the subjective, self-serving, and non-verified opinion of therapists and their notes.

Talk has been considered the cure-all for major dysfunctions and referral problems.This vehicle of communication and healing is still dominant in this century. It will take time to disperse its magical qualities. I have argued (L'Abate, 1997, 1999a, 1999b) that talk is an inefficient medium of communication and healing because it can be distorted, forgotten, and abused by both professionals and participants. It may be effective. There is no denying its positive outcome in many cases (Interchange, 2004-05; Wampold, 2001). However, how efficient is it? What does it cost to pay for f2f tb contact with a professional? Are there better, more efficient and less costly ways to obtain the same or even better results? Given two methods of treatment that produce the same results, one chooses the less expensive one. One does not need to be a rocket scientist to make that choice. Let's not forget that the majority of our population relies on medications to help their problems rather than on psychotherapy (Consumer Reports, 2004).

### *Personal Presence of Professionals*

The person and presence of the therapist is considered as paramount, leading to the therapeutic alliance at the expense of improvements in methods of treatment. What makes us think that talking with a professional f2f will produce improvement? Yet, most changes in participants, at least in the medical field, occur because of medications and operations that take place either at a distance from a professional or while the patient is asleep. The idea that the presence, personality, and good manners of the therapist will produce changes is a vestige left from the likes of Sigmund Freud, Carl Rogers, and the charismatic pioneers of family therapy, who propagated notions of exemplary practices through workshops, where they seemingly performed feats of magic worthy of joining the exclusive Pantheon of Therapists. Countless individually-oriented therapists seemingly believe in their personal power to change people for the better. Fortunately, this factor seems practically absent in current family therapy practices, because couples and families require more than presence, personality, or good manners to profit from treatment (Sexton, Weeks, & Robbins, 2003). Method rather than presence is the necessary ingredient to help troubled conditions.

### *Therapeutic Alliance*

As noted above, this alliance may be relevant in individual psychotherapy (Horvarth & Symonds, 1991; Martin, Garske, & Davis, 2000) as well as in family thereapy (Robbins, Liddle, Turner, et al., 2006). However, countless personal and possibly therapeutic alliances are built every day on the Internet among complete strangers, as evidence by chat-rooms, support groups, and blogs. Hence, one does not need f2f contact or talk to develop a helping relationship with someone else. Furthermore, as long as the personal alliance between professionals and participants is held as the basis for change, it will be impossible to find what factors do produce reliable and lasting change and which factors do not. The personal alliance may cloud the issue of what factors produce valid and reliable change and which do not.

Meta-analyses of the relationship between the therapeutic relationship and outcome have produced values that range from 0.11 (Stevens, Hynan, & Allen, 2000) to 0.26 (Horvath & Symonds, 1991), with most values averaging around 0.24 (Beutler, Kim, Davison, et al, 2003; Martin, Garske, & Davis, 2000). Those values are not high enough to justify the presence of a professional. Furthermore, how about the level of education and experience of the therapist? Are these qualities necessary and significant?

### *Subjective Impressions*

The triumph of subjective impressions at the expense of objective evidence, either in evaluation or in accounting for results, is still present. Because of emphasis on the subjective, as exemplified by the extensive use of tb interviews, rather than objective tests, there have been widespread failures to link practice with theory, to the point that most therapists describe themselves as "eclectic" to justify what amounts to an idiosyncratic, unsystematic mish-mash of theories and therapies that makes it impossible to validate any or all of them.

### *Anti-empirical Stance*

An anti-empirical stance is usually maintained, where anecdotes, case studies, and war stories are favored over method and outcome to attest to the therapist's acumen, astuteness, and sensitivity. Because of this stance, there are inadequacies in linking evaluation with treatment to the point that no such connection is made in actual practices. Those practices either discourage objective psychodiagnostic evaluation or even view them as counter-therapeutic (L'Abate, 1994). The subjective interview is the only way to evaluate participants and no additional objective measures are necessary.

One aspect of this anti-empirical stance is seen in the anti-medical stance present in many psychotherapists who criticize and reject labeling participants according to psychiatric nosology, even though they use this labeling to collect fees from insurance companies. The so-called "medical model" is used as a straw horse to show one's distinct and unique, high and ideal values that go beyond categorizing and labeling people -- supposedly to treat participants as special individuals, to justify using the same f2f tb approach without any differentiation from one case to another. How is that differentiation possible as long as talk is the vehicle of intervention? As Norcross noted on this regard:

> "The accumulated research indicates that adapting or tailoring the therapy relationship to specific patient needs and characteristics (in addition to diagnosis) enhances the effectiveness of treatment. For example, clients presenting with high resistance have been found, in 80% of the studies, to respond better to self-control methods and minimal therapist directiveness, whereas patients with low resistance experience improved outcomes with therapist directiveness and explicit guidance. There are many other empirically supported matches. The point is that psychotherapy must be tailored to the individual person, not simply diagnosis. And research tells us how that can be done in a systematic manner that improves the effectiveness of psychotherapy." ((Interchange, 2004-05, pp. 51).

I would go one step further, declaring and arguing that as long as psychotherapy is based on f2f tb contacts, it will be very difficult and expensive to obtain a match between evaluation and treatment. It may be obtained in research centers funded by external sources, but it will be impossible to implement and evaluate in private practice settings.

### *Practices without Theories*

This lack of connection between theory and practice is evident in evaluations as well as in interventions (Adams, 1995, Leigland, 1995). This failure is evident in the creation of great many models that are not connected with each other and with interventions (Liddle, Santisteban, Levant, & Bray, 2002). Furthermore, as long as psychotherapy is based on talk, how will it be possible to link practices with theory? The emphasis on empirical evidence has effected the whole profession of clinical psychology, to the point that even evaluation of couples and families are methodologically sound and frequent, but, except for few instances, lacking in any connection to any reasonable theory or model (Sperry, 2004). When psychotherapists are asked about their theoretical orientation, most of them profess and plead "integrationism" or "eclecticism", since they do no have any specific theory to fall back to or to justify their practices (Norcross, 2002; Norcross, Karpiak, & Lister, 2005; Norcross, Karpiak, & Santoro, 2005). Consequently, "eclecticism" becomes a catch-all to justify whatever arbitrary and undocumented mish-mash of practices therapists feel justified in using. The sad fact is that there is no theory that could encompass the multitude of therapeutic practices now in existence. Even if such a theory existed and therapists claimed to follow it, it would be difficult if not impossible to extract connections between what has been written in theory and what has been talked in practice (L'Abate & Cusinato, 2007).

### *Successes without Evidence*

All the foregoing models bring about the complete denial of accounting for one's failures. Assumed or claimed success on the part of the professional without any objective evidence to document claims is still the norm (Lilienfeld, Fowler, Lohr, & Lynn, 2005). Yet, the same professional would demand and require objective methods of treatment for his or her pet. Even if successful, as already discussed above and elsewhere (L'Abate, 2007a) at its best, psychotherapy based on the f2f talk is a drop in the bucket for helping all the people who need help, as argued earlier in this chapter. There is no way that psychotherapeutic practices, as traditionally performed, are going to help the millions of people who need help. We need to rely on repeatable, documented practices that can be used on a massive basis rather than on the expensive one-to-one f2f tb contact between professionals and participants.

In spite of these models, psychological interventions are becoming more and more differentiated. To wit, they are changing from unstructured toward more structured interventions. There is an increasing formalization of most psychological interventions, that is, they tend to become more structured, from vaguely general to extremely specific, with differential guidelines, plans, and instructions to treat a given condition. Rather that general textbooks about treatment of psychopathological conditions, there are now a variety of textbooks to treat only one specific condition, be it depression, anxiety, obsessive-compulsive disorder, etc. rather than overall textbooks to treat all conditions equally. More and more treatment approaches tend toward becoming more and more specific, giving step-by-step instructions on how to intervene. For instance, marriage family therapy is no longer researched as a general, overall approach. Instead, its effectiveness with various conditions (conduct disorders and delinquency, substance abuse, childhood behavioral and emotional disorders, alcohol abuse, marital problems, relationship enhancement, domestic violence, severe mental illness, affective and physical disorders (Pinsof & Wynne, 1995; Sexton, Weeks, & Robbins, 2003; Sprenkle, 2002). The same process is occurring in the field of individual psychotherapy. The empirically based psychotherapies are the direct outcome of these changes, as discussed below. This formalization has been augmented by the increasing use of homework assignments (Kazantzis, Deane, Ronan, & L'Abate, 2004; Kazantzis & L'Abate, 2007), as discussed in greater detail below.

## The Empirically-Validated Treatments Movement

This movement is the natural and evolutionary extension of psychotherapy becoming more and more specific to match an intervention with a specific clinical condition (Chambless & Ollendick, 2001; Beutler, Malik, Alimohamed, et al, 2003; Norcross,2001; Lambert & Barley (2001). It is also a needed, critical reaction to those very models of practice reviewed above.

Of course, such a movement has not been free of controversy, a topic that is outside of the focus of this chapter. For one instance, among the many, Westen and Morrison (2001) asserted that scientific studies do not study real or representative samples of patients. Against this position, there are many studies that refute such an assertion (Beutler, Kim, Davison, et al, 1997; Lipsey & Wilson, 1993; Shadish, Matt, Navaro, & Phillips, 2000). There is still agreement that clinical judgment can be erroneous and varying from one clinician to another. Errors are made because even clinicians are human beings (Garb, 1998). An egregious example of an erroneous clinical judgment on my part is given below.

### Writing as the Next Revolution in the Delivery of Mental Health Services

Writing could be more cost-effective than talk by minimizing professional contacts, that is: seeing a professional f2f should be contingent on completion of homework assignments (L'Abate, 2006a, 2006b; L'Abate, 2006c, 2006d). Writing, either with a pen, pencil, typewriter, or computer, serves as an adjunct or as an alternative to traditional mental health services based either on physical or on psychological treatment, either para-preventively (in parallel with preventive approaches) or para-therapeutically (in parallel with therapeutic approaches). The use of distance writing in prevention and psychotherapy has come of age recently (Esterling, L'Abate, Murray, & Pennebaker, 1999; L'Abate, 2007a; Lepore & Smyth, 2002), including autobiographies (Demetrio & Borgonovi, 2007), journaling and diaries (Levine and Calvanio, 2007), expressive writing or Pennebaker's paradigm (Kacewicz, Slatcher, & Pennebaker, 2007), and self-help mental health workbooks (L'Abate & Goldstein, 2007). Distance writing has become even more important with the increasing use of the Internet (Pulier, Mount, McMenamin, & Maheu, 2007). Consequently, given the high costs of psychiatric and psychological treatments, and the sheer masses of people needing help, writing is and will become the most cost-effective, mass-oriented, versatile form and vehicle of health promotion, treatment, rehabilitation, and prevention in the not-too-distant future (L'Abate, 2005).

An inmate (incarcerated for ten years for "self-defense" murder) whom I have never met but who participated in completing written protocols to decrease depression through the mail, answered with this admittedly personal testimonial to the question of whether distance writing had been helpful to him without tb meeting f2f with the writer:

> "I feel as though I was helped *more* this way. I felt more comfortable. I feel I thought my answers through more thoroughly, and I feel my answers came more from my heart this way. I'm sure we could have discussed things more in depth face-to-face, but I don't feel

like my answers would have been as honest, would not have been thought out as deeply, and I would not have felt as comfortable with the worry of what you think of my answers or with the thought of my time running out."

One cannot help wonder about how many inmates, who are languishing in prisons and penitentiaries not receiving any help throughout the USA, could be helped through distance, programmed writing as in protocols or workbooks (L'Abate, 2007b; McMahan & Arias, 2004; Reed, McMahan, & L'Abate, 2001).

## Greater Reliance on Homework Assignments

By the same token of empirically -based and validated treatments, the field of psychotherapy is following what research suggests (Kazantzis, Deane, & Ronan, 2000), and that is, increasing assertiveness in requiring participants to be more actively involved in the process of change by completing "in-between-sessions" homework assignments (Kazantzis, Deane, Ronan, & L'Abate, 2004; Kazantzis & L'Abate, 2007). Presently, most schools of psychotherapy are using some type of homework assignment, even though, at this juncture, these assignments are administered in less than systematic ways. Eventually, the variance due to personal contact and to homework assignments will be disentangled (L'Abate, 2004c).

Overlooked in previous publications (Kazantzis et al., 2005; Kazantzis & L'Abate, 2007) was Brown-Stanbridge's paradigm for the construction of family therapy tasks. She developed a scheme based on three major dimensions: (1) direct-indirect; (2) behavioral/non-behavioral; and (3) paradoxical/non-paradoxical. From permutations of these three dimensions, she expanded them to a definitive classification of tasks that transcends couples and families to include also individuals. However, this paradigm was based strictly on f2f tb therapy and did not include the other two media of communication, written and nonverbal. Together with a classification of written protocols (L'Abate, 2004b) Brown-Stanbridge's paradigm can be used as a practical springboard for the classification of most homework assignments.

Homework assignments have been studied extensively in psychotherapy research (Kazantzis, Deane, Ronan, & L'Abate, 2005; Kazantzis & L'Abate, 2007). However, there is little evidence on the way in which homework is transferred in clinical practice. A survey of 827 practicing psychologists nationwide regarding their use and attitudes toward homework showed that 68% of this sample that they "often" or "almost always" used homework assignments. A factor analysis of their attitudes indicated a range that varied from homework having a negative impact on in-sessions therapeutic work to a positive effect on therapy outcomes. This range of attitudes, from negative to positive, and the use of homework even by psychoanalytic-oriented psychotherapists (Stricker, 2007), suggests that more theoretical and empirical work is required to examine homework's effects in a range of psychotherapy approaches (Kazantzis, Lampropoulos, & Deane, 2005).

For instance, the relationship between treatment outcome and extent to which participants completed homework assignments was evaluated among 60 cocaine-dependent individuals assigned to cognitive-behavioral therapy. Homework as assigned in 72% of all sessions and initiated by participants in 48% of the sessions in which it was assigned.

Completion of homework was unrelated to participants' baseline characteristics and several indicators of treatment compliance. Participants who completed more homework assignments demonstrated significantly greater increases in the quantity and quality of their coping skills and used significantly less cocaine during treatment and through a one-year follow-up.

These results suggest that the extent to which participants are willing to complete extra-session assignments may be an important mediator of response to cognitive-behavioral therapy (Carroll, Nich, & Bull, 2005).

## Matching Diagnosis with Treatment: The Use of Self-help Mental Health Protocols

The meteoric rise of self-help mental health workbooks in the field of psychotherapy attests to the need to have participants use them as homework assignments (L'Abate, 2004a, 2004c). What is relevant to their use lies in their matching whatever clinical or non-clinical condition has been ever invented or created with interventions. At least five major publishing houses, among many others, have been involved in the production and advertising of self-help, mental health protocols or workbooks to be administered by mental health professionals and psychotherapists (L'Abate, 2004a, 2004c). Wiley (NJ) has produced "documentation" manuals, i.e., "treatment planners" that contain "handouts" or "work-sheets" that are equivalent to written protocols, in some cases, including a CD-Rom with the manual. Guilford (NY) has published quite a few books with "easy reproducible materials" that are also equivalent to written protocols. New Harbinger Publications (Oakland, CA) has produced also quite a few workbooks for many psychiatric and non-psychiatric conditions. Haworth (Binghamton, NY) has produced many "notebooks" full of handouts around a variety of topics, also equivalent to workbooks. Finally, Springer is publishing a major collection of protocols for individuals, psychiatric conditions, conflicting couples and families, non-clinical individual and relational enrichment and life-long learning, as well as protocols derived from single- or multiple-score tests and factor analyses of signs, symptoms, and behaviors (L'Abate, 2007b).

The cost-effective advantage I trumpeted from my clinical work using workbooks received a severe correction when this advantage was evaluated by comparing individuals, couples, and families who had been involved in outpatient psychotherapy without workbooks with similar participants who did receive workbooks as homework assignments (L'Abate, L'Abate, & Maino, 2005). The only dependent variable that could be evaluated in this research was the number of psychotherapy sessions, predicting that the number of sessions would decrease by the administration of written homework assignments, as indicated by the results of Kazantzis, Deane, and Ronan (2000). This prediction was completely inaccurate. Indeed, the use of written homework assignments for all three groups of individuals, couples, and families increased to a statistically significant level the number of psychotherapy sessions compared to participants who did not receive homework assignments.

Contradictory results, however, were obtained by Goldstein (L'Abate & Goldstein, 2007) using a problem-solving, cognitively-oriented workbook with hospitalized, decompensating women with certified personality disorders in Buenos Aires, Argentina. The use of this workbook cut in half the number of days spent in the hospital in comparison to a control group that did not receive this workbook. Hence, we are facing the empirical issue that workbooks may produce different results, at least in the number of sessions or days in the hospital, according to: (1) nature and composition of written protocol; (2) setting (inpatient versus outpatient); and (3) severity or type of condition (personality disorders versus problems in adjustment versus severe psychopathology).

Three analogies that have determined the course of research and writing on self-help, mental health protocols or workbooks: (1) they serve as software for computer-assisted interventions; (2) they are to psychological interventions what medications are to psychiatric interventions; and (3) they are now part of the therapeutic and preventive armamentarium of many mental health professionals (L'Abate, 2004a, 2004c, 2007a, 2007c). There is no need to elaborate on points 1 and 3. They have been elaborated here and elsewhere (L'Abate, 1992, 2004c, 2007a, 2007c). Point Number 2 needs elaboration in its analogy of protocols with medications. Most medications for psychiatric disorders are administered on a trial-and-error basis (Consumer Reports, 2004). If one medication for a particular condition, say depression, does not work, perhaps another will. By the same token, given the availability of more than one protocol for many clinical conditions, the same process can occur in homework assignments. If one protocol does not work for a particular condition, say depression, there are now more than half a dozen protocols that deal with the same condition (L'Abate, 2004a, 2007c). In spite of their questionable cost-effectiveness, as noted above, protocols are much more specific than any f2f tb interventions, because there is no way of controlling the latter. In addition, like medication, protocols can be mass-administered and are versatile. They can be used in classrooms, clinics, and hospitals in public and private practice with individuals, couples, and families.

## Working at a Distance from Participants

One implication of the LM that will be discussed at greater length in Chapter 19 of this volume relates to professionals learning to work at a distance from participants. One does not need to see or even meet (unless for insurance purposes) a participant. If that participant had received and completed a full battery of tests administered by trusted and reliable technicians, what is relevant is the consistency (or inconsistency) of various measures of functioning in various domains of interest to the referral source. If an entire battery of tests has been completed and interpreted, the resulting report would also give recommendations for whatever treatment may be necessary, that is, according to a stepped sieves design, whether a self-help group, a psychosocial skill training program administered by middle-levels professionals, or whether the participant should be seen f2f immediately by a professional or even a physician for treatment. By the same token, many psychological interventions can be administered by semi-professional personnel, and in some cases, as in self-help protocols, by para-professionals.

## OBSTACLES TO THE LABORATORY METHOD

There are at least three major obstacles that are antithetical to the LM: (1) the private health versus the public health practice model; (2) the clinical practice versus the research model; and (3) the solo versus the hierarchical model.

### Private versus Public Practice

Private practice is a perfectly legitimate, necessary professional activity that exists for the privilege of participants who can pay for services received, usually calculated on the hourly fee established by professionals themselves. Public health, on the other hand, means helping as many people as possible at the least possible cost but with the same effective methods used in private practice. That means also that a great many people in need of help who cannot afford to pay for it have to rely on publicly supported institutions. Public institutions rely on professionals who are paid a monthly salary, regardless of how many participants they see, even though usually 20 hours of f2f contacts are considered the norm. Their practices, however, as far as this writer knows, are not too different from those used in private practice. There is no uniformity of operations and no hierarchical structures of personnel. The professional does it all. He or she are responsible for rendering clinical services in the same way as a private practitioners. Hence, the private f2f tb practice model is also present in public institutions.

### Clinical versus Research Practice

Clinical practice means that operations for both evaluation and treatment vary from participant to participant, including different test batteries for different individuals and, even more importantly, supposedly different treatments taylor-made to the different needs to different participants. However, whether that specificity really exists is difficult to demonstrate since treatment remains in the privacy of professionals and, even if it could be demonstrated, very difficult to rely only on the professional's self-serving notes. As long as talk is the major if not the only medium of communication, as repeated here and elsewhere, it will be impossible to demonstrate what happened in the privacy of a professional's office. By the same token, professionals in public institutions also practice different approaches for participants without any uniformity of practices. In other words, being in a public institution does not guarantee that the evaluation of treatment outcome will be conducted. Consequently, research is left to professionals in academic settings where the norm of publishing or perishing through research grants is necessary for promotion and tenure. Therefore, neither private nor public institutions contribute to research efforts because their major goals are immediate help to participants either for pay or for needed services. Hence, the gap between practitioners and researchers continues unabated.

### Solo versus Group or Hierarchical Practice

The majority of private and public clinical practice is in the hands of professionals who are responsible for providing evaluation, treatment, or recommendations for treatment. Professionals perform technical and professional duties without differentiating between the two. Consequently, especially in evaluation, a great deal of professional time is spent on administrations of tests that could be administered at lesser costs by technical, paraprofessional personnel. The hierarchical structure found in other professions is not found in clinical psychology. Lawyers have para-professionals, physicians have physician assistants, nurses, and x-way technicians, as well as laboratories to examine blood samples, etc. These professions incidentally, rely on the written or printed word to reach final decisions left to the professional and not to the underlying personnel. Therefore, a great part of clinical psychologist's time is taken by activities that could be delegated and relegated to the hands of para-professionals. In this fashion, costs could decrease and efficiency could increase. Professional could see more participants for unit of their time than if it would be possible if all clinical activities were not left in his or her hands.

The LM, therefore, is wedded to a public health model with clinical practice and research going together tie-by-tie. A hierarchical structure in personnel would provide the best possible services that can be administered to as many people as possible who vary in the ability to pay, who cannot pay, or who can pay only portions of the costs involved.

## Conclusion

The LM does not claim to be a cure-all or panacea for all the shortcomings of clinical psychology and psychotherapy. Nor can it claim to cure all the ills of humankind. It is only an evolutionary step in attempting to make clinical psychology more accountable for its practices, lowering the costs of those very practices, and enlarging the populations of potential participants who could profit by psychological evaluations and treatments. Whether this volume will succeed in reaching this goal remains to its readers to decide.

## References

Adams, H. E. (1995). The relevance of psychological theories to standards of practice. In S. C. Hayes, V. M. Follette, R. M. Dawes, & K. E. Grady (Eds.), *Scientific standards of psychological practice: Issues and recommendations* (pp. 251-260). Reno, NV: Context Press.

Albee, G. W. (2000). Critique of psychotherapy in American society. In C. R. Snyder & R. E. Ingram (Eds.), *Handbook of psychological change: Psychotherapy processes & practices for the 21st century* (pp. 689-706). New York: Wiley.

Barrera, M., & Sander, I. N. (2006). Prevention: A report of progress and momentum into the future. *Clinical Psychology: Science and Practice*. 13, 221-226.

Bergin, A. E., & Garfield, S. L. (Eds.). (1994). *Handbook of psychotherapy and behavior change*. New York: Wiley.

Beutler, L. E. & Castonguay, L. G. (Eds). (2004). *Empirically supported principles of therapy change*. New York: Oxford University Press.

Beutler, L. E., & Davison, E. H. (1995). What standards should we use? In S.C. Hayes, V. M. Follette, R. M. Dawes, & K. E. Grady (Eds.), *Scientific standards of psychological practice: Issues and recommendations* (pp. 11-24). Reno, NV: Context Press.

Beutler, L. E., Kim, E. J., Davison, E., Karno, M., & Fisher, D. (1996). Research contributions to improve managed health care outcomes. *Psychotherapy*, *33*, 197-206.

Beutler, L. E., Malik, M., Alimohamed, S., Harwood, T. M., et al. (2003). Therapist variables. In M. J. Lambert (Ed), *Handbook of psychotherapy and behavior change* (5th ed.)(pp. 227-306). New York: Wiley.

Bracy, O. L. (1992). Q & A. *Computer Assisted Rehabilitation Therapy*, *1*, 2.

Bradley, V. A., Welch, J. L., & Skilbeck, C. E. (1993). *Cognitive retraining using microcomputers*. Hillsdale, NJ: LEA.

Brown-Stanbridge, M. D. (1989). A paradigm for construction of family therapy tasks. *Family Process*, *28*, 471-489.

Butcher, J. N. (2006). Assessment in clinical psychology: A perspective on the past, present challenges, and future prospects. *Clinical Psychology: Science and Practice*. 13, 205-209.

Carroll, K. M., Nich, C., & Bull, S. A. (2005). Practice makes progress? Homework assignments and outcome in treatment of cocaine dependence. *Journal of Consulting and Clinical Psychology*, *73*, 749-755.

Chambless, D. L., & Ollendick, T. H. (2001). Empirically supported psychological interventions: Controversies and evidence. *Annual Review of Psychology*, *52*, 685-716.

Cone, J. D. (1995). Assessment practice standards. In S. C. Hayes, V. M. Follette, R. M. Dawes, & K. E. Gracy (Eds.), *Scientific standards of psychological practice: Issues and recommendations* (pp. 201-224). Reno, NV: Context Press.

Consumer Reports (2004). Drugs vs. talk therapy: 3,079 readers rate their care for depression and anxiety. *Consumer Reports*, October, 22-29.

Davison, G. C., & Lazarus, A. A. (1995). The dialectics of science and practice. In S.C. Hayes, V. M. Follette, R. M. Dawes, & K. E. Grady (Eds.), *Scientific standards of psychological practice: Issues and recommendations* (pp. 95-). Reno, NV: Context Press.

DeMaria, R. (2003). Psychoeducation and enrichment: Clinical considerations for couple and family therapy. In T. L. Sexton, G. R. Weeks, & M. S. Robbins (Eds.), *Handbook of family therapy* (pp. 411-430). New York: Rutledge.

Demetrio, D., & Borgonovi, C. (2007). Teaching to remember ourselves: The autobiographical methodology. In L. L'Abate, (Ed.), *Handbook of low-cost interventions to promote physical and mental health: Theory, research, and practice* (pp. 251-270). New York: Springer.

Dineen, T, (1998). *Manufacturing victims: What the psychotherapy industry is doing to people*. Montreal, Canada: Robert Davies Multimedia Publishing.

Dobson, K. S., & Craig, K. D. (Eds.).(1998). *Empirically supported therapies: Best practice in professional psychology*. Thousand Oaks, CA: Sage.

Elliott, R., & Bradely, C. M. (1994). Developing a working marriage between psychotherapists and psychotherapy researches: Identifying shared purposes. In P. F.

Talley, H. H. Strupp, & S. F. Butler (Eds.), *Psychotherapy research and practice: Bridging the gap* (pp. 124-142). New York: Basic Books.

Esterling, B. A., L'Abate, L., Murray, E., & Pennebaker, J. M. (1999). Empirical foundations for writing in prevention and psychotherapy: Mental and physical outcomes. *Clinical Psychology Review, 19*, 79-96.

Follette, W. C. (1995). Correcting methodological weaknesses in the knowledge base used to derive practice standards. In S. C. Hayes, V. M. Follette, R. M. Dawes, & K. E. Grady (Eds.), *Scientific standards of psychological practice: Issues and recommendations* (pp. 229-247). Reno, NV: Context Press.

Garb, H. N. (1998). *Studying the clinician.* Washington, DC: American Psychological Association Press.

Gelso, C. J. (1985). Rigor, relevance, and counseling research: On the need to maintain our course between Scylla and Charybdis. *Journal of Counseling and Development, 63*, 551-553.

Hayes, S. C. (1995). What do we want from scientific standards of professional practice? In S. C. Hayes, V. M. Follette, R. M. Dawes, & K. E. Grady (Eds.), *Scientific standards of psychological practice: Issues and recommendations* (pp. 49-66). Reno, NV: Context Press.

Hayes, S. C., Follette, V. M., Dawes,R. M., & Grady, K. E. (Eds.).(1995). *Scientific standards of psychological practice: Issues and recommendations*. Reno, NV: Context Press.

Hayes, S. C., Barlow, D. H., & Nelson-Gray, R. O. (1999). *The scientist-practitioner: Research and accountability in the age of managed care: Second Edition*. Boston, MA: Allyn & Bacon.

Heppner, P. P., & Anderson, W. P. (1885). On the perceived non-utility of research in counseling. *Journal of Counseling and Development, 63*, 545-547.

Hersen, M., Kazdin, A. E., & Bellack, A. S. (Eds.).(1991). *The clinical psychology handbook: Second Edition*. New York: Pergamon.

Horvath, A. O., & Symonds, B. D. (1991). Relation between working alliance and outcome in psychotherapy: A meta-analysis. *Journal of Counseling Psychology, 38,* 139-149.

Howard, G. (1985a). Can research in the human sciences become more relavant to practice? *Journal of Counseling and Development, 63*, 539-544.

Howard, G. (1985b). Some thoughts I can't help thinking. *Journal of Counseling and Development, 63*, 554-555.

Howard, G. (1985c). The role of values in the science of psychology. *American Psychologist, 40*, 255-264.

Hsiung, R. C. (Ed.).(2002). *E-therapy: Case studies, guiding principles, and the clinical potential of the Internet.* New York: W. W. Norton.

Hunsley, J., & Mash, E. J. (2007). Evidence-based assessment. *Annual Review of Clinical Psychology, 3*, 29-51.

Huppert, J. D., Bufka, L. F., Barlow, D. H., Gorman, J. M., Shear, M. K.,, & Woods, S. W. (2000). Therapist, therapist variables, and cognitive-behavioral therapy outcome in a multi-center trial for panic disorder. *Journal of Consulting and Clinical Psychology, 69*, 747-755.

Interchange : The safety and efficacy of psychotherapy. *The Scientific Review of Mental Health Practice, 3*, 48-59.

Kacewicz, E., Slatcher, R. B., & Pennebaker, J. W. (2007). Expressive writing: An alternative to traditional methods. In L. L'Abate (Ed.), *Low-cost approaches to promote physical and mental health: Theory, research, and practice* (pp. 271-254). New York: Springer.

Kazantzis, N., Deane, F.P., & Ronan, K. R. (2000). Homework assignments in cognitive and behavioraltherapy: A meta-analysis. *Clinical Psychology: Science and Practice, 7*, 189–202.

Kazantzis, N., Deane, F. P., Ronan, K. R., & L'Abate, L. (Eds.).(2004). *Using homework assignments in cognitive behavior therapy*. New York: Rutledge.

Kazantzis, N., & L'Abate, L. (2007). *Handbook of homework assignments in psychotherapy: Theory, research, and prevention*. New York: Springer.

Kazantzis, N., Lampropoulos, G. K., & Deane, F. P. (2005). A National Survey of practicing psychologists' use and attitudes toward homework in psychotherapy. *Journal of Consulting and Clinical Psychology, 73*, 742-748.

Keen, E. (2000). *Ultimacy and triviality in psychotherapy*. Westpost, CT: Greenwood.

Keeney, B. P., & Morris, J. (1985). Implications of cybernetic epistemology for clinical research: A reply to Howard. *Journal of Counseling and Development, 63*, 548-550.

Kendall, P. C. (2006). The present and future of clinical psychology. *Clinical Psychology: Science and Practice*. 13, 203-204.

Kiesler, d. J. (1994). Standardization of interventions: The tie that binds psychotherapy research and practice. In P. F. Talley, H. H. Strupp, & S. F. Butler (Eds.), *Psychotherapy research and practice: Bridging the gap* (pp. 143-143). New York: Basic Books.

Kihlstrom, J. F. (2002). To honor Kraeplin…: From symptoms to pathology in the diagnosis of mental illness. In L. E. Beutler & M. L. Malik (Eds.), *Rethinking the DSM: A psychological perspective* (pp. 279-303). Washington, DC: American Psychological Association.

Kihlstrom, J. F., & Kihlstrom, L. C. (1998). Integrating science and practice in an environment of managed care. In D. K. Routh & R. J. DeRubeis (Eds.), *The science of clinical psychology: Accomplishments and future directions* (pp. 281-293). Washington, DC: American Psychological Association.

Kochalka, J., Buzas, H., L'Abate, L., McHenry, S., & Gibson, E. (1987). Structured enrichment: Training and implementation with paraprofessionals. In L. L'Abate, *Family psychology II: Theory, therapy, enrichment, and training* (pp. 279-287). Lanham, MD: University Press of America.

L'Abate, L. (1964). Il metodo di laboratorio nella psicodiagnosi (The laboratory method in psycho-diagnosis). *Bollettino di Psicologia Applicata, 63-64*, 36-39.

L'Abate, L. (1968a). Screening children with cerebral dysfunctions through the laboratory method. In C. H. Haywood (Ed.), *The diagnosis of brain-damage in school-age children* (pp. 128-158). Washington, DC: Council for Exceptional Children.

L'Abate, L. (1968b). The laboratory method as an alternative to existing mental health models. *American Journal of Orthopsychiatry, 38*, 296-297.

L'Abate, L. (1968c). The laboratory method in clinical psychology: An attempt at innovation. *The Clinical Psychologist, 21*, 183-184.

L'Abate, L. (1968d). Una stanza da giuoco automatizzata (An automated playtherapy room). *Bollettino di Psicologia Applicata, 88-90*, 43-54.

L'Abate, L. (1969). The continuum of rehabilitation and laboratory evaluation: Behavior modification and psychotherapy. In C. M. Franks (Ed.), *Behavior therapy: Appraisal and status* (pp. 476-494) New York: McGraw-Hill

L'Abate, L. (1971a). Three applications of the laboratory method in clinical psychology. *Bollettino di Psicologia Applicata, 109-111*, 33-39.

L'Abate, L. (1973a). The laboratory method in clinical child psychology: Three applications. *Journal of Clinical Child Psychology, 2*, 8-10.

L'Abate, L. (1973b). Valutazione della famiglia nel laboratorio (Laboratory evaluation of families). *Bollettino di Psicologia Applicata, 118-120*, 19-26.

L'Abate, L. (1974). Family enrichment programs. *Journal of Family Counseling, 2*, 32-38.

L'Abate, L. (1979). Aggression and construction in children's monitored playtherapy. *Journal of Counseling and Psychotherapy, 2*, 137-158.

L'Abate, L. (1986). *Systematic family therapy*. New York: Brunner/Mazel.

L'Abate, L. (1990). *Building family competence: Primary and secondary prevention approaches*. Newbury Park, CA: Sage.

L'Abate, L. (1992). *Programmed writing: Self-administere d applications for individuals, couples, and families*. Pacific Grove, CA: Brooks/Cole.

L'Abate, L. (1994a). *A theory of personality development*. New York: Wiley.

L'Abate, L. (1994b). *Family evaluation: A psychological perspective*. Newbury Park, CA: Sage.

L'Abate, L. (1996). Workbooks for better living. <*www.mentalhealthhelp.com*>

L'Abate, L. (1997). The paradox of change: Better them than us! In S. R. Sauber (Ed.), *Managed mental health care: Major diagnostic and treatment approaches* (pp. 40-66). Bristol, PA: Brunner/Mazel.

L'Abate, L. (1999a). Decisions we (mental health professionals) need to make (whether we like them or not): A reply to Cummings and Hoyt. *The Family Journal: Counseling and Therapy for Couples and Families, 7*, 227-230.

L'Abate, L. (1999b). Taking the bull by the horns: Beyond talk in psychological interventions. *The Family Journal: Counseling and Therapy for Couples and Families, 7*, 206-220.

L'Abate, L. (Ed.).(2001). *Distance writing and computer-assisted interventions in psychiatry and mental heath*. Westport, CT: Ablex.

L'Abate, L. (2002). *Beyond psychotherapy: Programmed writing and structured computer-assisted interventions*. Westport, CT: Ablex.

L'Abate, L. (2003a). *Family psychology III: Theory-building, theory-testing and psychological interventions*. Lanham, MD: University Press of America.

L'Abate, L. (2003b). Monitored play therapy revisited: Proposal for a virtual reality playroom. Unpublished manuscript. Author.

L'Abate, L. (2003c). Treatment t hrough writing: A unique new direction. In T. L. Sexton, G. Weeks, & M. Robbins (Eds.), *The handbook of family therapy* (pp. 397-409). New York: Brunner-Routledge.

L'Abate, L. (2004a). *A guide to self-help workbooks for mental health clinicians and researchers*. Binghamton, NY: Haworth.

L'Abate, L. (2004b). Family psychology as laboratory science. *The Family Psychologist, 20*, 21-22.

L'Abate, L. (2004c). The role of workbooks in the delivery of mental health services in prevention,psychotherapy and rehabilitation. In L. L'Abate (Ed.), *Workbooks in prevention, psychotherapy, and rehabilitation: A resource for clinicians and researchers* (pp. 3-64). Binghamton, NY: Haworth.

L'Abate, L. (2004d). Systematically written homework assignments: The case for homework based treatment. In L. L'Abate (Ed.), *Workbooks in prevention, psychotherapy, and rehabilitation: A resource for clinicians and researchers* (pp. 65-102). Binghamton, NY: Haworth.

L'Abate, L. (2005). *Personality in intimate relationships: Socialization and psychopathology*. New York: Springer..

L'Abate, L. (2007a). A completely preposterous proposal: The dictionary as an initial vehicle of change in the family. *The Family Psychologist, 23*, 39-43.

L'Abate, L (2007b). Introduction to Section IV. Writing. In L. L'Abate (Ed.), *Low-cost approaches to promote physical and mental health: Theory, research, and practice* (pp. 3-39). New York: Springer.

L'Abate, L. (2007c). (Ed.). *Low-cost approaches to promote physical and mental health: Theory, research and practice*. New York: Springer.

L'Abate, L. (2008). *Sourcebook of self-help protocols in mental health*. New York: Springer.

L'Abate, L. (in press).Proposal to introduce distance writing in couple therapy. *Journal of Relatioship and Couple Therapy,*

L'Abate, L. (2007). What I really believe about family therapy. *Journal of Family Psychotherapy*, 18, 33-44. .

L'Abate, L., Boyce, J., Fraizer, L., & Russ, D. (1992). Programmed writing: Research in progress. *Comprehensive Mental Health Care, 2*, 45-62.

L'Abate, L., & Cusinato, M. (2007). Linking theory with practice: Theory-derived interventions in prevention and family therapy. *The Family Journal: Counseling and Therapy for Couples and Families, 15,* 318-327.

L'Abate, L., & De Giacomo, P. (2003). *Intimate relationships and how to improve them: Integration of theoretical models with prevention and psychotherapy applications*. Westport, CT: Praeger.

L'Abate, L., & Goldstein D. (2007). Workbooks to promote mental health and life-long learning. In L. L'Abate (Ed.), *Handbook of low-cost interventions to promote physical and mental health: Theory, research, and practice* (pp. 285-302). New York: Springer.

L'Abate, L., & Jessee, E. (1981). Enrichment role-playing as a step in training of family therapists. *Journal of Marriage and Family Therapy, 7*, 507-514.

L'Abate, L., L'Abate, B. L., & Maino, E. (2004). A review of 25 years of part-time professional practice: Workbooks and length of psychotherapy. *American Journal of Family Therapy*, 33,19-31.

L'Abate, L., & Weinstein, S. E. (1987). *Structured enrichment programs for couples and families*. York: Brunner/Mazel.

L'Abate, L., & Young, L. (1987). *Casebook of structured enrichment programs for couples and families* New York: Brunner/Mazel.

Lambert, M. J., & Barley, D. E. (2001). Research summary on the therapeutic relationship psychotherapy outcome. *Psychotherapy: Theory/Research/Practice/Training, 38*, 357-361.

LeCroy, C. W. (Ed.).(1994). *Handbook of child and adolescent treatment manuals*. New York: Lexington Books.

Leigland, S. (1995). On the relation between clinical practice and psychological science. In S. C. Hayes, V. M. Follette, R. M. Dawes, & K. E. Grady (Eds.), *Scientific standards psychological practice: Issues and recommendations* (pp. 67-71). Reno, NV: Context Press.

Lepore, S., & Smyth, J. M. (2002). *The writing cure*. Washington, DC: American Psychological Association

Levine, M., & Calvanio, R. (2007). Patient recording of personal information as treatment and as electronic disease management. In L. L'Abate (Ed.), *Low-cost approaches to promote physical and mental health: Theory, research, and practice* (pp. 227-250). New York: Springer.

Liddle, H. A., Santisteban, D. A., Levant, R. F., & Bray, J. H., (2002). *Family psychology: Science-based interventions*. Washington, DC: American Psychological Association.

Lilienfeld, S. O., Fowler, K. A., Lohr, J. M., & Lynn, S. J. (2005). Pseudoscience, nonscience, and nonsense in clinical psychology: Dangers and remedies. In R. H. Wright & N. A. Cummings (Ed.), (pp. 187-218). *Destructive trends in mental health: The well-intentioned path to harm* (pp. 187-218). New York: Rutledge.

Lilienfeld, S. O., Lohr, J. M., & Lynn, S. J. (Eds.).(2003). *Science and pseudoscience in contemporary clinical psychology*. New York: Guilford.

Lipsey, M. W., & Wilson, D. B. (1993). The efficacy of psychological, educational, and behavioral treatment: Confirmation from meta-analyses. *American Psychologist, 48,* 1181-1209.

Martin, D. J., Garske,, J. P., & Davis, M. K. (2000). Relation of the therapeutic alliance with outcome and other variables: A meta-analytic review. *Journal of Consulting and Clinical Psychology, 68,* 438-450.

Maruish, M. E. (Ed.).(1999). *The use of psychological testing for treatment planning and outcomes assessment*. Mahwah, NJ: LEA.

McFall, R. M. (1995). Models of training and standards of care. In S. C. Hayes, V. M. Follette, R. M. Dawes, & K. E. Grady (Eds.), *Scientific standards of psychological practice: Issues and recommendations* (pp. 125-137). Reno, NV: Context Press.

McFall, R. M.(1996). Manifesto for a science of clinical psychology. *The Clinical Psychologist, 44*, 75-88.

McMahan, O., & L'Abate, L. (2001). Programmed distance writing with seminarian couples. In L. L'Abate (Ed.), *Distance writing and computer-assisted interventions in psychiatry and mental heath* (pp. 137-156). Westport, CT: Ablex.

McMahan, O., & Arias, J. (2004). Workbooks and psychotherapy with incarcerated felons: Replication of research in progress. In L. L'Abate (Ed.), *Using workbooks in mental health: Resources in prevention, psychotherapy, and rehabilitation for clinicians and researchers* (pp. 204-213).Binghamton, NY: Haworth.

Nathan, P. E., & Gorman, J. M. (Eds.).(1998). *A guide to treatments that work*. New York: Oxford.

Norcross, J. C. (2001). Purposes, processes, and products of the Task Force on Empirically Supported Therapy Relationships. *Psychotherapy: Theory/Research/Practice/Training, 38*, 345-356.

Norcross, J. C. (Ed). (2002). *Psychotherapy relationships that work: Therapist contributions and responsiveness to patient needs*. New York: Oxford University Press.

Norcross, J. C., Karpiak, C. P., & Lister, K. M. (2005). What's an integretionist? A study of self-identified integrative and (occasionally) eclectic psychologists. *Journal of Clinical Psychology, 61*, 587-594.

Norcross, J. C., Karpiak, C. P., & Santoro, S. O. (2005). Clinical psychologists across the years: The division of clinical psychology from 1960 to 2003. *Journal of Clinical Psychology, 61*, 1467-1483.

Persons, J. B. (1995). Why practicing psychologists are slow to adopt empirically-validated treatments. In S. C. Hayes, V. M. Follette, R. M. Dawes, & K. E. Grady (Eds.), *Scientific standards of psychological practice: Issues and recommendations* (pp. 142-157). Reno, NV: Context Press.

Pinsof, W., & Wynne, L. (Eds.).(1995). *Family therapy effectiveness: Current reseach and theory*. Washington, DC: AAMFT

President's New Freedom Commission on Mental Health (2003). *Achieving the promise: Transforming mental healthcare in America: Executive summary*. Rockville, MD: DHHS Publication No. SMA-03-3831.

Reed, R., McMahan, O., & L'Abate, L. (2001). Workbooks and psychotherapy with incarcerated felons: Research in progress. In L. L'Abate (Ed.), *Distance writing and computer-assisted interventions in psychiatry and mental health* (pp. 157-167). Newport, CT: Ablex.

Robbins, M. S., Liddle, H. A., Turner, c. W., Dakof, G. A., Alexander, J. F., & Kogan, S. M. (2006). Adolscent and parent therapeutic alliances as predictors of dropout in multidimensional family therapy. *Journal of Family Therapy, 20*, 108-116.

Roth, A., & Fonagy, P. (1996). *What works for whom? A critical review of psychotherapy research*. New York: Guilford.

Sajatovic, M., & Ramirez, L. F. (2001). *Rating Scales in Mental Health*. Hudson, OH: Lexi-Comp. Inc.

Schwartz, M. D. (1984). *Using computers in clinical practice: Psychotherapy and mental health applications*. New York: Haworth.

Sexton, T. L., Weeks, g. R., & Robbins, M. S. (2003). *Handbook of family therapy*. New York: Rutledge.

Shadish, W. R., Matt, G. E., Navarro, A. M., & Phillips, G. (2000). The effects of psychological therapies under clinically representative conditions: A meta-analysis. *Psychological Bulletin, 126*, 512-529.

Smyth, J., & L'Abate, L. (2001). A meta-analytic evaluation of workbook effectiveness in physical and mental health. In L. L'Abate (Ed.), *Distance writing and computer-assisted interventions in psychiatry and mental heath* (pp. 77-90). Westport, CT: Ablex.

Sperry, L. (Ed.).(2004). *Assessment of couples and families: Contemporary and cutting edge strategies*. New York: Brunner/Routledge.

Sprenkle, D. H. (Ed.).(2002). *Effectiveness research in marriage and family therapy*. Washington, DC: AAMFT.

Stevens, S. E., Hynan, M.T., & Allen, M. (2000). A meta-analysis of common factor and specific treatment effects across the outcome domains of the phase model of psychotherapy. *Clinical Psychology: Science & Practice*, *7*, 273-290.

Stiles, W. B. (1994). Views of the chasm between psychotherapy research and practice. In P. F. Talley, H. H. Strupp, & S. F. Butler (Eds.), *Psychotherapy research and practice: Bridging the gap* (pp. 154-180). New York: Basic Books.

Stricker, G. (1992). The relationship of research to clinical practice. *American Psychologist*, *47*, 543-549.

Stricker, G. (2007). Psychodynamic therapies. In N. Kazantzis & L. L'Abate (Eds.), *Handbook of homework assignments in psychotherapy; Research, practice, and prevention* (pp. 101-111). New York: Springer.

Sykes, C. J. (1992). *A nation of victims: The decay of the American character*. New York: St. Martin Press.

Tieyber, E., & McClure, F. (2000). Therapist variables. In C. R. Snyder & R. E. Ingram (Eds.), *Handbook of psychological change: Psychotherapy processes & practices for the 21st century* (pp. 62-87). New York: Wiley.

Touliatos, J., Perlmutter, B. F., & Straus, M. A. (Eds.).(1990). *Handbook of family measurement techniques*. Newbury Park, CA: Sage.

Treat, T. A., Bootzin, R. R., & Parker, T. B. (Eds.).(2007). *Psychological clinical science: Papers in honor of Ricahrd McFall*. Mahwah, NJ; LEA.

United States Public Health Service Office of the Surgeon General (1999). *Mental health: A report of the Surgeon General*. Rockville, MD: Department of Health and Human Services.

Van Hasselt, V. B., & Hersen, M. (Eds.).(1996). *Sourcebook of psychological treatment manuals for adult disorders*. New York: Lexington Books.

Walker, C. E. (Ed.).(1983). *The handbook of clinical psychology: Theory, research, and practice*. Homewood, IL: Dow Jones-Irwin.

Wampold, B. E. (2001). *The great psychotherapy debate: Models, methods, and findings*. Hillsdale, NJ: LEA.

Watters, E., & Ofshe, R. (1999). *Therapy's delusions: The myth of the unconscious and the exploitation of today's walking worried*. New York: Scribner.

Wilson, G. T. (1995). Empirically validated treatments as a basis for clinical practice: Problems and prospects. In S. C. Hayes, V. M. Follette, R. M. Dawes, & K. E. Grady (Eds.), *Scientific standards of psychological practice: Issues and recommendations* (pp. 163-196). Reno, NV: Context Press.

Woody, R. H. (Ed.).(1980). *Encyclopedia of clinical assessment*. Volumes I & II. San Francisco, CA: Jossey-Bass.

# Section I. The Laboratory Method in Evaluation and Treatment of Children and Families

In: Toward a Science of Clinical Psychology
Editor: Luciano L'Abate, pp. 37-55
ISBN: 978-1-60456-062-6


*Chapter II*

# SYSTEMATIC ASSESSMENT AND INTERVENTION WITH CHILDREN AND YOUTH

***Eleonora Maino***

## ABSTRACT

This contribution discusses the relevance of assessment and its objectives as well as the features that make it crucial for the diagnosis and treatment of children with a disability. We are of the opinion that a broad multidisciplinary evaluation, which integrates both qualitative and quantitative information and also takes into account the child and young person's contexts of development is the most suitable approach to take in order to define the child's rehabilitation route and to evaluate its efficacy.

This contribution describes the model used at a Medical Centre, situated in northern Italy, which was founded to meet the rehabilitation requirements of disabled children and their families and has recently become a reference centre for child neuropsychiatry and a centre of excellence for the diagnosis and treatment of children with autism.

In this model, the diagnosis and evaluation, which are carried out according to the World Health Organization Family of International Classification, are two distinct, yet co-present processes. The diagnosis is aimed at identifying, recognising and classifying the constant features of a disease or a condition, while the evaluation is aimed at detecting the peculiarities of the person's global functioning, both as an individual and within a given context.

In this perspective, evaluation is understood to be a broad evaluation process based on replicable operational procedures, which relies on the contributions of different specialists working within multidisciplinary teams. It also integrates subjective data, i.e. the examiners' opinions filtered by their own expertise, experience and training, and objective data obtained from the assessment, i.e. a formal process consisting of an interview and specific rating measures (L'Abate, 1994).

Such an evaluation must look not only at the minor but also explore her context of life, first and foremost her family and school.

This contribution thus discusses the methodology that is applied in order to involve the child's family in the assessment and outlines the effects, within the rehabilitative plan, of a comprehensive evaluation process which considers the child's limitations and resources alongside the family's limitations and resources.

## Diagnosis and Evaluation According to the World Health Organization Family of International Classification

In the study of disability, the need for increasingly more appropriate and specific language and measures that are shared among practitioners is a recent one. This common ground can help practitioners address the complex issues raised by disabilities in rehabilitation and socio-educational settings (Buono and Zagaria, 2003; Soresi, 1998, 2001; Zoccarato, 1996). The search for standardized and shared languages regarding disabilities, as well as measures which enable practitioners to detect and evaluate the outcomes of specific health conditions as consistently as possible involved numerous international teams coordinated by the World Health Organization (WHO).

In an attempt to pursue this objective and to improve the quality of the diagnosis of existing conditions, during the second half of the last century the WHO began to develop a classification system based on the observation and evaluation of organic, psychic and behavioural pathologies, now known as the Family of International Classification. Classifications such as this were, and still are, used as reference models to codify a wide range of health information and produce a common standardized language which enables this information to be shared between and across disciplines and branches, all over the world.

There are numerous advantages to relying on such an internationally accepted classification system. First of all, it offers the opportunity to compare data describing different situations in several regions across the world, and this is important, not to mention essential, when common goals are pursued. Not only does the comparison of data mean that the impact of an illness on a population can be understood in qualitative and quantitative terms, it also enables practitioners to make assumptions regarding its etiopathogenesis, as it is not equally distributed in the world.

Secondly, understanding the distribution of a disease enables practitioners to devise common preventive and/or therapeutic measures that are as effective as possible. In this regard, the availability of health evaluation measures which also monitor the changes due to the interventions is important for improving health (Leonardi and Ustun, 2002). Furthermore, a proper classification of diseases and correlated events (treatment, care, etc.) has recently led to the definition of health utilization parameters which are essential for the development of appropriate health economics policies, essential in every modern country. All this clarifies the usefulness and the significance of an increasingly comprehensive and explanatory common classification system and warrants the commitment and the energy invested by international and national organisations. This should come as no surprise as the need for a standardised and correct description of events in view of their classification was felt by health practitioners and statisticians as early as the 18$^{th}$ century (Fallone, 2004).

Historically, this need was perceived mainly by physicians processing health statistics as they needed an overview of the main causes of death across different populations. The first traceable attempts at producing a classification of diseases were mainly local in scope and only rarely did they achieve national significance. The first international classification of the causes of death was recognised at the First International Statistical Congress (Brussels, 1855) but it was only in 1893 that the International Institute of Statistics in Chicago proposed a classification (i.e. Bertillon Classification of Causes of Death and later International List of Causes of Death) which was met with acclaim and was fully accepted by the international community concerned.

Starting from 1900, this international classification underwent many revisions, both in content and assumptions, leading to the current WHO Family of International Classification. At least three important turning points which took place during this time need to be mentioned. The first turning point, which marked the beginning of a new era for medical statistics, took place in 1948 when the first World Health Assembly approved a new classification based on the indications of the International Conference for the Sixth Revision of the International List of Diseases and Causes of Death. This classification was named "Manual of the International Statistical Classification of Diseases, Injuries and Causes of Death" and was to be used not only for the causes of death, but also for diseases, which were not necessarily followed by the death of the person involved.

The second important turning point took place in 1975 when the International Conference for the Ninth Revision of the International Classification of Diseases (ICD-9, 1977) made a number of amendments which led to a more detailed classification, useful not only as a list of diseases, but also as a nosographic model that focused on the etiological origins of diseases and provided, for each symptom or disorder, a description of the main clinical features and indications for diagnosis. So, additional classifications correlated to the ICD were published: "Impairments and Handicaps" and "Procedures in Medicine".

Now in its tenth revision (ICD-10, 1992), this tool allows for the systematic detection, evaluation, interpretation and comparison of data about mortality and morbidity in different countries or regions, even at different times.

The third important turning point was linked to the recent realisation that the ICD does not provide a reliable overview of current health and disease issues, because it focuses exclusively on diseases – it is inadequate for describing what is happening in health and diseases nowadays. Medical care progressively improved over the last century, and instead of acute diseases for which an approach based on a single episodic diagnostic and short treatment intervention would suffice, there is now an increase in chronic diseases, also associated with a longer life expectancy, and the consequent need to provide long-term treatment.

For this reason, practitioners are now concentrating not only on the disease (or disability) understood as a limited entity in itself but also on the sequaele of the disease, namely how the child and her family and her caregivers cope with the disease.

Therefore, at the centre of the new WHO classification, i.e. the International Classification of Impairments, Disability and Handicap (ICIDH, 1980), there is a concept of disease seen as both an entity in itself and an event which seriously affects an individual's life.

Unlike the ICD, the ICIDH is focused on an individual's health and any changes that can interfere with daily living and raise the need for the individual to be referred to the health services. The ICIDH also looks at the individual from three different points of view: the body, the person and her social skills, in a so-called "biological-psychic-social" perspective. This approach offers a comprehensive view of the biological, psychological and social features of an individual and attempts to overcome the distinction between purely "medical" models and purely "social" models of disability by integrating them into a single concept.

Like any classification, the ICIDH underwent many reviews over time, according to the issues and doubts that emerged from its practical application. So, the 54th World Health Assembly approved a new WHO classification, namely the International Classification of Functioning, Disability and Health (ICF, 2001), in May 2001.

The ICF evolved from the ICIDH, and the new title reveals the desire to take into account positive experiences as well, by considering the individual's global functioning and focusing on the elements that concur to determine an individual's health rather than merely looking at the disease sequaele.

The ICF takes a neutral stance on aetiology and its main objective is to provide indications regarding an individual's global functioning by identifying her limitations and resources, and enabling practitioners to detect different functioning levels associated to a disease and similar functioning levels associated to different health conditions. On this assumption, there is a need for an increasingly more accurate and broader evaluation.

The ICF consists of two parts: Part I explores health domains and investigates the person as an individual, Part 2 explores health domains and investigates the person as a social entity influenced by environmental factors acting as obstacles or facilitators.

The WHO is currently completing the first classification of health and disability for children and young people (ICF – CY: ICF version for Children and Youth) that will be officially presented in Venice on 25-26 October, 2007.

Together with the ICD and the ICHI (International Classification of Health Intervention), the ICF is part of the aforementioned WHO Family of International Classification.

The WHO advocates the importance of using both classifications – ICD and ICF – in a complementary manner to investigate and understand the health and well-being of an individual in broad terms through the integration of the etiological data with an analysis of the impact that such a disease can have on the individual and her environmental context. In this regard, the ICD-10 provides the guidelines for making a diagnosis and describes the process and the aetiology of the disease, while the ICF describes and assesses the individual's global functioning, taking into consideration her limitations and resources.

Based on these considerations and this short historical overview, it is easy to understand how, despite their frequent use as synonyms, diagnosis and evaluation are distinct, yet co-present, processes.

Diagnosis may be defined as a process which enables the constant features of a pathology or condition to be detected, recognised and classified, while evaluation stands for the process which reveals the peculiarities in the functioning of a given individual, "differentiating" the people who, although they have the same pathology, can show a different development and functioning (thus skills, resources and limitations) dependent on time, context and rehabilitation.

This leads us to conclude that the more integrated diagnosis and evaluation are, the easier it is to define a targeted and individualised intervention. A clinical diagnosis is not sufficient for the purpose of developing an appropriate rehabilitation plan and understanding the needs and the resources of a child with a disability. An assessment pathway is essential in order to detect the child's specific functioning characteristics. This assessment should take into account individual differences and the fact that two children may not present with the same level of development and functioning, even though they may share the same diagnosis.

In this regard, the diagnosis is a starting point and needs to be integrated with the information obtained from a functional evaluation which:

- is specific and individualised, free of general definitions and which evaluates an individual based on her functioning within a certain context;
- evaluates the child's functioning based on norm comparisons (Vig and Kaminer, 2003);
- identifies the child's functional deficits and the potentials that can be leveraged;
- helps people to develop appropriate expectations for their child's development (Meisels and Atkins-Burnett, 2000);
- is interdisciplinary: a single practitioner is not likely to identify all the rehabilitation needs of a person within her context;
- is dynamic and is subject to regular adjustments according to the child's pathological picture;
- uses objective measures to quantify/verify/compare the data obtained;
- points to the most significant intervention and enables an outcome assessment to be made.

This is the only methodology which facilitates an understanding of the complexity of the variables at stake, provides an accurate picture of the child's situation, enables information to be shared among all the practitioners involved, identifies and plans the most appropriate intervention and assesses its outcome.

In this perspective, carrying out an assessment means that results may be verified. On the one hand, the assessment enables the practitioner to understand the situation as it is at the beginning, whereas on the other, it enables the practitioner to verify the efficacy of the intervention by comparing the intervention goals with the change achieved.

## Multidisciplinary Evaluation and Team Work

It is now clear that an evaluation is a broad, complex and interdisciplinary process. And it could not be otherwise, especially where disability is concerned.

If the needs and the development of a healthy child are complex, the needs and the development of a child with a disability are even more complex. Furthermore, there is a wide variability in disability that needs to be taken into account in terms of skills, needs and resources. It can be expected that a child with multiple disabilities and complex neurological problems (i.e. a typical cerebral palsy picture) has needs which are different from those of a child with a specific disability and a moderately severe impairment such as controllable epilepsy or a mild hemiplegia.

Furthermore, the more complex the disability, the more difficult it is for a single practitioner to identify all the needs and problems of the child and her family. Therefore it is advisable to work in multidisciplinary teams as this ensures that an intervention will be as comprehensive, flexible and integrated as possible (Robards, 1994).

With regard to service access, the families of a disabled child are referred to many different service agencies (social and health services, educational services, no-profit organisations, etc.). It is estimated that families meet 10 different practitioners and make more than 20 visits to hospitals or clinics every year (Sloper and Turner, 1992). Unfortunately, these agencies are not always well coordinated and parents report difficulties such as understanding when services are available, how they can be accessed, what the role of the different departments and practitioners is, and they feel they are not understood by practitioners and do not obtain what they need (Sloper, 1999). To overcome these difficulties, many studies stress the importance of relying on key workers who can help parents keep in touch with these agencies (Sloper, Greco, Beecham and Webb, 2006) and experience a greater integration and coordination of services.

With regard to evaluation, the "model recommended by the Division for Early Childhood of the Council for Exceptional Children (Hemmeter, Joseph, Smith and Sandall, 2001) involves a transdisciplinary approach. Team members are interdependent and release professional roles, based on discipline-specific skills, to one another. The team includes parents and may also include other individuals (paediatricians, relatives) who are part of a child's life" (Vig and Kaminer, 2003, p. 342).

It is important that the multidisciplinary teams involved in the assessment or provision of rehabilitation services are well integrated and work in synergy, with ranks being defined according to background, expertise and experience: "just as skyscrapers are not built by architects and engineers alone, so, in the mental health field, we need to start practicing according to different credentials, competencies, and capacities at various levels (lattices or ladders) of human endeavour" (L'Abate, 1994, p. 95).

Within these teams, practitioners (child neuropsychiatrists, physiatrists, pharmacologists, psychologists, physical therapists, assistants, nurses, etc.) first make their own assessment by applying specific methodologies and measures, and then work as a team in order to make a diagnosis and a functional evaluation and develop a rehabilitation plan.

For this methodology to be effective, it is important that practitioners share a common language, which does not mean a single approach. On the contrary, it involves a knowledge of the cultural models and the approaches that direct the other team members' work (Sorrentino, 2006).

To this end, assessment procedures should make a synergistic use of qualitative and quantitative measures. Qualitative measures are indeed an advantage because they enable practitioners to increase their knowledge base and share it with others (Clerici and Bertrando, 1993), thus contributing to the creation of a common language.

Within these teams, practitioners must be aware that, by playing a well-defined role, they contribute to a consistent assessment and intervention. It would be detrimental for the team, as well as for the child and her family, if each single practitioner made an assessment or proposed an intervention without considering the other team members' opinions and verifying whether there is consistency of judgment (Sorrentino, 2006).

In this perspective, as a fundamental resource and the first life context for the child, the family must necessarily be involved in the assessment and care pathway.

Over the last 10 years there have been many legislative and sociocultural changes, and the families' relationship with service agencies has changed. Parents now have more influence in deciding what services are best for their children. Because of a lack of health resources, their involvement has grown and they are now involved in the coordination of services and the implementation of rehabilitation programmes at home. In light of this, family-centred services (FCSs) were set up in North American hospitals and community-based service organizations (Law, Teplicky, King, King, Kertoy, Moning, Rosenbaum and Burke-Gaffney, 2005).

FCS is a method and philosophy of service delivery that emphasizes the partnership between parents and service providers (Hostler, 1994). In this approach, each family is given the opportunity to decide how involved they want to be in the services and decision-making for their child (Brown, Humphry and Taylor, 1997; Rosenbaum, King, Law, King and Evans, 1998). The strengths, resources and needs of all family members are considered (Allen and Petr, 1998; Rosembaum et al., 1998). There is evidence that FCS leads to improved outcomes for children and families (King, King, Rosembaum and Goffin, 1999; King, Teplicky, King and Rosembaum, 2004), and that parents are more satisfied with services that are perceived to be family-centred (King et al., 1999; Law, Hanna, King, Hurley, King, Kertoy, and Rosembaum, 2003).

## INVOLVING THE FAMILY IN DIAGNOSIS AND EVALUATION

Involving the parents in the child's management has many different advantages for child and parents alike and bodes well for the rehabilitation success.

In point of fact, it is usually the parents who take their children to a service even when their concerns are downplayed by friends, relatives, teachers, paediatricians, etc., and they are told that their child's difficulties will disappear with time. At other times, parents are urged, yet not persuaded, by other family members or other acquaintances. In both cases, and especially in the latter case, it is advisable for parents to be involved in the evaluation process.

The evaluation can give parents an opportunity to observe their child from different perspectives: the routine questions on the developmental milestones and the behaviours of the child and the observations carried out in their presence help them identify behaviours, limitations and resources which had gone unnoticed.

To this end, the clinician should try to understand what the parents think and know about their child's difficulties, listen attentively, spend time with them in order to understand how they see their child, what their greatest concerns are and what they expect from the evaluation. Seeing the child with different eyes is particularly useful even when parents and clinicians have different concerns, as is usually the case at the beginning of diagnosis and evaluation.

It sometimes happens that parents have a concern that reveals a different problem (Vig and Kaminer, 2003). Even in this case, the evaluation process can help them reflect on the fact that their child's problems are greater than expected. For example, a referral for a language delay could lead to a diagnosis of deafness, autism or mental retardation.

This once again stresses the importance of a comprehensive multidisciplinary evaluation of the child's functioning in order to help parents form a truer-to-life picture of her limitations, resources and future development. So they can develop a different awareness of their child and learn how to interact with her in new and more appropriate ways.

It must not be forgotten that forming a clear idea of the child's resources is an important stage in the assessment, in spite of the fact that parents want to verify whether their doubts are founded and identify their child's limitations, the aetiology and severity of her disease, and know the prognosis and the therapeutic indications.

All children, including those with significant developmental delays, have resources that can be leveraged by both practitioners and families alike. Practitioners should therefore help parents understand the child's problems and, at the same time, highlight her resources in order to increase the parents' acceptance of her abilities and limitations.

This is especially important after the diagnosis has been given, when the parents' concerns are confirmed.

This is a painful experience for parents, especially when it is unexpected, or when they realise that the difficulties they had reported were a warning of much more serious problems. At this time, when pain, confusion and often denial prevail, it is important to help parents give vent to, and express their pain and re-establish a connection with their child.

To this end, a broad interdisciplinary evaluation which focuses the parents' attention not only on the "diagnostic label" and the child's limitations, but also on her resources and potential for development, can lead them to accept their child as she is and slowly abandon the idea of the child they would have wanted her to be.

On the other hand, the parents also feel relieved as they can now pool their efforts towards rehabilitation, especially when the time between the first observation of the child's difficulties and diagnosis is long and the child has undergone several specialist examinations. Not all parents, however, are eager to know their child's diagnosis. Some families want to know what the diagnostic label is, whereas others are more interested in the rehabilitation options available and want to experience them before knowing the diagnosis. In both cases, however, an accurate diagnosis with indications on the future child's development can be an important part of the intervention. According to Werner (2000), diagnosis and evaluation are the first step in early intervention. This is even truer if the assessment is seen as a valuable opportunity to increase the parents' compliance with the child's therapies and follow-ups, besides establishing a partnership with the practitioners.

Clinical practice has shown that, the more confidence a family has in the intervention, the more successful this will be. This is another reason why the evaluation process should also rely on a partnership between parents and practitioners.

To provide an indication of what this means in practice, the remainder of this chapter will present the diagnosis and evaluation process that takes place within a Rehabilitation Centre for children and adolescents, with particular emphasis given to the diagnosis and evaluation for children referred for a suspected generalised developmental disorder.

# A Rehabilitation Centre for Children and Adolescents

The "Eugenio Medea" Scientific Institute of La Nostra Famiglia Association is situated in northern Italy. The Association, which has many other Rehabilitation Centres in Italy, was set up to provide services for the diagnosis, treatment and rehabilitation of children with disabilities and counselling for their families.

La Nostra Famiglia Association, which has a high attendance record, is the largest in Italy providing services to children and adolescents. It is attended each year by around 16,000 patients, generally children and adolescents (age 0-18 years) with organic pathologies (genetic diseases, rare syndromes, mental retardation, neuromotor disorders, brain tumours and infantile brain tumours) or psychopathological disturbances.

In 1985, the Association founded the "Eugenio Medea" Scientific Institute, drawing from its varied and solid experience in the field of disability in order to meet the need to implement validated preventive and rehabilitation methodologies and practices in a better way.

The priority goals of the Centre include broadening the knowledge and the skills which have an immediate effect on daily clinical practice with regard to both prevention and rehabilitation and preventive, educational, psychoeducational and therapeutic interventions in the family and the community.

The Centre counts many specialist departments where practitioners with different backgrounds can work together in teams and cooperate with other services and units. A brief description of each department is given below:

Neurorehabilitation 1 is attended by patients with early-onset neurological pathologies (above all, brain diseases, epilepsy and headache, mental retardation and neuropsychological deficits, neurovisual disorders, rare syndromes involving the CNS). Diagnosis and evaluation are carried out, and indications for rehabilitation are provided.

Neurorehabilitation 2 is attended by patients with psychopathological disorders. For more specific intervention lines, the department is organized in multidisciplinary working groups for patients with Autism and Generalised Developmental Disorders, Rett syndrome, Cornelia de Lange syndrome and Wolf-Hirschhorn syndrome; Learning disabilities and Attention Deficit Hyperactivity Disorder (ADHD); Language Disorders; Emotional disorders and Depression; Eating disorders.

Neurorehabilitation 3 is responsible for the clinical management and rehabilitation of post-traumatic patients, patients with a brain tumour or other CNS lesions, from the subacute phase up to re-entry into the community.

Functional rehabilitation carries out a functional evaluation of, and provides rehabilitation to, patients with neuromotor disability, congenital and acquired motor disabilities which may persist into adulthood. In particular, rehabilitation is provided to patients with infantile cerebral palsy, neuromuscular diseases, severe skeletal deformities, osteogenesis imperfecta.

In each department, the multidisciplinary teams are formed by the following practitioners: a physician (neurologist, child neuropsychiatrist, psychiatrist, physiatrist, orthopedist, paediatrician, dietologist, radiologist, etc.), a psychologist (with different orientations and specialisations), a pedagogist, a social worker, a nurse, a rehabilitation therapist (speech therapist, psychomotor therapist, assistant, etc.).

The child is referred to the department that is most appropriate for the rehabilitation of her pathology or her suspected diagnosis. She then undergoes diagnostic tests and assessment or receives the necessary rehabilitation.

For the purpose of diagnosis and evaluation the child is hospitalised or attends the Centre in day-hospital regimen. This requires about 1-2 weeks, during which time a physician becomes the key coordinator of the process and decides which tests need to be performed.

The physician then communicates the outcome of these tests to the parents and, if possible, she makes a diagnosis and outlines a functional evaluation together with the most appropriate interventions. Rehabilitation can then be provided on an outpatient basis at the Centre or at other local service agencies.

As the evaluation and management of children with disabilities are not only focused on the child's pathology but also on her context of life (mainly her family), a Family Psychology Service was set up in 1998.

The Family Psychology Service is a cross-departmental unit responsible for the evaluation of family dynamics, providing counselling and family therapy as well as carrying out research, which is closely linked to clinical practice. The presence of a Family Psychology Service – which also provides counselling to parents – within a medical and rehabilitation centre is certainly an innovative approach in Italy. In point of fact, medical intervention in Italy usually focuses on the patient and sometimes on the disease or the affected part of the body, disregarding other equally fundamental aspects such as the family of origin or significant relationships, especially in childhood and adolescence.

The theoretical approach applied in our Service is the systemic relational approach according to Mara Selvini Palazzoli and colleagues (Selvini Palazzoli, Boscolo, Cecchin, and Prata, 1975; Selvini, 1985; Selvini Palazzoli, Cirillo, Selvini, and Sorrentino, 1988; Selvini Palazzoli, Cirillo, Selvini, and Sorrentino, 1998).

This model is most in line with the management provided in our Institute as it takes into account the individual with her needs, intentions and goals as well as the relational system to which she belongs. It integrates both systemic/relational patterns and individual patterns according to the intrapsychic functioning model proposed by authors such as Bowlby (1988), Kouth (1987), Miller (1981), Fairbain (1952) and the current family structure (triad) and family history (the last three generations).

In recent years, there has been a considerable increase in the number of referrals of children with autism. While in 1998 we had 7 children participating in an intensive rehabilitation program, we now have around 100 children. We also have 300 children each year – and their number is on the increase – who are referred to us for diagnosis and evaluation, or for follow-up.

This led us to improve our diagnostic and evaluation methodology as well as our intervention approaches. Due to this progressive specialisation our Centre has recently been recognised as a centre of excellence for the diagnosis and management of children with autism.

## DIAGNOSIS AND EVALUATION OF CHILDREN WITH AUTISM

Infantile autism is a behavioural disturbance characterised by deficits in social interaction (Frith, 1989; Rogers and Pennington, 1991; Sigman and Ruskin, 1999) and communication (Paul and Cohen, 1984; Tager-Flusberg, 198la; 1981b; 1999) and restricted interests. Some authors also report the presence of a particular cognitive trait (Baron-Cohen, Leslie and Frith, 1985).

Despite the fact that autism is present at birth, it is usually diagnosed late as until age 2-3 years it is difficult to recognise it and distinguish it from normal development, pragmatic disorders of communication or mild mental retardation.

At present there is no single comprehensive examination for the diagnosis of infantile autism which must therefore rely on an accurate search for symptoms through ad-hoc scales and questionnaires, accessory examinations and an assessment of developmental milestones.

As a diagnosis of autism relies on purely behavioural parameters, it is essential to observe the child in standardised settings and administer objective assessment scales that have been validated against the diagnostic criteria of DSM-IV (1994) and ICD-10 (1992) (i.e. the guidelines of the American Academy of Neurology and the Child Neurology Society). Furthermore, a diagnosis of autism must also include a number of clinical examinations in order to identify the various features of the disease and any possible comorbidities. The guidelines of the American Academy of Neurology and the Child Neurology Society suggest the routine examinations and the tests that need to be performed upon medical prescription, when autism is suspected. While the final diagnosis is made by the physician, the diagnostic and functional evaluation process should involve other practitioners such as psychologists, rehabilitation therapists and assistants who have a fair knowledge of the pathology and work together in a multidisciplinary team.

According to the American Academy of Neurology and the Child Neurology Society, the functional evaluation should target the following areas:

- Speech and language
- Cognitive level
- Adaptive behaviour
- Psychoeducational evaluation
- Neuropsychological picture
- Family resources

The coordinating physician (generally the child neuropsychiatrist) is responsible for the whole process, from the most appropriate tests to the length of hospitalisation. Both qualitative and quantitative measures are used to form a picture that is as accurate as possible. Usually the physician coordinates the diagnostic testing, while all the other practitioners carry out the functional assessment.

In particular, to make a diagnosis, the child neuropsychiatrist has interviews with parents, observes the child during play and also administers assessment scales that are relevant for diagnosis, including the Childhood Autism Rating Scale (CARS, Schopler, Reichler, DeVellis, and Daly, 1980), the Autism Diagnostic Observation Schedule (ADOS, Lord, Risi,

Lambrecht, Cook Jr., Leventhal, DiLavore, Pickles and Rutter, 2000) and the Autism Diagnostic Interview – Revised (ADI-R, Lord, Rutter, and Le Couteur, 1994).

**Table 1. Lists the main examinations and diagnostic tests performed at Eugenio Medea Institute.**

| DIAGNOSTIC FRAMING AND FUNCTIONAL EVALUATION FOR CHILDREN WITH AUTISM | | |
|---|---|---|
| DIAGNOSTIC FRAMING | | |
| | CHILD NEUROPSYCHIATRIST (responsible for the child's diagnosis and evaluation) | **ADMISSION INTERVIEW, CLINICAL INSTRUMENTAL EVALUATION SCHEDULE** (sleep EEG, haematology, FRAXA/FRAXE, audiometric testing, ophthalmologic examination, etc.) |
| | | **CLINICAL NEUROPSYCHIATRIC ASSESSMENT** Interview, collection of personal and familial history, neurological examination, objective testing (CARS/ADOS-G/ADI-R) |
| FUNCTIONAL EVALUATION | | |
| | EDUCATIONAL PSYCHOLOGIST | **PSYCHOLOGICAL AND PSYCHOEDUCATIONAL ASSESSMENT** Parent interview, individual observation, objective testing (PEP-3, Vineland) |
| | TESTING PSYCHOLOGIST and EDUCATOR | **PSYCHOMETRIC ASSESSMENT** Age-appropriate testing (Griffiths, Leiter or Wisc-R) |
| | SPEECH THERAPIST | **SPEECH THERAPY EVALUATION** Receptive/expressive language examination, analysis and recording of spontaneous speech, study of communication pragmatics |
| | PSYCHOMOTOR THERAPIST | **PSYCHOMOTOR EVALUATION** Individual observation and outline of a psychomotor profile |
| | NEUROPSYCHOLOGIST | **NEUROPSYCHOLOGICAL EVALUATION** Executive function testing and administration of NEPSY II |
| | FAMILY PSYCHOLOGIST | **FAMILY DYNAMICS EVALUATION** 2 interviews with both parents and self-report measures (FES and PSI) |

The CARS is a 15-item behavioural rating scale that allows the practitioner to assess and collect information about various contexts and from multiple informants. The 15 domains include: relating to people, imitation, emotional response, body use, object use, adaptation to change, visual response, listening response, taste/smell/touch response and use, fear or nervousness, verbal communication, nonverbal communication, activity level and consistency of intellectual response, general impressions.

Widely used for the diagnosis of autism, the ADOS is complementary to the structured interview for parents (ADI-R). It is based on direct observation and consists of a number of modules targeting social behaviour in natural communication contexts. The ADI-R is a semi-structured interview for parents, which includes a list of questions on the behaviours belonging to the symptomatological triad of autism and the type of games the child plays.

The child's functional profile is also outlined by the results of other two widely applied measures, namely the Psycho-Educational Profile – Third Edition (PEP-3, Schopler, Lansing, Reichler, and Marcus, 2005) and the Vineland Adaptive Behaviour Scales (VABS, Sparrow, Balla, and Cicchetti, 1984). These measures are usually administered by a psychologist with the help of an assistant in the framework of the child's psychological and psychoeducational assessment.

The PEP-3 assesses the skills and behaviours of children with autism in order to outline a detailed developmental picture and devise an individualised intervention plan based on observation of the child. The VABS is a semi-structured interview for parents and is considered to be the best psychometric scale. It assesses the adaptive behaviour of an individual while she performs daily life activities and the tasks related to her social role, against the community's expectations for an individual of the same age and from the same cultural context.

Together with other qualitative and quantitative measures used in the framework of the functional assessment, these measures outline a detailed picture of the child's functioning, one that is predictive of the most appropriate rehabilitation interventions which can be shared within the team and with the parents.

Here special attention must not only be given to the child but also to her context of life through what is generally known as an "assessment of family dynamics", the goals of which are to identify the main concerns of the parents, verify the needs and resources of each single family member and the family as a whole, understand the impact that an often invalidating organic pathology has on the family, establish a partnership with parents and favour their compliance with the diagnostic and evaluation process as well as verify the advisability for an individual or a group intervention based on the child's symptoms, the family dynamics, and their resources and needs.

At present the assessment, which is made by a psychologist of the Family Psychology Service, relies on a protocol including clinical interviews and self-report measures. This enables information to be collected from multiple informants in order to provide a more complete and comprehensive assessment.

The family dynamics is usually evaluated through two interviews with parents (usually with both, sometimes separately). There may be a third interview at which it is considered appropriate to involve siblings or grandparents or significant adults.

The collection of information usually starts with the child and her history, paying particular attention on the symptom/problem as is perceived currently and in her history. The parents' concerns and their –sometimes different– views of the child's unease and/or disease aetiology are targeted. The meaning that each family member gives to the child's symptom/unease is shared in order to achieve a relational interpretative key of the actual unease, if possible.

The evaluation then includes the family subsystems, first of all the parent-parent dyad and the parent-child dyad, and the sibling subsystem. Each subsystem contributes to the family functioning in specific ways. Therefore, the assessment looks at the child's history, primary care giving and attachment, the parents' role, the couple dynamics and the history of the couple relationship as well as the quality of the relationship between the child and her siblings.

Howells' (1971) dimension of group properties is then considered. The family is seen as a system within which each member exerts an influence on others and is influenced by others. It is thus important to collect information on the history of the family as such, on the perceived family climate and on the way each member feels and is considered within the family.

Lastly, the quality of the relationship of the family system with the families of origin of both spouses – paying particular attention to the presence of defined generational barriers – is evaluated, as is their capacity to integrate within the community to which they belong.

With regard to the self-report measures included in the evaluation protocol used by the Family Psychology Service, a few of them enable practitioners to detect the information pertinent to the evaluation process and the issues covered by the clinical interviews. These measures operationalise variables concerning the parent-child relationship, the couple relationship and family functioning.

Abidin's *Parenting Stress Index* (1983) is applied in order to explore some areas of the parent-child relationship. This measure established the stress levels of fathers and mothers. The child's adjustment, her ability to complete tasks vs. being disorganised and hyperactive or showing frequent mood changes is compared with the parents' difficulties and responsibilities (e.g. they may feel isolated, unable to regulate the distance from their child, they may suffer the restrictions imposed by their parenting role, they may feel more or less skilled, etc.) and the stress caused by factors external to the parent-child relationship such as the death of a relative, the loss of a job, moving somewhere else, etc.

This measure outlines the stress felt by the parents, separately for the mother and the father, and provides useful clues as to the assessment results and the most appropriate intervention. For example, it reveals which of the two parents is coping worse and in what areas. At the same time, this unease provides an indication of the parent's resources.

The family climate and some relational aspects are investigated through the Italian adaptation of the *Family Environment Scale* by Moos, Insel and Humphrey (1974). This self-report measure consists of 100 items divided into 10 subscales tapping three important dimensions of family functioning and climate: 1) the Relationship dimension provides clues to the quality and quantity of the relationships within the family in terms of cohesion, expressiveness and conflict; 2) the Personal growth dimension provides clues to the importance given by the family to the development processes necessary for the individual to achieve independence, decision-making and responsibility-taking; 3) the System Maintenance dimension showing to which extent the family attempts to keep the *status quo* unchanged or, in contrast, whether they attempt to change the balance in terms of organisation and control.

This measure is particularly useful because at a descriptive level it reveals the perception of the family climate and relational dynamics by all members, at a predictive level it allows for assumptions on the development of the family system, the change that can be achieved and the family's strengths and weaknesses, and at a prescriptive level it allows the practitioner to discriminate between families along the continuum of functional-dysfunctional behaviour and throughout life stages, while at the same time providing valuable indications for intervention.

## COMMUNICATING THE OUTCOME TO THE FAMILY

The outcomes of the single evaluations made by the different practitioners are then discussed with the coordinating physician who informs the parents, at the end of the child's hospital stay, of each single test result and communicates the diagnosis, when possible, with indications on the child's functional profile and the most appropriate intervention.

The discussion with the family is generally conducted by the coordinating physician only. Sometimes, the conclusions are drawn separately or together by the coordinating physician and the psychologist responsible for the psychoeducational evaluation or the psychologist responsible for the evaluation of family dynamics. This usually happens when the team deems it best for the family to receive support or when there is a need to discuss with them an intervention involving the family.

With regard to family dynamics, the evaluation outcome is also detailed in writing. The report describes the family functioning in light of the information collected through interviews and measures. This report thus provides: 1) valuable clinical information and meets the criterion for objectivity; 2) a multifaceted description of the family; 3) an indication of possible discrepancies between informants and measures used (clinical interviews *versus* objective measures).

The report also specifies whether there are dysfunctional relationships that can affect the child and the family's well-being. At the same time, when needed and in agreement with the coordinating physician, it provides indications for: 1) a follow-up on the family situation; 2) family counselling; 3) family therapy (for the couple or individual); 4) a structured intervention programme or parent training; 5) management of the family by local service agencies.

A copy of the report is handed to the coordinating physician and to the child's parents. The report is first and foremost an opportunity for the family to retrace, based on a written document, what has been done and said so far, what intervention was proposed, based on which reasons and resources are available (Maino and Fara, 2005).

## Conclusions

The discussion above shows how the diagnostic and evaluation process can rightfully be considered as the starting point for any effective intervention which meets the child and the family's needs. Only a clear picture of the child's disability can enable practitioners to devise the most appropriate rehabilitation plan with the lowest margin of error and resource expenditure.

Here "resource" is used in a broad sense: in an economic perspective, since an accurate diagnostic and evaluation process can avoid ineffective interventions, and in an emotional perspective, since parents are given a limited time to orient themselves and understand their child's difficulties, and build a more functional relationship with her.

Given its importance, this process must be as ordered, integrated and as wide-ranging as possible, and be able to integrate information collected from qualitative and quantitative measures, taking into consideration the child and her contexts of life (first of all, the family context) as well.

In this perspective, the evaluation is an inventory of the child and family's resources and limitations as well as an opportunity for the parents to build a truer-to-life picture of their child and more effective interaction styles. It also favours the compliance and the partnership with practitioners for the child's well-being.

Lastly, a structured and replicable diagnostic and evaluation process can be used by practitioners working at different sites and can therefore become generalised. On the other hand, it can be repeated during and after the rehabilitation to monitor its outcome and efficacy so as to enhance the actual rehabilitation interventions.

## References

American Psychiatric Association (1994). Diagnostic and Statistical Manual of Mental Disorders – Fourth Edition (DSM-IV), Washington, D.C: American Psychiatric Association

Abidin, R. R. (1983). *Parenting Stress Index, Third Edition Professional Manual.* Odessa, FL: Psychological Assessment Resources, Inc.

Allen, R. I., and Petr, C. (1998). Rethinking family-centered practice. *American Journal of Orthopsychiatry, 68*, 4-15

Baron-Cohen S., Leslie, A. M., and Frith, U. (1985). Does the autistic child have a "theory of mind"? *Cognition*, *21*, 37-46.

Bowlby, J. (1988). *A Secure Base: Parent-child Attachment and Health Human Development.* New York: Basic Books. Tr. It. *Una base sicura.* Milano: Raffaello Cortina Editore, 1989.

Brown, S. M., Humphry, R., and Taylor, E. (1997). A model of the nature of family-therapist relationships: Implications for education. *American Journal of Occupational Therapy, 51*, 597-603

Buono, S., and Zagaria, T. (2003). ICF – Classificazione internazionale del funzionamento, della disabilità e della salute. *Ciclo evolutivo e disabilità /Life Span and Disability*, *6*,

121-141

Clerici, M., and Bertrando P. (1993), *Strumenti di valutazione familiare*. In A.S. Gurman, D.P. Kniskern (eds.), *Handbook of Family Therapy*. Brunner/Mazel, New York, 1991. Trad. It. *Manuale di terapia della famiglia* (pp. 707-734). Torino: Bollati Boringhieri.

Fairbairn, W. R. D. (1952). *An object-relations theory of the personality*. New York: Basic Books.

Fallone, R. (2004). *L'approccio multicausa nell'analisi della mortalità in Italia*. Tesi di laurea non pubblicata. Università degli studi di Roma "La Sapienza".

Frith, U. (1989). *Autism: Explaining the enigma.*Oxford: Blackwell.

Hemmeter, M. L., Joseph, G. E., Smith, B. J., and Sandall, S. (2001). *DEC recommended practice*. Denver, CO: DEC.

Hostler, S. L. (1994). *Family-Centered Care: An approach to implementation*. University of Virginia, Charlottesville, VA, Canada.

Howells, J. G. (1971), *Theory and Practice of Family Psychiatry*. New York: Brunner/Mazel.

Kohut, H. (1987). *The Kohut Seminars*. New York – London: Norton.

King, G., King, S., Rosembaum, P., and Goffin, R. (1999). Family-centered caregiving and well-being of parents of children with disabilities: linking process with outcome. *Journal of Pediatric Psychology*, *24*, 41-53.

King, S., Teplicky, R., King, G., and Rosembaum, P. (2004). Family-centered service for children with cerebral palsy and their families: a review of the literature. *Seminars in Pediatric Neurology*, *11*, 78-86.

Law, M., Hanna, S., King, G., Hurley, P., King, S., Kertoy, M. and Rosembaum, P. (2003). Factors affecting family-centred service delivery for children with disabilities. *Child: Care, Health and Development*, *29*, 357-366.

Law, M., Teplicky, R., King, S., King, G., Kertoy, M., Moning, T., Rosenbaum, P., and Burke-Gaffney, J. (2005). Family-centered service: moving ideas into practice. *Child: Care, Health and Development*, *31*, 633-642.

L'Abate, L. (1990). *Building Family Competence*. Newbury Park, CA: Sage.

L'Abate, L. (1994). *Family Evaluation. A Psychological Approach*. Thousand Oaks, CA: Sage.

Leonardi, M., and Ustun, T. B. (2002). The Global Burden of Epilepsy. *Epilepsia, 43*, 21-25.

Lord, C., Rutter, M., and Le Couteur, A. (1994). Autism Diagnostic Interview-Revised: A revised version of a diagnostic interview for caregivers of individuals with possible pervasive developmental disorders. *Journal of Autism and Developmental Disorders*, *24*, 551-692.

Lord, C., Risi, S., Lambrecht, L., Cook Jr., E. H., Leventhal, B. L., DiLavore , P., Pickles A., and Rutter M. (2000). The Autism Diagnostic Observation Schedule—Generic: A Standard Measure of Social and Communication Deficits Associated with the Spectrum of Autism. *Journal of Autism and Developmental Disorders*, *30*, 181- 266.

Maino, E., and Fara, D. (2005). Un servizio di psicologia della famiglia in una struttura sanitaria per l'età evolutiva. In M. Cusinato & M. Panzeri (Eds.), *Interventi e valutazione nel lavoro con le famiglie* (pp. 81-99). Bologna: Il Mulino.

Meisels, S. J., and Atkins-Burnett, S. (2000). The elements of early childhood assessment. In J. P. Shonkoff & S. J. Meisels (Eds.), *Handbook of early childhood intervention* (pp.

231-257). New York: Cambridge University Press.

Miller, A. (1981). *Du sollst merken: Variationen über das Paradies-Thema.* Frankfurt am Main: Suhrkamp Verlag. Trad. It. *Il bambino inascoltato. Realtà infantile e dogma psicoanalitico.* Torino: Bollati Boringhieri, 2004.

Moos, R. H., Insel, P. M., and Humphrey B. (1974). *Combined Manual for Family, Work and Group Environment Scales.* Palo Alto, CA: Consulting Psychologist Press.

Paul, H., and Cohen, D. J. (1984). Responses to contingent queries in adults with mental retardation and pervasive developmental disorders. *Applied Psycholinguistics, 5,* 349 - 357.

Robards, M., F. (1994). *Running a team for disabled children and their families.* London: MacKeith Press.

Rogers, S.J., and Pennington, B.F. (1991). A theoretical approach to the deficits in infantile autism. *Development & Psychopathology, 3,* 137-162.

Rosenbaum, P., King, S., Law, M., King, G., and Evans, J. (1998). Family-centered service: A conceptual framework and research review. *Physical and Occupational Therapy in Pediatrics, 18,* 1-20.

Selvini, M. (1985). *Cronaca di una ricerca. L'evoluzione della terapia familiare nelle opere di Mara Selvini Palazzoli.* Roma: La nuova Italia Scientifica.

Selvini Palazzoli, M., Boscolo, L., Cecchin, G., F., and Prata, G. (1975). *Paradosso e controparadosso.* Milano: Feltrinelli.

Selvini Palazzoli, M., Cirillo, S., Selvini, M., and Sorrentino, A., M. (1988). *I giochi psicotici nella famiglia.* Milano: Raffaello Cortina Editore.

Selvini Palazzoli, M., Cirillo, S., Selvini, M., and Sorrentino, A., M. (1998). *Ragazze anoressiche e bulimiche.* Milano: Raffaello Cortina Editore.

Sigman, M., and Ruskin, E. (1999). *Change and continuity in the social competence of children with Autism, Down syndrome, and developmental delays.* Monograph of the Society for Research in Child Development. London, England: Blackwell.

Schopler, E., Reichler, R. J., DeVellis, R. F. and Daly, K. (1980). Toward objective classification of childhood autism: Childhood Autism Rating Scale (CARS). *Journal of Autism and Developmental Disorders, 10,* 91-103.

Schopler, E., Lansing, M.D., Reichler, R.J. and Marcus, L.M. (2005). *Psychoeducational Profile - 3rd Edition (PEP-3).* Austin, TX: PRO-ED.

Sloper, P. (1999). Models of service support for parents of disabled children; What do we know? What do we need to know? *Child: Care, Health and Development, 25,* 85-89.

Sloper, P., and Turner, S. (1992). Service needs of families of children with severe physical disability. *Child: Care, Health and Development, 18,* 259-282.

Sloper, P., Greco, V., Beecham J., and Webb, R. (2006). Key worker services for disabled children: what characteristics of services lead to better outcomes for children and families? *Child: Care, Health and Development, 32,* 147-157.

Soresi, S. (1998). *Psicologia dell'handicap e della riabilitazione.* Bologna: Il Mulino.

Soresi, S. (2001). Riflessioni a margine della seconda edizione della Classificazione Internazionale delle Menomazioni, delle Disabilità e degli Handicap. *Giornale Italiano delle Disabilità, 1,* 5-22.

Sorrentino, A. M. (2006). *Figli disabili. La famiglia di fronte all'handicap.* Milano: Raffaello

Cortina Editore.

Sparrow, S. S., Balla, D. A., and Cicchetti, D. V. (1984). *Vineland Adaptive Behavior Scales.* Circle Pines, MN: American Guidance Service.

Tager-Flusberg, H. (1981a). Sentence comprehension in autistic children. *Applied Psycholinguistics, 2*, 5-24.

Tager-Flusberg, H. (1981b). On the nature of linguistic functioning in early infantile autism. *Journal of Autism and Developmental Disorders, 11*, 45-56.

Tager-Flusberg, H. (Ed.), (1999). *Neurodevelopmental disorders.* Cambridge MA: MIT Press/Bradford Books (Series on Cognitive Science of Development).

Vig, S., and Kaminer, R. (2003). Comprehensive interdisciplinary evaluation as intervention for young children. *Infants and Young Children, 4*, 342-353.

Zoccarato, M. (1996). I sistemi internazionali di classificazione delle disabilità psichiche e comportamentali *Difficoltà di apprendimento 2*, 79-101.

Werner, E. E. (2000). Protective factors and individual resilience. In P. Shonkoff & S. J. Meisels (Eds.), *Handbook of early childhood intervention* (pp. 115-132). New York: Cambridge University Press.

World Health Organization (1948). Manual of the International Statistical Classification of Disease, Injuries, and Causes of Death (Sixth Revision). Geneva, Switzerland: Office of Publications, World Health Organization.

World Health Organization (1977). *Manual of the International Statistical Classification of Disease, Injuries, and Causes of Death (Ninth Revision)* – based on the recommendations of the Ninth Revision Conference, 1975. Geneva, Switzerland: Office of Publications, World Health Organization.

World Health Organization (1980). *International Classification of Impairments, Disabilities and Handicaps: A Manual of Classification Relating to Consequences of Disease.* Geneva. Switzerland: Office of Publications, World Health Organization.

World Health Organization (1992). *International Statistical Classification of Diseases and Related Health Problems, (Tenth Revision).* Geneva. Switzerland: Office of Publications, World Health Organization.

World Health Organization (2001). *International Classification of Functioning Disability and Health.* Geneva, Switzerland: Office of Publications, World Health Organization.

In: Toward a Science of Clinical Psychology
Editor: Luciano L'Abate, pp. 57-77

ISBN: 978-1-60456-062-6


*Chapter III*

# BEHAVIORAL SKILLS TRAINING FOR DEPRESSED MOTHERS OF CHILDREN WITH ADHD

***Andrea Chronis-Tuscano and Tana L. Clarke***

## ABSTRACT

Attention-deficit/hyperactivity disorder (ADHD) is a chronic disorder beginning early in development (i.e., before age 7) that is characterized by age-inappropriate levels of inattention, impulsivity, and hyperactivity (American Psychiatric Association, 1994). The behavior of children with ADHD is typically associated with impaired family interactions (Johnston & Mash, 2001). Indeed, parent-child interactions are more negative (Cunningham & Barkley, 1979; Barkley, 1985; Mash & Johnston, 1982), parenting is more stressful (Fischer, 1990), and marital distress is common in families of children with the disorder (Johnston & Mash, 2001). Moreover, parents of children with ADHD are far more likely than parents of non-disordered children to experience psychopathology themselves (Chronis, Lahey, Pelham, Kipp, Baumann, & Lee, 2003a). It has been theorized that parental stress, psychopathology, and marital distress may negatively impact parenting, which in turn exacerbates child behavior problems, creating a reciprocal pattern of negative parent-child interactions within families of children with ADHD (Cummings & Davies, 1999; Patterson, 1982). Indeed, there are data pointing to this relationship between maternal psychopathology, especially depression, and parenting cognitions and behaviors in mothers of children with ADHD (Chi & Hinshaw, 2002). Furthermore, emerging evidence suggests that parental psychopathology and early parenting behavior predict the future course of conduct problems in children with ADHD (Chronis, Lahey, Pelham, Williams, Baumann, Kipp, & Jones, 2007), underscoring the important implications parental psychopathology and parenting have for the developmental outcomes of children with ADHD.

It is also valuable to consider the role of parental psychopathology in outcomes following evidence-based treatments for children with ADHD. Given that both of the evidence-based treatments for ADHD—behavior therapy and stimulant medication- rely on parents (most often mothers) to obtain and consistently administer treatment, it is no surprise that parental psychopathology, particularly maternal depression, predicts poorer outcomes for children with ADHD across behavioral and pharmacological treatment modalities (Owens, Hinshaw, Kraemer, Arnold, Abikoff & Cantwell, 2003).

Depression is the most common disorder among mothers of children with ADHD. Our own prior research suggests that mothers of children with ADHD are three times more likely than mothers of non-disordered children to be depressed and at least 40% have experienced a major depressive episode in their lifetime (Chronis et al., 2003). Indeed, depressed mothers may lack the energy, motivation, patience, and organization to consistently implement complex behavioral programs. Furthermore, the well-studied link between depression and negative parenting (Lovejoy et al., 2000) evokes an additional rationale for consideration off maternal depression in behavioral treatments aimed at improving parenting. Yet, existing evidence-based treatments for children with ADHD largely fail to directly address maternal psychological problems and are therefore less beneficial for this subgroup of families (Chronis, Chacko, Fabiano, Wymbs, & Pelham, 2004). It may be that concurrent treatment of maternal depression would remove some barriers to positive treatment outcomes.

With this in mind, we developed a novel, integrated approach to behavioral parent training for mothers of children with ADHD with elevated depressive symptoms in order to facilitate successful outcomes across three domains: maternal depression, parenting, and child behavior. In this chapter, we will describe the ongoing development of our treatment which integrates an empirically-supported, cognitive-behavioral depression intervention with behavioral parent training for depressed mothers of children with ADHD. We will also present preliminary results based on twelve families who participated in the pilot phase of this NIMH-funded treatment development project.

## Theoretical Model

Research findings suggesting that mothers of children with ADHD are more likely to experience psychopathology, particularly depression, and studies pointing to the detrimental effects of maternal depression on developmental and treatment outcomes set the stage for a transactional model in which child externalizing behavior and parental psychopathology exert reciprocal influences on one another (see Cummings & Davies, 1999; Patterson, 1982). This transactional model (depicted in Figure 1) can also be understood in terms of Lewinsohn's integrated theory of depression (Lewinsohn, Hoberman, Teri, & Hautizinger, 1985), which suggests that depression is the result of "environmentally-initiated" changes in behavior, affect and cognitions. Within this model, environmental antecedent risk factors, such as parenting a difficult child, may influence the onset of depression. This environmental stressor may lead to an elevation in the situational causes of depression (e.g., less engagement in pleasurable activities, feelings of hopelessness related to parenting, negative cognitions related to one's child or one's own parenting), which contributes to aversive interpersonal experiences (e.g., negative parent-child interactions) and eventually has a negative impact on the person's quality of life. In this case, it can be hypothesized that mothers of children with ADHD may experience depression in part as a result of negative child behavior, which may contribute to the use of maladaptive interpersonal coping skills and parenting practices, and exacerbate child behavior problems (Patterson, 1982).

This process has important implications for the development, maintenance, and/or exacerbation of co-occurring conduct problems in children with ADHD. Children with ADHD often have associated propensities that are linked to antisocial behavior, such as difficult temperament (Lahey & Waldman, 2003), cognitive impairments (Nigg, 2001; Moffit & Silva, 1988), or genetic vulnerabilities (Martin, Levy, Peika, Hay, 2006; Rhee & Waldman, 2002). These child characteristics may both evoke and interact with environmental stressors to elicit antisocial behavior. It has been amply demonstrated that ADHD and co-occurring conduct disorder (CD) are associated with additive negative effects (King, Waschbusch, et al., 2005), and that these children are at risk for a multitude of negative outcomes such as more severe and persistent antisocial behavior (Lynam, 1996; Manuzza, Klien, Abikoff, & Mouton, 2004) and substance abuse problems (Marshall & Molina, 1996). Thus, because children with ADHD are at risk for CD, it is crucial to intervene early in the hopes of preventing the occurrence or exacerbation of conduct problems. Maternal depression and maladaptive parenting are examples of environmental factors that may evolve from, and contribute to, this cycle. For example, if a hyperactive child with the propensity for antisocial behavior begins to act out, external control in the form of consistent, responsive, and proactive parenting will be important in preventing the development of additional behavior problems. However, if the primary caretaker is overwhelmed or depressed, her personal resources may not allow for the effective management of difficult child behavior. A depressed mother may alternatively "give in" more easily when a child misbehaves, or discipline the child in a harsh or inconsistent manner. This type of maladaptive parenting may not only fail to regulate child behavior, but may exacerbate the oppositionality or volatility that goes along with aggression and rule-breaking behaviors. Once parents and children are caught in this "negative spiral," both the child's negative behavior and mother's stress/depression levels worsen. Consistent with this model, maternal stress/depression can be viewed as both an antecedent and a consequence of child attention and behavior problems. Thus, it can be argued that, because antisocial behavior arises out of a multitude of risk factors, including ADHD and maternal psychopathology, successful treatments must attempt to target multiple risk factors in the child's environment.

Although there are undoubtedly biological contributions to both ADHD and depression, a large body of research demonstrates the importance of environmental factors in maintaining and exacerbating the course, impairment and symptomatology associated with both disorders (e.g., Joiner, 2000; Patterson, 1982). Thus, it follows that focusing on more malleable environmental factors in the treatment of each disorder may be the most effective point of intervention.

We will now turn to a review of evidence-based psychosocial treatment approaches for ADHD and depression, and then describe our integrated intervention for depressed mothers of children with ADHD.

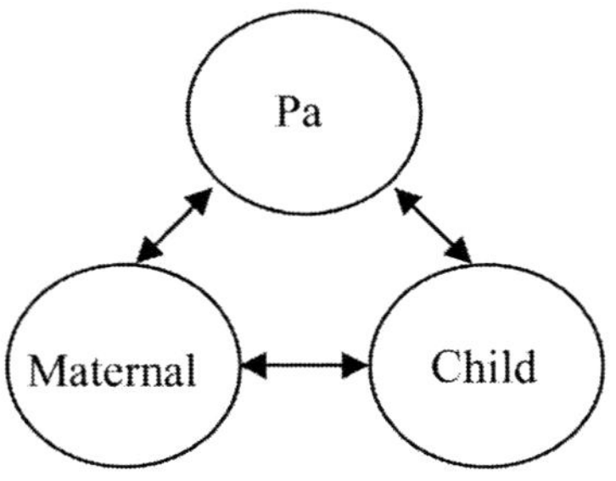


Figure 1. The reciprocal relationship between parent and child behavior.

## Behavioral Parent Training

As reviewed herein, the child behaviors that characterize ADHD are associated with impairments in parent-child interactions and overall family functioning (Johnston & Mash, 2001) and parents may develop maladaptive and counterproductive parenting strategies that serve to maintain or exacerbate existing behavioral difficulties over time (Patterson, DeBaryshe, & Ramsey, 1989). It follows that one critical component of comprehensive treatment for ADHD involves working directly with parents to modify their parenting behaviors in order to increase positive outcomes with their children (Pelham et al., 1998). Effectively enhancing positive parenting and modifying poor parenting practices is of utmost importance, as both positive and negative parenting are among the more robust predictors of negative long-term outcomes in children with behavior problems (Chamberlain & Patterson, 1995; Chronis, Lahey et al., 2007). Parent training, then, is one of the most effective ways to change parenting and therefore treat ADHD (Pelham et al., 1998) and co-occurring behavior problems (Brestan & Eyberg, 1998).

Indeed, behavioral parent training (BPT) has a long, successful history as a treatment for children with ADHD (Pelham et al., 1998), and ODD/CD (Brestan & Eyberg, 1998), as well as many internalizing disorders (e.g., Silverman, Kurtines, Ginsburg, Weems, Rabian, & Serafini, 1999). BPT explicitly provides parents with behavior modification techniques that are based on social learning principles. Specifically, parents are taught to identify and manipulate the antecedents and consequences of child behavior, target and monitor problematic behaviors, reward prosocial behavior through praise, positive attention, and tangible rewards, and decrease unwanted behavior through planned ignoring, time out, and other non-physical discipline techniques. In order for these strategies to be effective, they must be implemented consistently and over the long-term_(Chronis et al., 2001).

Parents are the agents by which behavior management skills taught in BPT programs shape child behavior and the consistent administration of the strategies described above require adequate psychological resources on the part of the parent. Thus, it is no surprise that maternal depression consistently emerges as a predictor of poorer treatment compliance and outcomes following BPT for children with ADHD (e.g., Owens et al., 2003; Sonuga-Barke, Daley, & Thompson 2002) and noncompliant/aggressive behavior problems (Griest & Forehand, 1982; McMahon, Forehand, Griest, & Wells, 1981; Webster-Stratton, 1985;

Webster-Stratton, 1992a). Indeed, stressed or depressed individuals often lack the motivation and persistence to consistently implement the behavioral management techniques taught in BPT. It is for this reason that we have developed our integrated intervention to enhance the effects of parent training for depressed mothers of children with ADHD.

## Cognitive-Behavioral Therapy: The Coping with Depression Course

The cognitive model of depression holds that depressed individuals have unrealistically negative views of themselves, others, and their futures, and a predisposition to negative, automatic thinking (Beck, 1976). Cognitive and cognitive-behavioral therapies are based on the perspective that the way in which an individual interprets an event is an important factor in determining the individual's response to the event (Hollon & Beck, 1994). Thus, cognitive and cognitive-behavioral interventions attempt to change distortions in the thoughts/beliefs of depressed individuals in order to foster changes in affect and behavior.

It is also important to note the growing body of literature implicating the causal role of maternal cognitions and attributions in the development of negative parent-child interactions. This is especially important in families of children with ADHD and behavior problems (see Johnston & Ohan, 2005 for review). Because depression is also associated with negative interpretations of one's environment (Beck, 1976), it follows that negative attributions about a child and one's own parenting would exist at higher levels in mothers of children with ADHD who also struggle with depression. Thus, treatment components directly addressing maternal negative cognitions about their child and his/her behavior may prove especially fruitful in this population.

A wealth of evidence exists supporting the efficacy of cognitive and cognitive-behavioral treatments for depression (Hollon & Beck, 1994; Hollon, Shelton, & Loosen, 1991; Dobson, 1989). Cognitive therapy based on Beck's model (Beck, Rush, Shaw, & Emery, 1979) has been shown to be more effective than no treatment and behavior therapy alone in reducing depressive symptoms measured by the Beck Depression Inventory-II (BDI-II; Owens et al., 2003, Dobson, 1989). Studies comparing the efficacy of cognitive or cognitive-behavioral therapy (CBT) and antidepressant medication have found CBT to be at least as effective as medication (Hollon & Beck, 1994) and in some cases, superior (Rush, Beck, Kovacs, & Hollon, 1977; Blackburn, Bishop, Glen, Whalley, & Christie, 1981).

Lewinsohn and colleagues developed a psychoeducational program based upon the principles of CBT, the Coping with Depression Course (CWDC; Lewinsohn, Antonuccio, Steinmetz, & Teri, 1984). The CWDC is based upon a social learning model that holds that depression results from an imbalance between positive and negative interactions with one's environment. The treatment emphasizes the relationship between thoughts, feelings, and behaviors, and each of the treatment modules highlights coping skills to address each of these areas. The four treatment modules include: relaxation training, increasing pleasurable activities, cognitive restructuring, and social skills/assertiveness training. Given its psychoeducational format, the CWDC is thought to be less stigmatizing than traditional cognitive therapy.

The CWDC has empirical support in the treatment of unipolar depression (Cuijpers, 1998; Lewinsohn, Hoberman, & Clarke, 1989). Relative to a waitlist control group, the

CWDC has been shown to significantly reduce BDI scores and to lead to a greater recovery rate from depressive episodes (Lewinsohn et al., 1989). The CWDC is equally effective in group, individual, and minimal contact formats (Brown & Lewinsohn, 1984), and thus represents a cost-effective alternative to traditional cognitive therapy. Furthermore, it has been used as an effective method of prevention in individuals at risk for depression (e.g., Kühner, Angermeyer, & Veiel, 1996), and has been adapted for use with diverse populations, including adolescents (e.g., Lewinsohn, Rohde, & Seeley, 1998), the elderly (Breckenridge, Zeiss, & Thompson, 1987), minority groups (e.g., Organista, Muñoz, & Gonzalez, 1994), and caregivers for the elderly (Lovett & Gallagher, 1988). These adaptations have taken into account the unique needs of the target population and suggest that the treatment package may be applicable to a range of individuals with varying levels of depression.

Taken together, these studies support the efficacy of cognitive-behavioral interventions in the treatment and prevention of depression. The CWDC appears to be a non-stigmatizing, cost-effective alternative to traditional CBT that has been shown to be effective with a variety of patient populations including both depressed individuals and individuals at risk for depression. The CWDC has also been effectively applied for different populations and for use in different contexts and lends itself to administration in a group format.

## The CWDC as an Add-On to Parent Training

Our research team previously conducted a 3-year treatment outcome study evaluating the efficacy of a cognitive-behavioral intervention for mothers of children with ADHD, a group that is at risk for depression (Chronis, Gamble et al., 2006). In this study, 51 mothers of 6-12 year old children with ADHD who had recently completed the Children's Summer Treatment Program (STP; Chronis et al., 2004; Pelham, Greiner, & Gnagy 1997; Pelham et al, 2005) were initially assessed using the Structured Clinical Interview for the DSM-IV, Non-Patient Edition (SCID; First et al., 1996) and the Modified Hamilton Rating Scale for Depression (MHRSD; Miller, Bishop, Norman, & Maddever, 1985). At this initial assessment point, approximately 50% of the mothers reported a history of Major Depressive Disorder (MDD) on the SCID-IV (48% of mothers in the treatment group and 52% of mothers in the control group), the mean MHRSD score was 5.4 (SD = 4.5), and the mean BDI-II score was 10.2 (SD = 5.9).

In this pilot study, 60 participants were randomly assigned to receive the CWDC (Lewinsohn et al., 1989) immediately following the intensive STP or after a waitlist period. For the purpose of this study, the CWDC was adapted to increase its relevance for mothers of children with ADHD and was referred to as the "Maternal Stress and Coping Group." Parallels were drawn between this program and the social learning principles taught in the STP BPT sessions, examples related to ADHD children were provided, and the term "depression" was replaced with "stress" and "distress" to enhance its applicability to mothers with a broad range of depressive symptoms. This adaptation of the CWDC manual for mothers of children with ADHD was used as the basis for the development of the Integrated Parent Intervention for ADHD (IPI-A) manual described in the next section.

Improvements in depressive symptoms, self-esteem, and cognitions about child behavior were found for mothers who received treatment relative to those in the waitlist group

(Chronis et al., 2006). Neither maternal history of MDD nor child comorbid ODD/CD moderated treatment response. However, when the magnitude of treatment effects on maternal depressive symptoms was computed separately for initially symptomatic (BDI > 9 ), and nonsymptomatic individuals, we found an effect size of 0.63 for the symptomatic group, which is comparable with the average effect size reported for the CWDC (Cuijpers, 1998), while the effect size for the non-symptomatic group was only 0.02. Mothers in the treatment group also reported improvements in self-esteem, and fewer depressive attributions and negative expectations regarding child behavior following treatment relative to controls. That is, they felt better about themselves, were less likely to make internal, global, and stable attributions for their children's misbehavior, and were less likely to expect noncompliance from their children. Considering reports from the Multimodal Treatment Study of Children with ADHD (MTA) indicating that parental self-esteem, parenting efficacy, and attributions for child noncompliance were associated with poorer response to ADHD treatments, including pharmacological treatments (Hoza et al., 2000), findings from this study suggest that the CWDC may be useful for mothers of children with ADHD, and may serve to enhance child treatment response (Chronis, Gamble, et al., 2006).

Direct effects of the intervention were not found on several of the outcome measures, including the parent-child relationship, the marital relationship, and parent and teacher ratings of child behavior. We speculate that these negative findings may be attributed to the fact that the children had just completed the comprehensive, 8-week STP that intensively targeted the parent-child relationship and child behavior. In fact, parent and teacher ratings of child behavior at the end of the STP were in the normative range of functioning, leaving little to no room for additional improvement as a result of the CWDC. At the same time, one would only expect improvements in child behavior, the parent-child relationship, and the marital relationship for mothers who experienced improvements in depressive symptoms. Indeed, results suggested that improvement in maternal depressive symptoms was associated with improvements in maternal ratings of child behavior, parent-child warmth, and the parent-child relationship.

Although the results of this study were promising, this preliminary study was limited in many regards. First, the CWDC intervention followed the intensive and highly specialized STP, making it difficult to detect unique changes that resulted from the CWDC intervention. Additionally, since CWDC skills are relevant to the implementation of BPT skills, it may be that concurrent, rather than sequential, presentation of relevant skills may enhance positive changes in the parenting domain.

In an effort to increase the generalizability of the findings to more widely-available treatments for ADHD and to allow an examination of the impact of this intervention on child behavior, in Phase II of our current project we are comparing the integrated treatment to a once-weekly outpatient BPT program that is more widely available in real-world clinical settings than the STP. The combined intervention utilized in our prior study lasted 20 weeks and included over 400 hours of intensive treatment. In the current study, we have integrated these BPT and CBT interventions into a 14-week outpatient treatment program in order to make the application of CWDC skills to parenting situations more explicit and to increase the transportability of the integrated intervention by offering a more time-limited treatment.

Another important limitation of this initial pilot study was that all of the outcome measures relied on maternal report, which can be influenced by maternal depressive symptoms (Richters, 1992). Thus, in the current study we are collecting observational data, as well as more direct measures of parenting behavior. This pilot study also did not select mothers based on a history of MDD or current elevated depressive symptomatology. Since results suggest that the intervention is most effective and potentially most useful for mothers experiencing current elevated levels of depressive symptoms, the study we are describing here targets mothers with BDI-II scores at or above 10, which is the point at which mothers in the pilot study exhibited increased a treatment outcome effect size.

Finally, the use of a no-treatment control group rather than comparing the intervention under investigation to an already-established treatment resulted in our inability to parse apart the unique effects of the CWDC intervention from the amount of treatment/therapist attention. For this reason, Phase II of the current study includes standard BPT as the comparison condition, given that BPT has been identified as an empirically-supported treatment for ADHD (Pelham et al., 1998) and is more widely available in real-world, clinical settings. Both the standard BPT and the integrated treatment are matched on therapist contact time.

## Integrated Parent Intervention

As reviewed herein, both components of this IPI-A have been empirically validated: BPT for the treatment of ADHD (Pelham, Wheeler, & Chronis, 1998) and CBT, specifically the CWDC, for the treatment of adult depression (Cuijpers, 1998; Lewinsohn & Clarke, 1984). In our prior work, we developed and tested a modification of the CWDC manual for mothers of children with ADHD as an adjunct that followed BPT (Chronis, Gamble, Roberts, & Pelham, 2006); however, we have now *integrated* the CWDC treatment components into a BPT program in a more efficient and purposeful manner. The skills included in the CWDC were mapped onto BPT skills in the manner displayed in Table 1. This integrated format facilitates the use of CBT coping skills in parenting situations in an effort to directly highlight and address the negative impact of maternal depression on parenting and parent training outcomes. Furthermore, this integrated intervention allows child and maternal problems, which exert reciprocal negative effects on one another, to be addressed simultaneously.

## Development and Evaluation of the Integrated Parent Intervention for ADHD

The first phase of this project was designed to develop and then evaluate the efficacy of the IPI-A. Phase I refers to the pilot phase for the newly-designed IPI-A. During the pilot phase, we concentrated on manual development, piloting with a small group of participants, and refinement through the solicitation of feedback from both participants and professionals. Treatment outcome was also assessed in the Phase I participants assessing three primary outcome domains: maternal depression, parenting, and child behavior.

**Table 1: Related Parent Training and CWDC Topics**

| Behavioral Parent Training Skill | Relevant CWDC Skill |
|---|---|
| Psychoeducation about ADHD | Social learning model of depression |
| ABCs of behavior change | Relations between thoughts, feelings, and behaviors |
| Spending quality time with child | Pleasant (social) activities |
| Structure and routines | Time management |
| Praise and Rewards | Quantity of positive vs. negative thoughts; cognitive restructuring |
| Ignoring minor misbehavior | Relaxation techniques |
| Effective commands | Assertiveness training |
| Time out/removal of privileges | Assertiveness, relaxation training |
| Working with schools | Social skills and assertiveness; constructive thinking |

*CWDC = Coping with depression course

*Participant recruitment and selection.*

Participants were included if they were the biological mother of a child age 6-12 who met DSM-IV criteria for ADHD. Children were excluded if they had an estimated IQ of 70 or below. Mothers were excluded if they currently met criteria for any Axis I psychopathology that would warrant alternative treatment (substance abuse, psychosis, or bipolar disorder) and they were required to have a BDI-II score of 10 or above across two administrations. In addition, mothers and children were asked to refrain from any additional psychosocial treatment for the duration of their participation in the treatment group and to remain on a stable dose of medication for the time period of the group, unless failing to do so was clinically contraindicated.

The group originally consisted of 12 mothers recruited through local elementary and middle schools, as well as local treatment providers. The average age of mothers was 39.5 years old and the average age of the target child was 8.1 years old. All children included in this pilot phase were male and 50% were taking stabilized doses of stimulant medication. Mothers were primarily Caucasian (83%) and 25% were taking stabilized doses of antidepressant medication. Of note, one participant discontinued her attendance to the treatment group after 2 sessions due to the lengthy commute required for her to attend. Thus, manual refinement results will be presented without the input of this participant; however, post-treatment outcome results do include data from this mother and child based on an intent-to-treat approach.

*Procedure.*

Interested parents called our clinic and were screened over the phone. If they met preliminary inclusion criteria at that time, they were invited to come in for an initial assessment (IA) session. As part of the assessment, the parents completed diagnostic interviews and self-report measures of their own psychopathology, their child's behavior, and their parenting. Once it was determined that participants met criteria for inclusion in the study, they were admitted into the IPI-A pilot group. Medication status and psychosocial treatment attendance were carefully monitored throughout the course of the group to ensure that these were kept constant. Outcome assessments were conducted at post-treatment (PA) and at a three-month follow-up (FA) period.

*Assessments.*

Every effort was made to utilize multi-informant and multi-method assessments of child and mother characteristics in each of the three outcome domains. Initially, maternal depression and other forms of psychopathology were assessed using the SCID-IV. Also, maternal depression severity was assessed with the MHRSD, which is also a clinician rated interview, and a self-report measure of depressive symptoms, the BDI-II.

Child diagnostic status was arrived at through the compilation of information from both the child's mother and teacher. Trained clinicians interviewed mothers about their child's behavior using the Schedule for Affective Disorders for School-Aged Children (K-SADS; Orvaschel & Puig-Antich, 1995). Both the child's mother and teacher completed the Disruptive Behavior Disorders Rating Scale (DBD; Pelham et al., 1992) as a measure of child symptoms of ADHD, ODD and CD, and the Children's Impairment Rating Scale (CIRS; Fabiano et al., 2006) as a measure of associated impairment. A symptom of ADHD, ODD, or CD was counted as clinically significant if it was endorsed by either the mother on the K-SADS or DBD, or the teacher on the DBD. Finally, child IQ was screened using the Vocabulary and Block Design subtests of the Weschler Intelligence Scale for Children, 4th Ed. (WISC-IV; Weschler, 2003).

Parenting was measured through several self-report indices of parenting, including the Alabama Parenting Questionnaire (APQ; Shelton, Frick, & Wooton; 1996) and the Parenting Stress Index–Short Form (PSI-SF, Abidin, 1986). Due to possible biases inherent in self-report measures of parenting, observational measures of parenting were also obtained. For this, mother-child dyads underwent a 20-minute parent-child interaction consisting of a clean-up, free play, and homework task where the mother assisted the child with these activities. These interactions were recorded and will be coded at a later date by trained coders using a well-validated behavioral rating system.

Outcome assessments utilized repeated administration of the self-report measures of maternal depression (BDI-II), parenting (APQ, PSI-SF), and child behavior (DBD). The Longitudinal Interval Follow-up Evaluation (LIFE; Keller et al., 1987) was used at post-treatment and follow-up to evaluate syndromal or diagnostic changes in the mothers since the last interview and to probe for the occurrence of new disorders. The MHRSD was administered to the mothers during the PA and FA and the parent-child interaction was also completed to obtain outcome assessments of depression severity and observed parenting, respectively.

At the conclusion of the administration of the pilot group, participants attended focus groups where systematic and free-response feedback was obtained. Questions focused on applicability and usefulness of the techniques provided, therapist competence, and sensitivity to cultural and minority issues. Due to the importance of anonymity in giving feedback regarding the treatment, participants were also asked to complete an anonymous satisfaction survey designed to reflect the issues discussed in the focus groups. Satisfaction and focus group data were used to refine the treatment manual for Phase II.

*IPI-A Treatment.*

As described previously, the 14-week IPI-A is a manualized intervention that integrates standard BPT techniques (described above) with treatment components from Lewinsohn's CWDC in an integrated and efficient manner that explicitly promotes the application of CBT techniques to parenting situations. Like BPT, the CWDC is based upon social learning principles. As applied to depression, the social learning model emphasizes the relationship between thoughts, feelings, and behaviors and each of the four CWDC treatment modules highlights skills that allow the participant to intervene in one of these three areas. As mentioned above, the four treatment modules include: relaxation training (progressive muscle relaxation and deep breathing), increasing pleasurable activities, cognitive restructuring (improving the quantity of positive vs. negative thoughts and changing patterns of distorted thinking), and social skills/assertiveness training.

In our adaptation of the CWDC for mothers of children with ADHD, we hypothesized that each of these treatment components could enhance the delivery of behavioral parenting strategies (Chronis, Gamble et al., 2006). Specifically, the relaxation component may help mothers remain neutral during punishment situations and ignore mildly inappropriate behaviors (e.g., fidgeting, excessive talking). The pleasant activities component is relevant because mothers of children with ADHD often describe spending the majority of their time fulfilling parenting or work obligations, with little time to do things that they enjoy. Additionally, the first step in BPT programs involves parents setting time aside to play with their children, in an effort to create a positive foundation between mother and child. This "special time" can be framed as increasing pleasant (social) activities with one's child. As reviewed herein, many mothers of children with ADHD hold detrimental negative expectations and attributions about their children's behavior that may influence their parenting, so the cognitive restructuring module may be helpful in changing these patterns of negative thinking. The CWDC skill of increasing positive thoughts (and decreasing negative thoughts) can also assist mothers in "catching their children being good" (e.g., praising appropriate behavior) rather than focusing exclusively on the child's negative behavior. Finally, mothers of children with ADHD are required to be assertive (rather than passive or aggressive) in discipline situations with their children, in advocating for their children's educational needs, and in responding to critical family members. Thus, they may benefit from assertiveness training. These four skills map onto the BPT skills in the manner depicted in Table 1.

Of note, each skill was not only presented during the allotted session (as outlined in Tables 1 and 2), but was also reviewed throughout the treatment program in a dynamic fashion. For example, relaxation techniques were presented initially during the planned ignoring session, but were revisited during the time out session since time out is most often used in high-intensity discipline situations when it is particularly important for parents to remain calm. Likewise, social skills and assertiveness training applied to many of the BPT skills, including commands, time out, and working with schools, and were therefore discussed repeatedly as appropriate. Finally, based on our experience applying the CWDC skills to this population in our pilot work, participant comments during the group sessions often prompted a review or discussion of prior topics. For example, during a discussion of time out procedures, a mother may say "Time out *never* works for Johnny," for which the therapist would prompt group members to identify cognitive distortions (e.g., fortune telling, overgeneralization), as well as the impact that these negative expectations may have on the mother's feelings and parenting behavior.

The IPI-A treatment is provided in a group format with 10-12 participants per group. Within this approach, participants receive all aspects of BPT, with a unique focus on applications of CWDC/CBT techniques to parenting situations and the utilization of behavioral parenting techniques. As with standard BPT and the CWDC, homework exercises are assigned to encourage practice of each skill outside the treatment session and integration of these coping behaviors in participants' everyday lives. Session topics are presented in Table 2.

### *Phase I Results: Treatment Outcomes.*

As described above, outcomes were assessed in the three domains of maternal depression, parenting, and child behavior. Repeated measures analyses were used to assess changes in these domains. Results indicated statistically significant reductions in maternal depression (See Figure 2) from pre- to post-treatment on both the BDI-II, $F\ (1, 10) = 5.859$, $p < .05$, and the MHRSD, $F\ (1, 11) = 5.239$, $p < .05$. While the average BDI-II score of participants at the IA was originally in the moderate range of depression, at PA the average score moved to the mild range of depression. Similarly, the average MHRSD score was in the mild range at IA, and was in the normal range at PA. Of note, at the 3-month FA the BDI-II evidenced maintenance of these improvements, while the MHRSD indicated a slight increase in depression severity. Thus, while it is clear that statistically significant treatment gains were evident at post-treatment, data related to maintenance of these gains were less clear.

An important caveat to these findings is that statistically significant differences in outcome do not necessarily indicate *clinically* significant differences (Beutler, & Moleiro, 2001). Because of this, we also evaluated categorical diagnoses of MDD to determine if clinician-rated levels of symptoms and impairment evidenced clinically significant reductions. At the initial assessment, 33.3% of mothers met current DSM-IV criteria for MDD. At the follow-up assessment 16.6% of the mothers met criteria. Thus, there was a substantial portion of participants (about half of mothers who initially met criteria for MDD) who experienced noteworthy changes in depression during the course of treatment.

In terms of parenting, we will be presenting only the self-report data here, as the observed parent-child interactions have yet to be coded. A review of Figure 2 reveals increases in positive parenting and involvement and a decrease in the corporal punishment and poor monitoring/supervision scales on the APQ. A closer examination of these data reveals that the changes in involvement were statistically significant from pre- to post-treatment and these gains were maintained at follow-up, $F\ (2, 14) = 5.030$, $p < .05$. Furthermore, the poor monitoring scale evidenced a trend toward improvement from pre- to post-treatment and continued improving from the PA to FA, resulting in overall statistically significant change, $F\ (2, 14) = 5.676$, $p < .05$. While the corporal punishment and positive parenting scales indicated adaptive changes in parenting, these changes were not significant. Finally, inconsistent discipline was not significantly modified during the course of treatment. When parenting stress was measured with the total score on the PSI-SF, significant reductions in stress were found from pre- to post-treatment, $F\ (2, 12) = 12.39$, $p < .05$, and these improvements were maintained through the 3-month follow-up period, $F$ (2, 12) = 10.34, $p < .05$ (see Figure 2).

**Table 2: Proposed Session Content**

| Session | Standard Behavioral Parent Training (BPT) | Integrated Parent Intervention (IPI-A) *(CWDC Skills in italics)* |
|---|---|---|
| 1 | Psychoeducation about child misbehavior: Child, parent, environmental characteristics | Psychoeducation about child misbehavior: Child, parent, environmental characteristics<br>*Mood Monitoring: How does your mood affect parenting?* |
| 2 | Special time with child: Improving Relationship Differential Attending/Ignoring | *Social learning model of depression*<br>*Relationship between thoughts, feelings, behaviors* |
| 3 | Giving Commands/Increasing Compliance | Special time with child: Improving Relationship<br>*Increasing pleasant activities alone/with child* |
| 4 | House Rules<br>Structure/Routines<br>Increasing Parental Monitoring | Preparation for Positive Parenting Strategies: *Constructive Thinking: Recognizing & Changing parenting cognitive distortions; Increasing positive/decreasing negative thoughts about child* |
| 5 | Home Token/Point System I: Rewards | Differential Attending/Ignoring I: Praise<br>*Constructive Thinking; Increased focus on positive (rather than negative) aspects of child* |
| 6 | Home Token/Point System II: Response Cost<br>Time Out I: Time Out Basics | Differential Attending/Ignoring II: Ignoring<br>*Relaxation Techniques* |
| 7 | Time Out II: Extending Time Out to other Misbehavior | Preparation for Punishment Techniques:<br>*Social Skills and Assertiveness Training* |
| 8 | Managing Misbehavior in Public Places | Giving Commands/Increasing Compliance<br>*Assertiveness Training* |
| 9 | Misbehavior at School<br>Daily School Behavior Report Card | House Rules/Structure/Routines<br>Increasing Parental Monitoring<br>*Time Management/Setting Priorities* |
| 10 | Anticipating Future Behavior Problems | Home Token/Point System: Rewards and Response Cost |
| 11 | Peer Programming in Home and School (e.g., Setting up play dates)* | Time Out<br>*Assertiveness Training (review and application)*<br>*Relaxation Techniques (review and application)* |
| 12 | Parental Support with Homework* | Managing Misbehavior in Public Places<br>*Relaxation Techniques (review and application)*<br>*Planning Ahead* |
| 13 | Troubleshooting Daily School Behavior Report Card* | Misbehavior at School<br>Daily School Behavior Report Card<br>*Social Skills/Assertiveness Training (review and application)*<br>*Constructive Thinking (review and application)* |
| 14 | Review and Wrap-Up | Review and Wrap-Up |

* Supplemented from MTA Parent Training Manual (Abikoff et al., 1994).

As illustrated in Figure 2, there were no significant changes in child behavior as measured by ADHD, ODD, and CD symptoms during the course of treatment or at follow-up. When simple means were examined for the total amount of ODD/CD symptoms across assessment points, the mean ODD/CD symptoms at IA were 5, and the mean was decreased to 3.3 at PA and 2.6 at FA. Thus, it may be the case that the small sample used here did not allow for the power to detect significant differences in child behavior variables. The larger sample in Phase II will clarify the findings in this outcome domain. While this negative finding may be due to a lack of power, it is nevertheless important to consider the lack of findings in this domain since modifying child behavior is our ultimate goal. The IPI-A treatment directly addresses parenting and depression, whereas child behavior is a more peripheral outcome variable that may not evidence immediate change. However, both parenting and negative cognitions (that would be associated with depression) have been found to both moderate and mediate treatment outcome for children with ADHD (Hoza et al., 2000; Wells et al., 2000; Hinshaw et al., 2000). Therefore it would be expected that changes in parenting and negative cognitions would lead to eventual changes in child behavior.

Overall, these preliminary results suggest that the IPI-A program is helpful in improving maternal depression and parenting, while more peripheral measures of child behavior have yet to evidence improvements. Importantly, this was a very small sample without the benefit of a control group, so interpretations of these data should be extremely cautious. At this time, we cannot rule out the passage of time or repeated administration of the outcome measures as alternative explanations for these findings. However, Phase II of this treatment development study, the randomized controlled trial of the IPI-A, will directly address these methodological issues.

*Phase I Results: Manual refinement.*

The satisfaction survey was collected from all mothers who completed the treatment (11 of 12). Table 3 presents a summary of these measures. Generally, participants indicated that they were satisfied with the applicability and usefulness of the group content, as indicated by average ratings between four and five (with a scale ranging from 0 to 6; 1 = Not at all helpful, 3 = Somewhat helpful, 6 = Extremely helpful). Of note, participants found positive parenting components to be the most helpful and relevant of the parenting modules, and gave mood monitoring and social skills components the highest ratings out of the CWDC modules. The satisfaction survey revealed that the home token system was the least applicable (and perhaps overwhelming) to the mothers and the session focusing on managing misbehavior in public was not as helpful as the other parenting components. In terms of the CWDC modules, the sessions on time management and relaxation techniques received the lowest ratings. Of note, the mean for the lowest rated components was between a 3.4 and 4.1, indicating that these sessions were still viewed by participants as at least somewhat helpful.

The information collected during the focus groups was consistent with the questionnaire data, but provided additional insight into what the mothers wanted and needed. In several ways during the focus group, mothers revealed that they liked the integrated format of the group that allowed them to explore the links between their mood and their parenting. Mothers found both the mood and parenting components helpful. Most mothers indicated that at least some of the parenting components were useful (specifically commands and setting up house rules) and some participants indicated that they were interested in receiving additional treatment for depression. Consistent with the satisfaction survey, the participants also enjoyed the positive parenting sessions that allowed them to refocus on the positive attributes of the child and encouraged them to plan special activities with their child.

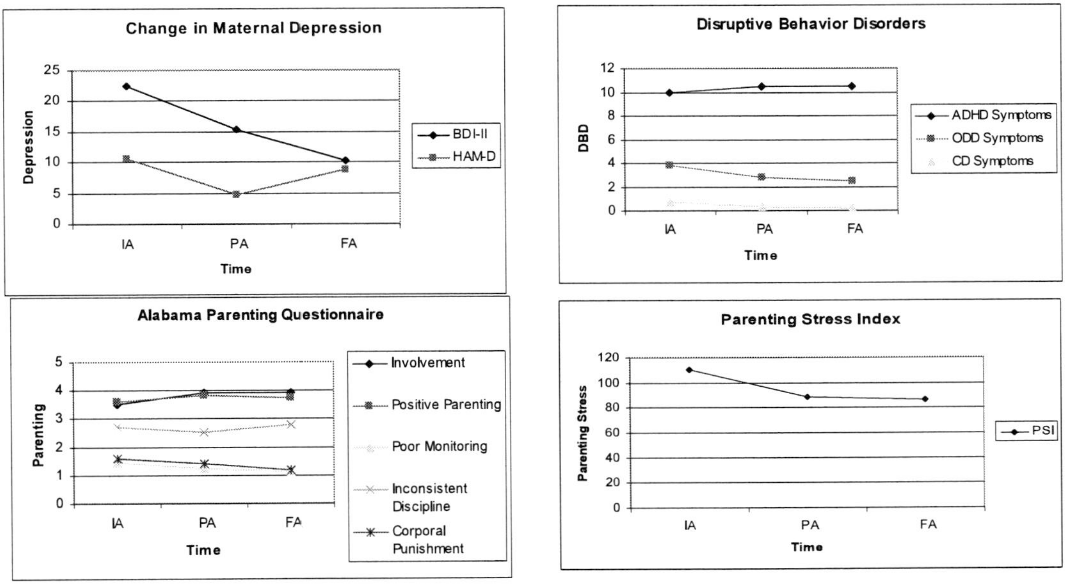


Note. IA = Initial Assessment, PA = Post-Assessment, FA = Follow-up Assessment

Figure 2. Treatment outcome changes in maternal depression, parenting, and child behavior

With the additional information from the focus groups, we obtained a cohesive picture of how we could modify the group to make it more valuable for this population of mothers with elevated levels of depression. With regard to the lower-rated sessions on the satisfaction survey, participants reported that more time should have been spent on time management, and the token economy session was too overwhelming for them to effectively implement. Also, mothers felt overwhelmed with the amount of material covered and the quantity of changes they were encouraged to make. Given that we targeted stressed and overwhelmed mothers, this feedback fits with the population and manual revisions were made accordingly. Specifically, we removed some treatment components, such as the session on child behavior at school, and now focus exclusively on behavior modification in the home. This allowed us to slow down and elaborate our presentation of the rest of material. We also simplified the home point system procedures substantially and enhanced sessions where participants wanted more information. Mothers desired to involve their spouses more and wished that the group allowed for easier sharing of information with their spouses. Although it is beyond the scope of this study to include the involvement of spouses in treatment, future research within our laboratory will attempt to explore and address the characteristics and needs of fathers within these families.

**Table 3: Satisfaction Survey**

| | Mean (out of possible 6) |
|---|---|
| How helpful was the IPI-A course in improving your mood? | 4.00 |
| How well did you feel that the course applied to you? | 4.91 |
| How helpful was the IPI-A course in improving your parenting? | 4.36 |
| How well did you feel that the course applied to your parenting? | 5.00 |
| Would you recommend this course to other mothers of children with ADHD? | 5.18 |
| How well did you feel the course was sensitive to minority issues? | 3.56 |
| Highest Rated Components | |
| *Most helpful* mood component | Mood monitoring/ thoughts, feelings and behaviors |
| *Most relevant* mood component | Social skills and assertiveness |
| *Most helpful* parenting component | Special time with your child |
| *Most relevant* parenting component | Praise and positive parenting |
| Lowest Rated Components | |
| Least helpful mood component | Time management/setting priorities |
| Least relevant mood component | Relaxation techniques |
| *Least helpful* parenting component | Manage child misbehavior in public |
| *Least relevant* parenting component | Home token and point system |

Note. 1 = Not at all helpful, 3 = Somewhat helpful, 6 = Extremely helpful

*Phase II: Future directions*

In Phase II of this study, the IPI-A will be contrasted with standard BPT, in which CBT coping skills for parents will *not* be presented. Seventy-two mothers will be randomly assigned to receive either the IPI-A treatment or standard BPT and outcomes will be compared across treatment modalities. The same therapists will conduct both treatments and the groups will be matched on therapist time to eliminate any potential therapist contact or non-specific therapist-related confounds. The participant selection and study procedures described previously for Phase I will be utilized for this phase of the project as well. All outcome assessments will be conducted by independent evaluators who are blind to the treatment status of each participant. It is expected that participants randomized to the IPI-A condition will evidence enhanced incremental benefits in maternal depression, parenting, and child behavior compared to those receiving standard BPT.

## SUMMARY

We have reviewed evidence of a theoretical model in which maternal depression, negative parenting, and child behavior problems exhibit reciprocal and interactive effects on one another. This negative cycle can contribute to the maintenance and exacerbation of maternal negative mood and child conduct problems. Maternal depression not only contributes to the development, maintenance, and exacerbation of child conduct problems, but is also an important barrier to successful outcomes following empirically-based treatments for child ADHD. We have therefore described a program of research on the development of a novel, integrated treatment for depressed mothers of ADHD children that concurrently targets maternal stress/depression and maladaptive parenting, with the ultimate goal of improving the developmental and treatment outcomes of children with ADHD.

## REFERENCES

Abidin, R. (1986). The Parenting Stress Index. Charlottesville, VA: *Pediatric Psychology Press.*

Abikoff, H., Abramowitz, A., Courtney, M., Cousins, L., Del Carmen, R., Eddy, M., et al. (1994). Parent training manual: MTA study. *Unpublished manuscript.*

American Psychiatric Association (1994). *Diagnostic and Statistical Manual of Mental Disorders (4th edition).* Washington, D.C.

Barkley, R. A. (1985). The effects of methylphenidate on the interactions of preschool ADHD children with their mothers. *Journal of the American Academy of Child & Adolescent Psychiatry*, 27, 336-341.

Beck, A. T. (1976). Cognitive therapy and the emotional disorders. New York: *International Universities Press.*

Beck, A. T., Steer, R. A., & Brown, G. K. (1996). Manual for the Beck Depression Inventory-II. San Antonio TX: *Psychological Corporation.*

Beck, A. T., Rush, A. J., Shaw, B. F., & Emery, G. (1979). Cognitive therapy of depression. New York: *Guilford Press.*

Beutler, L. & Moleiro, C. (2001), Clinical versus reliable and significant change. *Clinical Psychology: Science and Practice*, 8(4): 441-445.

Biometrics Research Department (Producer). (1996). SCID-101 for DSM-IV: Training Video for the Structured Clinical Interview for DSM-IV Axis I Disorders, *New York State Psychiatric Institute.*

Blackburn, I. M., Bishop, S., Glen, A. I. M., Whalley, L. J., & Christie, J. E. (1981). The efficacy of cognitve therapy in depression: A treatment trial using cognitive therapy and pharmacotherapy, each alone and in combination. *British Journal of Psychiatry*, 139, 181-189.

Breckenridge, J. S., Zeiss, A. M., & Thompson, L. W. (1987). The life satisfaction course: An intervention for the elderly. In R. F. Muñoz (Ed.), *Depression prevention: Research directions.* Washington, D.C.: Hemisphere Publishing Corporation.

Brestan, E. V., & Eyberg, S. M. (1998). Effective Psychosocial treatments of conduct-disordered children and adolescents: 29 years, 82 studies, and 5, 272 kids. *Journal of Clinical Child Psychology,* 27, 180-189.

Brown, R. A. & Lewinsohn, P. M. (1984). A psychoeducational approach to the treatment of depression: Comparison of group, individual and minimal contact procedures. *Journal of*

*Consulting and Clinical Psychology*, 52, 774-783.

Chamberlain, P. & Patterson, G. R. (1995).Discipline and child compliance in parenting. In Bornstein, Marc H (Vol. Ed. 4), *Handbook of parenting: Applied and practical parenting* (pp. 205-225) . Lawrence Erlbaum Associates, Inc., Hillsdale, NJ, England .

Chi, T. C. & Hinshaw, S. P.(2002). Mother-child relationships of children with ADHD: The role of maternal depressive symptoms and depression-related distortions. *Journal of Abnormal Child Psychology,* 30(4), 387-400.

Chronis, A. M., Chacko, A., Fabiano, G. A., Wymbs, B. T., & Pelham, W. E. (2004). Enhancements to the behavioral parent training paradigm for families of children with ADHD: Review and future directions. *Clinical Child and Family Psychology Review*, 7, 1-27.

Chronis, A. M., Gamble, S. A., Roberts, J. E., & Pelham, W. E. (2006). Cognitive behavioral depression treatment for mothers of children with attention-deficit/hyperactivity disorder. *Behavior Therapy*, 37, 143-158.

Chronis, A. M., Fabiano, F. A., Gnangy, E. M. (2001). Comprehensive and sustained behavioral and pharmacological treatment for attention-deficit/hyperactivity disorder: A case study. *Cognitive and Behavioral Practice*, 8, 346-358.

Chronis, A. M., Lahey, B. B., Pelham, W. E., Kipp, H., Baumann, B, & Lee, S. S. (2003a). Psychopathology and substance abuse in parents of young children with ADHD. *Journal of the American Academy of Child & Adolescent Psychiatry*, 42, 1424-1432.

Chronis, A. M., Lahey, B. B., Pelham, W. E., Williams, S. H., Baumann, B. L., Kipp, H., & Jones, H. A. (2007). *Parental psychopathology and maternal positive parenting predict future conduct problems in young children with attention-deficit/hyperactivity disorder.*

Cuijpers, P. (1998). A psychoeducational approach to the treatment of depression: A meta-analysis of Lewinsohn's "Coping with Depression" course. *Behavior Therapy*, 29, 521-533.

Cummings, E. M. & Davies, P. T. (1999). Depressed parents and family functioning: Interpersonal effects and children's functioning and development. In T. Joiner & J. C. Coyne (Eds.) *The interactional nature of depression.* Washington, DC: American Psychological Association.

Cunningham, C. E. & Barkley, R. A. (1979). The interactions of normal and hyperactive children with their mothers in free play and structured tasks. *Child Development*, 50, 217-224.

Dobson, K. S. (1989). A meta-analysis of the efficacy of cognitive therapy for depression. *Journal of Consulting and Clinical Psychology*, 57, 414-419.

Fabiano, G. A., Pelham, W. E. Jr., Waschbusch, D. A. (2006), A Practical Measure of Impairment: Psychometric Properties of the Impairment Rating Scale in Samples of Children With Attention Deficit Hyperactivity Disorder and Two School-Based Samples. *Journal of Clinical Child and Adolescent Psychology*, 35(3), 369-385.

First, M. B., Gibbon, M., Spitzer, R. L. & Williams, J. B. (1996). *Structured Clinical Interview for DSM-IV Axis I Disorders*. New York: Biometrics Research.

Fischer, M. (1990). Parenting stress and the child with attention deficit hyperactivity disorder. *Journal of Clinical Child Psychology*, 19(4), 337-346.

Griest, D. L. & Forehand, R. (1982). How can I get any parent training done with all these other problems going on? The role of family variables in child behavior therapy. *Child and Family Behavior Therapy*, 4, 73-80.

Hinshaw, S. P., Owens, E. B., Wells, K. C., Kraemer, H. C., Abikoff, H. B., Arnold, L. E., et al. (2000). Family processes and treatment outcome in the MTA: Negative/ineffective parenting practices in relation to multimodal treatment. *Journal of Abnormal Child Psychology*, 28, 555-568.

Hollon, S. D. & Beck, A. T. (1994). Cognitive and cognitive-behavioral therapies. In A. Bergin, S. Garfield, et al. (Eds.), *Handbook of psychotherapy and behavior change* (4th ed., pp.428-466). New York: John Wiley & Sons.

Hollon, S. D., Shelton, R. C., & Loosen, P. T. (1991). Cognitive therapy and pharmacotherapy for depression. *Journal of Consulting and Clinical Psychology*, 59, 88-99.

Hoza, B., Owens, J. S., Pelham, W. E., Swanson, J., Conners, C. K., Hinshaw, S. P., et al. (2000). Effect of parent cognitions on child treatment response in attention deficit/hyperactivity disorder. *Journal of Abnormal Child Psychology*, 28, 569-583.

Johnston, C. & Mash, E. J. (2001). Families of children with attention deficit hyperactivity disorder: Review and recommendations for future research. *Clinical Child & Family Psychology Review*, 4, 183-207.

Johnston, C. & Ohan, J. L. (2005), The Importance of Parental Attributions in Families of Children with Attention-Deficit/Hyperactivity and Disruptive Behavior Disorders. *Clinical Child and Family Psychology Review*, 8(3), 167-182.

Joiner, T. E. (2000). Depression's vicious spree: Self-propogating and erosive processes in depression chronicity. *Clinical Psychology: Science and Practice*, 7, 203-218.

Keller, M. B., Lavori, P. W., Friedman, B., Nielsen, E., Endicott, J., & McDonald-Scott, P. A. (1987). The Longitudinal Interval Follow-up Evaluation: A comprehensive method for assessing outcome in prospective longitudinal studies. *Archives of General Psychiatry*, 44, 540-548.

King, S., Waschbusch, D. A., Fankland, B. W., Andrande, B. F., Thurston, D. M., McNutt, L., Terrio, B. (2004). Taxonomic examination of ADHD and conduct disorder comorbidity in elementary school: A cluster analysis. *Journal of Psychopathology and Behavioral Assessment*, 27, 77-88.

Kühner, C., Angermeyer, M. C., & Veiel, H. O. (1996). Cognitive-behavioral group intervention as a means of tertiary prevention in depressed patients: Acceptance and short-term efficacy. *Cognitive Research & Therapy*, 20, 391-409.

Lahey, B. B. & Waldman, I. D. (2003). A developmental propensity model of the origins of conduct problems during childhood and adolescence. In B. B. Lahey, T. E. Moffitt, & A. Caspi (Eds.), *Causes of conduct disorder and juvenile delinquency* (pp. 76-117). New York; Guilford Press.

Lewinsohn, P. M., Hoberman, H., Teri, L. & Hautizinger, M. (1985). An integrative theory of depression. In S. Reiss & R. Bootzin (Eds.), Theoretical issues in behavior therapy. NY: *Academic Press*, 331.359.

Lewinsohn, P. M., Antonuccio, D., Steinmetz, J., & Teri, L. (1984*). The Coping with depression course: A psychoeducational intervention for unipolar depression.* Eugene, OR: Castalia.

Lewinsohn, P. M., Hoberman, H. M., & Clarke, G. N. (1989). The coping with depression course: Review and future directions. *Canadian Journal of Behavioural Science*, 21, 470-493.

Lewinsohn, P. M., Rohde, P., & Seely, J. R. (1998). Major depressive disorder in older adolescents: Prevalence, risk factors, and clinical implications. *Clinical Psychology Review*, 18, 765-794.

Lewinsohn, P. M., & Clarke, G. N. (1984). Group treatment of depressed individuals: The "coping with depression" course. *Advances in Behaviour Research and Therapy*, 6, 99-114.

Lovejoy, M. C., Graczyk, P.A., O'Hare, E., & Neuman, G. (2000). Maternal depression and parenting behavior, A meta-analytic review. *Clinical Psychology Review*, 20(5), 561-592.

Lovett, S. & Gallagher, D. (1988). Psychoeducational interventions for family caregivers: Preliminary efficacy data. *Behavior Therapy*, 19, 321-330.

Lynam, D. R. (1996). Early identification of chronic offenders: Who is the fledgling psychopath? *Psychological Bulletin*, 120, 209-234.

Mannuzza, S., Klein, R. G., Abikoff, H., Moulton, J. L. (2004). Significance of child conduct problems to the development of later conduct disorder among children with ADHD: A prospective follow up study. *Journal of abnormal child psychology*, 32, 565-573.

Marshal, M. P., Molina, B. S. (2006). Antisocial behaviors moderate the deviant peer pathway to substance abuse in children with ADHD. *Journal of Clinical Child and Adolescent Psychiatry*, 35, 216-226.

Martin, N., Levy, F., Piek, J., and Hay, D. (In Press), *A genetic study of attention deficit hyperactivity disorder, conduct disorder, oppositional defiant disorder and reading disability: Aetiological overlaps and implications.*

Mash, E. J. & Johnston, C. (1982). A comparison of the mother-child interactions of younger and older hyperactive and normal children. *Child Development*, 53, 1371-1381.

McMahon, R. J., Forehand, R., Griest, D. L., & Wells, K. C. (1981). Who drops out of treatment during parent behavioral training? *Behavioral Counseling Quarterly*, 1, 79-85.

Miller, I. W., Bishop, S., Norman, W. H., & Maddever, H. (1985). The modified hamilton rating scale for depression: Reliability and validity. *Psychiatry Research*, 14, 131-142.

Moffit, T. E. & Silva, P. A. (1988), Self-reported delinquency: results from an instrument for New Zealand. *Australia and New Zealand Journal of Criminology*, 21, 227-240.

Nigg, J. T. (2001), Is ADHD a disinhibitory disorder? *Psychological Bulletin*, 127, 571-598.

Organista, K. C., Muñoz, R. F., & Gonzalez, G. (1994). Cognitive-behavioral therapy for depression in low-income and minority medical outpatients: Description of a program and exploratory analyses. *Cognitive Therapy & Research*, 18, 241-259.

Orvaschel, H. & Puig-Antich, J. (1995). *Schedule for Affective Disorders and Schizophrenia for School-Aged Children-Epidemiologic 5th Version*. Ft. Lauderdale, FL: Nova University.

Owens, E. B., Hinshaw, S. P., Kraemer, H. C., Arnold, L. E., Abikoff, H. B., Cantwell, D. P., et al. (2003). What treatment for whom for ADHD: Moderators of treatment in the MTA. *Journal of Consulting and Clinical Psychology*, 71, 540-552.

Patterson, G. R. (1982). Coercive family process. *Castalia*: Eugene, Oregon.

Patterson, G.R., DeBaryshe, B.D., Ramsey, E. (1989). A developmental perspective on anti-social behavior. *American Psychologist*, 44, 329-335.

Pelham, W. E., Gnagy, E. M., Greenslade, K. E.(1992), Teacher ratings of DSM-III---R symptoms for the disruptive behavior disorders, *Journal of the American Academy of Child & Adolescent Psychiatry*, 31(2), 210-218.

Pelham, W. E., Greiner, A. R., & Gnagy, E. M. (1997). Summer treatment program manual. Buffalo, NY: *Comprehensive Treatment for Attention Deficit Disorders, Inc.*

Pelham, W. E., Wheeler, T., Chronis, A. (1998). Empirically supported psychosocial treatments for ADHD. *Journal of Clinical Child Psychology*, 27, 190-205.

Rhee, S. H. & Waldman, I. (2002), Genetic and environmental influences on antisocial behavior: A meta-analysis of twin and adoption studies. *Psychological Bulletin*, 128(3), 490-529.

Richters J. E. (1992). Depressed mothers as informants about their children: A critical review of the evidence for distortion. *Psychological Bulletin*, 112, 485-499.

Rush, A. J., Beck, A. T., Kovacs, M., & Hollon, S. D. (1977). Comparative efficacy of cognitive therapy and pharmacotherapy in the treatment of depressed outpatients. *Cognitive Therapy and Research*, 1, 17-38.

Shelton, K. K., Frick, P. J., & Wooton, J. (1996). Assessment of parenting practices in families of elementary school-age children. *Journal of Clinical Child Psychology*, 25, 317-329.

Silverman, W. K., Kurtines, W. M., Ginsburg, G. S., Weems, C. F., Rabian, B., & Serafini, L. T. (1999). Contingency management, self-control, and education support in the treatment of childhood phobic disorders: A randomized clinical trial. *Journal of Consulting and Clinical Psychology*, 67, 675-687.

Sonuga-Burke, E., Daley, D., & Thompson, M. (2002). Does maternal ADHD reduce the effectiveness of parent training for preschool children's ADHD? *Journal of the American Academy of Child and Adolescent Psychiatry*, 41, 696-702

Wells, K. C., Epstein, J. N., Hinshaw, S. P., Conners, C. K., Klaric, J., Abikoff, H. B., et al. (2000) Parenting and family stress treatment outcomes in attention-deficit hyperactivity disorder (ADHD): An empirical analysis of the MTA study. *Journal of Abnormal Child Psychology*, 28, 543-553.

Webster-Stratton, C. (1985). Predictors of treatment outcome in parent training for conduct disordered children. Behavior Therapy, 16, 223-243.

Webster-Stratton, C. (1992a). Individually administered videotape parent training: "Who benefits?" *Cognitive Therapy and Research*, 16, 31-52.

Wechsler, D. (2003), Wechsler Intelligence Scale for Children – Fourth Edition: Manual. *San Antonio: The Psychological Corporation.*

# SECTION II. THE LABORATORY METHOD IN PREVENTION: PSYCHO-SOCIAL-EDUCATIONAL SKILLS TRAINING PROGRAMS

In: Toward a Science of Clinical Psychology
Editor: Luciano L'Abate, pp. 81-99
ISBN: 978-1-60456-062-6


*Chapter IV*

# Evolution of a Social-Skills Intervention for At-Risk Preschoolers in an Applied Setting

***Douglas W. Nangle, Erika Carpenter Rich, Elizabeth J. Shepherd and Jessica Fales***

## Abstract

Social skills are vital for academic success, effective interpersonal communication, and the establishment of positive peer relations for children of all ages (see Asher & Parker, 1989, for a review). Such skills may be of particular importance to preschoolers in helping to set a foundation for future relationships with peers, siblings, parents, and teachers (Eisenberg et al., 1999). This is illustrated in the findings of one study showing that spontaneous sharing among preschoolers predicted the exhibition of prosocial behaviors in childhood and early adulthood (Eisenberg et al., 1999). Discussions about the importance of social skills for children most often focus on their crucial role in the development of peer relationships and there is an abundance of research linking low peer acceptance and indices of maladjustment ranging from aggression, mental illness, failure to complete school, and criminal activity (e.g., Kupersmidt, Coie, & Dodge, 1990; Parker & Asher, 1987; Parker, Rubin, Price, & DeRosier, 1995).

Largely based on the predictive nature of poor peer relationships, social-skills intervention for children has emerged as a major treatment approach and an impressive literature base now exists supporting its efficacy (see McFadyen-Ketchum & Dodge, 1998, Nangle, Erdley, Carpenter, & Newman, 2002, for reviews). The vast majority of evaluative studies, however, have targeted elementary-aged children and the surprisingly few published interventions with preschoolers have been criticized for their lack of sensitivity to important developmental issues (Bierman & Montminy, 1993; Nangle et al., 2002; Price & Ladd, 1986). No doubt, the demonstrated hesitance to intervene with preschoolers is to some extent attributable to their less unified social behavior, more variable sociometric status, and propensity to base peer preferences on more recent interactions (Bierman & Montminy, 1993). The fluidity of their social knowledge and less crystallized peer status, however, would appear to make preschool children ideal candidates for prevention and/or intervention efforts. Furthermore, despite their apparent state of flux, relatively stable individual differences in social competence and peer acceptance are evident amongst preschoolers and those in need of intervention can be readily identified on the basis of their problematic social behavior (Mize & Ladd, 1990). Also arguing for early intervention is the fact that some problematic social behavior patterns, such as aggression, become fixed and stabilized as early as eight years of age (Tremblay, Masse, Pagani, & Vitaro, 1996). In further support, there is meta-analytic evidence suggesting that social skills training interventions are more effective with preschoolers than their school-aged counterparts (Schneider & Byrne, 1987).

In this chapter, we describe the use of the laboratory method in our attempts to transport evidence-based social skills assessment and treatment practices into an applied community setting. Over the past decade, we have developed a collaborative relationship with a community agency coordinating a number of Head Start centers in Eastern Maine. In our role as mental health consultants, we tested an early clinical observation by conducting a more formal analysis of referrals by Head Start teachers and determined that most of these involved peer interaction difficulties. In the ensuing years, we began the process of developing and refining an intervention capable of targeting multiple children to more systematically address these referral concerns. Following a brief review of the preschool literature, the chapter provides a detailed description of this process starting with overviews of the Head Start setting and the development of an intervention. Next, we review two effectiveness studies, emphasizing the challenges posed by the applied setting and lessons learned, and close with a summary and discussion of future directions. Evolution aptly captures the nature of this process. In adapting to the applied setting, we made a number of procedural modifications along the way. Unfortunately, illustrating the gaps between research and practice, the realities of the applied setting often pulled us away from the existing literature base. For example, structural variations across the Head Start centers made direct observation difficult, if not impossible, and attempts to pilot a parenting component met with a lack of acceptance and compliance.

## Social Skills Interventions with Preschoolers

The basic components of effective social skills interventions for preschoolers are quite similar to those used with older children. Based on operant learning principles, the *behavioral* approaches typically target overt responses and seek to control them via reinforcement and punishment linked to the occurrence of the response and/or the manipulation of its behavioral antecedents (see Elliott & Gresham, 1993, for a review). Example strategies include contingent attention and token reinforcement to increase desirable responding and response cost and differential reinforcement to decrease undesirable responding. Instruction and modeling are added to such contingency management strategies in order to teach children novel social behaviors (Bierman, 2004; Elliott & Gresham, 1993). *Cognitively-based* approaches often include behavioral strategies, but also focus on modifying the thought processes hypothesized to underlie overt behavioral responses (McFadyen-Ketchum & Dodge, 1998; Nangle et al. 2002). Example intervention strategies include coaching and problem solving skills training. In coaching interventions, the child is provided with a rationale for learning a skill, instruction on how or when to use it, practice opportunities, and specific feedback following enactment (e.g., Oden & Asher, 1977). Problem-solving interventions use a variety of instructional methods to teach children cognitive skills that presumably lead to more competent responding in difficult social situations (e.g., generating multiple alternative solutions, thinking about the consequences of actions, and pairing solutions and consequences; Spivack & Shure, 1974).

Interventions with preschoolers rarely fall neatly into one of these basic approach categories. Instead, most utilize some combination of these approaches and strategies. Some are designed to target specific populations, such as children with early onset conduct problems (e.g., Webster-Stratton, Reid, & Hammond, 2001), aggression (Barkley et al., 2000), developmental delays (e.g., Guglielmo & Tyron, 2001), or other behavioral handicaps (e.g., McConnell, Sisson, Cort, & Strain, 1991). Others target children who are low in social status (e.g., Mize & Ladd, 1990). Yet others target all children in a particular class using a curriculum-based approach (e.g., Cartledge & Kleefield, 1991; Factor & Shilmoeller, 1983). The following review is necessarily restrictive and is designed simply to familiarize the reader with the different types of evidence-based interventions for preschool children (for more complete reviews see Bierman, 2004, Mize & Ladd, 1990, and Nangle et al., 2002).

## Problem Solving Skills Interventions

In pioneering work, Spivack and Shure (1974) demonstrated the effectiveness of social problem solving skills (SPPS) training with preschool-aged children. Following instruction in prerequisite concepts and skills (e.g., listening to and observing others; perspective taking), their program uses the facilitated instruction (e.g., use of pictures, puppets) and practice (e.g., role plays) of problem-solving skills. Using similar procedures, Vaughn, Ridley, and Bullock (1984) targeted aggressive preschoolers identified using teacher ratings with a 50-session program. Compared to children in a story-reading control condition, those children receiving the SPPS training were able to generate more competent solutions to interpersonal problems at post and follow-up assessments. Shure and Spivack (1982) demonstrated the utility of SPPS training with a sample of low SES African-American children enrolled in federally-funded day care. Improvements in problem-solving skills and behavioral adjustment were found and maintained for one year following intervention. Improvements in targeted cognitive skills, however, have not always translated into overt behavior change (e.g., Rickel, Eshelman, & Loigman, 1983; Sharp, 1981).

## Interventions Targeting Early Conduct Problems

Webster-Stratton and her colleagues developed a comprehensive intervention targeting the social difficulties often experienced by young children with conduct problems (Webster-Stratton et al., 2001). The intervention combines more traditional social skills training and cognitive-behavioral approaches, such as problem-solving and anger-management training. To assist with maintenance and generalization, a parent component, group activities, and videotape role plays are also included. Compared to a control group, children receiving this intervention showed clinically significant improvements in SPPS and conduct problems (Webster-Stratton et al., 2001). For example, 80% of the children diagnosed with Attention-Deficit/Hyperactivity Disorder (ADHD) at baseline no longer met criteria at the follow-up assessment. A previous investigation found that this type of child-focused intervention was even more effective when a parent training component was added (Webster-Stratton & Hammond, 1997). Barkley and his colleagues, however, found parent training alone to be ineffective for a sample of preschoolers with aggressive and attention-related symptoms, although a comparison classroom-based treatment, that included group social skills and anger-management training, resulted in improved social behavior and decreased conduct problems (Barkley et al., 2000).

## Status-Specific Interventions

Mize and Ladd (1990) intervened with a group of low social status preschoolers identified through a combination of sociometrics ratings and behavioral observations. Once per week, the identified children met with adult coaches and received instruction in four verbal communication skills (i.e., leading, questioning, supporting, and commenting) associated with increased peer acceptance. In addition to modeling, rehearsal, and feedback, these authors used puppets to facilitate instruction and high status peer partners to assist with the skill rehearsal. In further attempts to enhance generalization, the coaches also assisted (e.g., identifying situations in which the skills could be used with peers) the low-status children as they participated in regular classroom activities with their classmates. The frequency of positive social skill use doubled for the treated children and resulted in concomitant sociometric improvements at a one-month follow-up assessment. Somewhat unexpectedly, the improvements in social skills were not accompanied by any decreases in aggression.

In a very brief classroom intervention more directly targeting aggression, Zahavi and Asher (1978) intervened with the eight most aggressive children by having the teacher pull each target child aside for a 10 minute period of verbal instruction focusing on three major concepts: aggression causes harm to others, aggression does not solve problems, and there are more positive ways to solve problems, such as sharing, taking turns, and playing together. Remarkably, behavioral observations indicated that this brief verbal, teacher-mediated intervention resulted in decreases in aggression and increases in positive behavior.

## Curriculum-Based Interventions

Curriculum-based interventions are more broad-based in that they target all of the children in a classroom and instruction is integrated into the typical daily schedule. For example, the Taking Part Curriculum (TPC) developed by Cartledge and Kleefield

(1991) incorporates instruction in three major domains of social skills thought to be critical for preschool-aged children: social communication, group play skills, and conflict resolution. McKinney and Rust (1998) compared the TPC with nonspecific social skill instruction (i.e., teachers provided with a list of skills to target, but no actual curriculum) with an African-American preschool sample. By the end of the 15-week intervention period, the TPC children improved on teacher-rated prosocial skills and problem behaviors, whereas the nonspecific intervention resulted in no detectable changes.

Factor and Shilmoeller (1983) also intervened with an entire classroom of preschool children. They used verbal instructions to teach skill concepts, similar to those used by Zahavi and Asher (1978), but also incorporated modeling, feedback, and rehearsal components. In a departure from more typical curriculum-based interventions, these authors taught the skills (i.e., communication, participation, cooperation, and validation/support) outside of the classroom to small groups of four children. Instruction was supplemented by prompts, modeling, and practice play periods. This relatively brief (i.e., 10 eight minute sessions) resulted in gains in sociability and decreases in aggression relative to a control group. A one week follow-up assessment, however, indicated inadequate generalization of the trained skills to the classroom setting.

In sum, this empirical literature base influenced all of our treatment development decisions. At the conceptual level, we were guided by the model underlying the Mize and Ladd (1990) investigation, a decision based on its thorough nature, developmental sensitivity, and close connections to treatment (Ladd & Mize, 1983a; 1983b). Regarding format, we set out to develop a curriculum-based intervention capable of targeting all of the children in the Head Start classrooms (e.g., Factor & Shilmoeller, 1983; McKinney & Rust, 1998). Procedurally, we decided to rely primarily on cognitive behavioral training methods, such as instruction, modeling, and coaching, in delivering the curriculum.

## Developing an Intervention for Head Start Preschoolers

We now turn to a description of our decade-long efforts to develop a social-skills intervention in the Head Start setting. Our application of the laboratory method began with an objective mental health referral review and continued as we based our initial interventions and subsequent modifications on the previously reviewed efficacy literature. To provide sufficient context, we first briefly describe Head Start and our relationship with the coordinating community agency. After a summary of our initial needs assessment, piloting, and conceptual basis for intervention development, we review two effectiveness studies with an emphasis on the difficulties encountered in the applied setting and lessons learned.

## Setting Overview

### *Head Start.*

Head Start is a federally-funded program started in 1965 for preschoolers from families living in poverty (Ripple, Gilliam, Chanana, & Zigler, 1999). Head Start students are considered to be at-risk for a variety of difficulties associated with economic disadvantage. For example, they begin the program with lower ability levels and are less likely to have a father in the home than students at other types of preschools (Lee, Brooks-Gunn, Schnur, & Liaw, 1990). In a comprehensive review of 64 centers, Webster-Stratton and Hammond (1998) found Head Start students to have higher base rates of social skills deficits, aggression, and disruptive behavior than typical preschoolers. Although academic readiness is its principal goal, Head Start strives to emphasize all aspects of development in its curriculum, including social competence. Results from longitudinal studies indicate that Head Start has a favorable impact on global measures of social competence, such as delinquency, teen pregnancy, special education placement, and school attendance (see Locurto, 1991, for a review), although specific measures of social skills are not included in this outcome research. Overall, the social development of these youngsters is considered to be an under-researched area (Ravler & Zigler, 1997).

#### *Penquis Community Action Program (CAP).*

For more than 25 years, the Psychological Services Center (PSC), the University of Maine's Psychology Department outpatient training clinic, has been contracted by Penquis CAP, a private nonprofit community health and social service agency, to provide mental health consultation services for the students in the more than 25 Head Start classrooms it coordinates. In fulfilling this contract, PSC personnel observe each classroom two times per year and provide objective feedback on the overall climate (e.g., safety, daily activities, facilitation of developmental skills, staff-children interactions). Also, at the request of center staff, specific children can be referred for further observation and treatment recommendations. Treatments come in the form of staff-initiated procedures (e.g., behavioral techniques, teaching peer interaction skills) and/or referrals to community providers for more intensive services (e.g., family therapy, developmental evaluations).

### Needs Assessment and Initial Piloting

In our work as consultants, we noted that many of the mental health referrals seemed to be either directly or indirectly related to problematic social interactions. A more formal follow-up review supported our observations, showing that 40% of the 177 children referred between fall of 1991 and spring 1999 had aggressive behavior as one of the principal precipitants (Carpenter & Nangle, 1999). Poor social functioning typically either contributed to the aggression indirectly (e.g., an inability to communicate leading to pushing a peer and taking a toy) or was a major concern in and of itself (e.g., social withdrawal). Rather than continuing to address these problems on a case-by-case basis, we presented these data to Penquis CAP administrators and asked for their cooperation in developing a more systematic method of intervention. Though more than willing to cooperate in these efforts, the agency was limited in its ability to provide much in the way of financial or personnel resources. Thus began our collaborative efforts to develop a time- and cost-efficient, curriculum-based intervention for eventual use in all of the classrooms.

Based on our prior experiences, we knew that we would confront some significant obstacles in trying to transport evidence-based procedures into the Head Start setting. For instance, although we recognized the need for a teacher-mediated approach, in order to enhance generalization and, more practically speaking, to proceed given our very limited personnel resources, we were also aware that the teachers were already strapped for time because of the large student-teacher ratios and long list of mandated activities. In this context, we decided to begin with a replication of the Zahavi and Asher (1978) study in one of the classrooms. Such a pilot study would allow not only for a test of the brief teacher-mediated procedures with a Head Start sample, but also help in determining the feasibility of working in this challenging setting.

As in the Zahavi and Asher (1978) study, we selected the eight most aggressive children in one classroom based on behavioral observations (Carpenter & Nangle, 2002). After some training on how to administer the verbal instructions, the teacher was asked to pull each child aside for a 10 minute period of instruction on the three concepts (aggression causes harm, aggression does not solve problems, and there are more positive ways to solve problems). Compared to a non-aggressive control group, the children receiving the instructions demonstrated significant improvements in teacher rated prosocial skills from pre- to post-treatment that were maintained at a one month follow-up assessment. Significant improvements in observed positive and negative behavior were also found between the post-treatment and follow-up. The absence of significant pre- to post-treatment changes, however, made it impossible to definitively determine whether or not the observed improvements were caused by the intervention, although it seemed plausible that they were delayed treatment effects (e.g., Bierman, Miller, & Staab, 1987).

## Guiding Conceptual Model

Encouraged by the ability of this brief intervention to result in noticeable improvements, we continued with our efforts to develop a more comprehensive curriculum-based approach. To help guide these efforts, we turned to the oft-cited Ladd and Mize (1983a, 1983b) social-cognitive learning model of social skill training. These authors contend that successful social-skills interventions must address all of the components described in their social cognitive learning model. In accordance with the social skills deficit hypothesis, a failure to demonstrate appropriate social skills could arise from deficits in any one of three areas: skill knowledge, skill performance, or knowledge of the appropriate contexts in which to employ the skill. As such, the model proposes that interventions should have three commensurate training goals: *enhancing skill concepts*, *promoting skill performance*, and *fostering skill maintenance and generalization*. Verbal and modeled instruction, rehearsal, and feedback are the recommended procedures to reach these training goals.

The social-cognitive nature of the model is most reflected in the first training goal. Enhancing skill concepts involves ensuring that children learn the appropriate concept underlying a skill, including its defining features (e.g., the behavioral components necessary to enact the skills). Ideally, these skill concepts will function as templates for future social behavior. In order to do so, however, instruction needs also to address their *functional relevance*. That is, children must understand the usefulness of the skill. This training goal is bet met through verbal and/or modeled instruction. The instructional component can also provide information regarding the generalizability of the social concepts. Generalizability is further enhanced when both positive and negative instances of skill usage are included. In other words, contexts or situations in which the use of the skill is appropriate versus inappropriate should be integrated into the instruction. Along these same lines, it is also important to provide an example of an ineffective way of solving a conflict, such as the use of aggression, prior to modeling the trained skill.

The second goal, enhancing skill performance, involves gaining mastery of the social concepts. The skills are recalled by the children to ensure that they have been properly encoded into memory. Through rehearsal, children attempt to behaviorally enact the skills, fleshing out their cognitive representations of the concepts. Early on in training, the environment should be structured to ensure success, but less structured trials are incorporated later on as the children approach mastery.

The third and final goal, skill maintenance and generalization, focuses on the use of the skills in the naturalistic environment. First, performance feedback is provided. It is either evaluative, providing praise for correct skill usage, or informative, providing correction or bolstering memory for the concept. Later on, children begin to use the skill more independently and they are encouraged to self-monitor performance. Training focusing on more realistic performance evaluation may be necessary. Ideally, children will eventually be able to modify performance based on such feedback.

## Resulting Curricula and Evaluative Studies

### Study One

#### *Curriculum*

Our initial intervention development efforts resulted in the Curriculum on the Management and Promotion of Appropriate Social Skills (COMPASS; Carpenter, 2002). With its conceptual basis in the Ladd and Mize (1983a, 1983b) model and applied format following that of Mize and Ladd (1990), the curriculum targets improved social concept knowledge, skill performance, and skill monitoring through instruction, feedback, and rehearsal. As in our pilot study, classroom teachers serve as the instructors, but, as a curriculum-based intervention, COMPASS targets all students in the classroom and requires a total of 12 sessions (two times per week for six weeks), with each session occurring across two daily activity periods.

The instructional component is designed to fit into the already scheduled "circle time." Targeted social skills include cooperation (i.e., sharing, taking turns, solving conflicts verbally with other children), participation, validation/support (i.e., helping others and having fun during play), and communication (i.e., talking, listening, questions, comments, and leads; Factor & Schilmoeller, 1983). Teachers model the skills using puppets, using appropriate and inappropriate exemplars, as well as counterexamples for each prosocial skill (e.g., aggression as a counterexample of cooperation). The children also engage in activities that focus on skill integration. In the rehearsal component, children initially role-play appropriate behaviors using hand puppets and then with actual play partners. These play partner rehearsals occur during cooperative activities, such as puzzle assembly and group drawing, as part of already scheduled "free play station" periods. The skill monitoring component also occurs during the play station period. Following peer partner rehearsal, children are asked questions about the interactions that specifically target skill use and effectiveness.

Our efforts to enhance maintenance and generalization dovetailed with our goal of developing an intervention that would "fit" into the applied setting. COMPASS training sessions are integrated into ongoing Head Start activities. This not only makes its implementation less disruptive for the teachers, but provides multiple durable stimulus cues (e.g., teachers, peers, classroom, and activities) for appropriate skill use for the children as well. Two COMPASS features, training across natural environmental stimuli and the inclusion of peers in training, have been recommended as effective generalization facilitation strategies (Stokes & Osnes, 1989). We considered these to be critical intervention features since the lack of maintenance and generalization has plagued the preschool and overall social skills training literatures (see Chandler, Lubeck, & Fowler, 1992, and Fox & McEvoy, 1993, for reviews).

### *Study design*

We evaluated the effectiveness of the COMPASS intervention by comparing two treatment classrooms (N=34) with two active control classrooms (N=46; Carpenter, 2002). Pre-, post-, and three-month follow-up assessments included teacher ratings (i.e., Social Skills Rating System, Preschool Level; Child Behavior Checklist, Caregiver-Teacher Report Form), peer acceptance ratings, and a puppet-facilitated analogue interview (Enactive Social Knowledge Interview). With blanket parental consent obtained through Penquis CAP, 100% of the children in the four classrooms participated in the assessments.

### *Results and lessons learned*

Children were included in the analyses if they had data from all three assessments and attended Head Start on at least 75% of the COMPASS session days (N=26 in the treatment group; N=37 control). Unfortunately, after controlling for site differences, no treatment effects were found. We considered a number of possible explanations for these null findings. First, in retrospect, our "control group" was probably more accurately described as an active treatment in that Head Start is in and of itself an early intervention that targets social and other functioning domains. Second, we observed much more variability across the classrooms than was expected. There were striking differences across the four classrooms at the pre-assessment period, which could be attributed to an interaction of various factors including class size, student composition, classroom environment, and/or teacher experience. Third, perhaps the "dose" of treatment was not sufficient. The 12 sessions across six weeks may not have been enough to add significantly to the already present Head Start intervention. A related factor was the absence of a parent component. Additional considerations included developmental appropriateness (e.g., perhaps there was too much reliance on verbal instruction) and lack of contingency management supports.

## Study Two

We set out to address some of these considerations in a revised curriculum and, given the observed variability across classrooms, also decided to use a different study design to test its effectiveness.

### *Curriculum*

The revised curriculum stayed true to the Ladd and Mize (1983a; 1983b) model and incorporated a number of elements found in the Mize and Ladd (1990) and COMPASS interventions (Shepherd, 2007). The "dose" of instruction was increased in a number of ways. A more constricted set of skills is targeted (i.e., sharing, taking turns, leads, and comments). With enhanced developmental sensitivity, instruction begins with non-verbally based skills (i.e., sharing, turn taking) and subsequently targets the more sophisticated verbally-based skills (i.e., leads, comments).

Another major change bolstering instruction is the introduction of both *universal* and *intensive* components. In the *universal* component, all children receive daily instruction on the targeted skills during regularly scheduled "circle time" (every day of the week for the duration of the intervention). Additional universal elements include the display of posters depicting the targeted skills and a simple contingency management plan (i.e., sticker charts rewarding appropriate skill usage). A subset of four children in each classroom exhibiting particular social difficulties (i.e., identified during the baseline assessment on the basis of a combination of low peer acceptance ratings and low rates of observed target skills) also receives the *intensive* component. Twice each week, they are pulled from the ongoing classroom activities and receive added instruction, modeling, rehearsal, and feedback from trained therapists (i.e., graduate students), who also act as "coaches" as they accompany the intensive children back into the classroom and provide prompts, additional instruction, and feedback during naturally occurring peer interactions.

Notably, we also piloted a parental component to add to this revised curriculum (Shepherd, Nangle, Rivera, Erdley, & Hecker, 2003). In a minimal therapist contact format, 34 parents of Head Start students received instruction in the use of targeted skills and how to best facilitate their use through self-administered videotaped modules and accompanying workbook exercises (e.g., Webster-Stratton, 1992). In addition, parents were asked to attend two therapist-led meetings and were provided with dinner and childcare to facilitate their participation. Compared to a matched control group, no significant treatment effects were found across a broad range of measures that included parent and teacher ratings of social behaviors, as well as self-reported perceptions of parenting competence. Likely contributing to these disappointing results were the lack of parental compliance with the intervention procedures. Considering these null findings and our very limited resources, we chose to proceed, at least temporarily, without a parent component.

### *Study design*

In attempting to address some of the limitations of the Carpenter (2002) investigation, we modified our study design. Recall that we had encountered tremendous baseline variability across classrooms in that study. One way to address this limitation would be to expand the number of classrooms to enhance statistical power, but our limited resources ruled out this option. Another factor we considered was the lack of direct measures of actual skill acquisition (i.e., direct observation). Without such measures, we could not determine whether the disappointing results stemmed from a failure for the children to learn the targeted skills or for the acquired skills to translate into concomitant improvements on the teacher and peer ratings.

We turned to a single-group, multiple baseline design, which is a variant of the single-subject, multiple baseline design. According to Kelly (1980), this design is particularly well suited for the evaluation of small group interventions in applied settings due to its ability to control for maturation effects, eliminate the need for an untreated control group, and enhance time and cost efficiency relative to repeated single-subject evaluations (see Lumpkin, Silverman, Weems, Markham, & Kurtines, 2002, for an example application with children diagnosed with anxiety disorders).

This design requires repeated measures capable of providing frequent and continuous measurements of the dependent variable(s). We used behavioral observations of the targeted skills for this purpose. Using a focal-child observation scheme (Altmann, 1974), trained observers were asked to locate specific children upon an audio signal transmitted via wireless headphones and record coded behaviors occurring within six five-second intervals (see Mize & Ladd, 1990). Observations occurred during free-play periods two days each week across the baseline, intervention, and follow-up assessment phases. Adjunct measures administered at pre-, post-, one- and three-month follow-up included peer acceptance and teacher ratings (i.e., Social Skills Rating System, Preschool Level; Aggressive Behavior Subscale of the Child Behavior Checklist, Caregiver-Teacher Report Form). In addition to serving as a continuous measure, the observations were combined with the peer acceptance ratings to identify the intensive intervention group at the baseline assessment (Mize & Ladd, 1990).

Following baseline assessments in the three participating classrooms (N=38 total; 12 in the intensive group; participation rate of 95%), the intervention was introduced sequentially in a time-lagged manner. In brief, upon a demonstrated improvement (via visual inspection of graphed data) in the observed combined use of the target skills by the intensive children within a classroom, the intervention was subsequently introduced into the next classroom, and so on. Similarly, within each classroom, three of the four intensive intervention children had to show demonstrable improvements in a targeted skill in order for the intervention to proceed to the next target skill. If such demonstrable progress did not occur within four sessions, the intervention proceeded to the next skill anyway.

### *Results and lessons learned*

Data collection for this study was completed just as this chapter was being written. As such, our results are considered preliminary and should be interpreted cautiously. One issue complicating interpretation was a much higher than expected degree of within child day-to-day variability on the primary continuous measure (i.e., % use of combined targeted skills). To help make sense of what graphically was a very complex picture, we modeled linear growth curves to predict change in the daily use of target skills for both the intensive and universal children (Raudenbush & Bryk, 2002) and the following summary is based primarily on these analyses (see Figure 1).

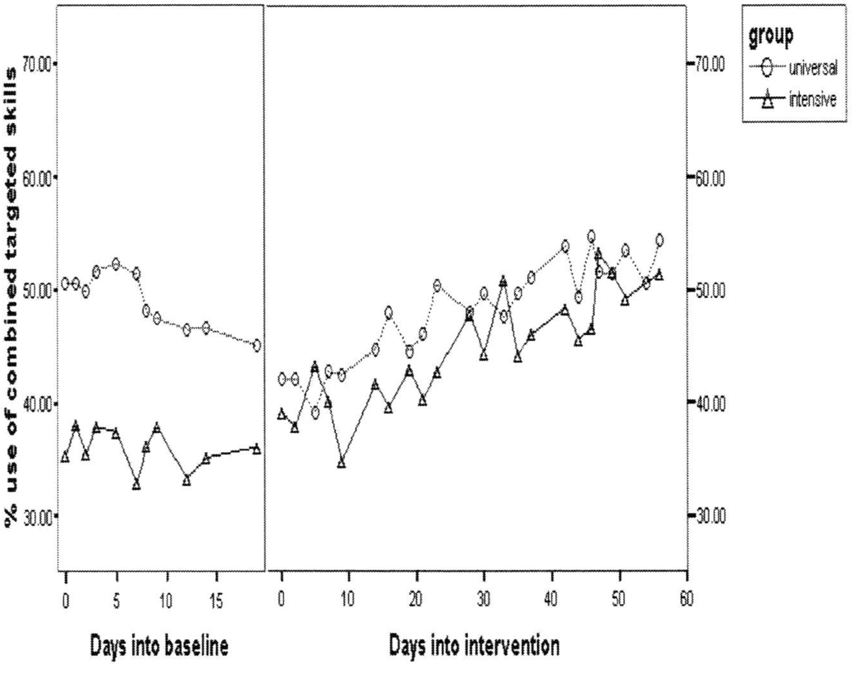


Figure 1. Mean predicted change in use of targeted social skills.

As expected given the identification method, the children receiving the intensive component began with significantly lower rates of observed target skill use and peer acceptance, as well as higher levels of teacher-rated problem behaviors, than their classmates. Interestingly, however, perhaps questioning the validity of our continuous measure to some extent, these children did not have significantly lower teacher ratings of social skills.

Relative to baseline, both groups evidenced modest but significant improvements in predicted target skill use across the intervention period (see Figure 1). In addition, seemingly supporting the added "dose" of instruction, the children receiving the intensive component were indistinguishable from their classmates in observed target skill use by the end of the active intervention phase, although it should be noted that the degree of within child day-to-day variability in this phase made it more difficult to detect a significant difference between the intervention groups. That is, there was an apparent difference between the groups in the rate of improvement over time (the universal group improving at a faster rate), but it was not large enough to be considered significant given the day-to-day variability of the continuous measure. In addition, there was some limited evidence of skill maintenance. Although the intensive children as a group once again fell below their classmates in target skill use by the follow-up assessment phase, this group difference did not remain significant when controlling for each child's predicted end-of-treatment outcome. That is, individual children displaying higher-than-average target skill use at the post assessment continued to engage in higher-than-average skill use across the follow-up assessment, regardless of treatment group.

Despite the improvements in observed skill use, the intervention failed to significantly impact the teacher ratings. Thus, the gains in target skill use were not sufficient to alter teacher perception. Perhaps with more time and exposure the gains would have been detected. In contrast, by the three month follow-up assessment, the children receiving the intensive component had, on average, similar peer acceptance ratings to their classmates. We, however, interpret these results with caution due to attrition in the intervention groups and changes in classroom student composition across the study period (changes common in Head Start classrooms).

We are encouraged by these preliminary results in that they provide some support for the effectiveness of both intervention components. First, it appears that the easier to implement universal component (i.e., group instruction by classroom teachers during already scheduled "circle time"; visual and verbal prompts; and simple contingency management procedures) was enough to result in significant social behavior improvements for most Head Start students. Second, though more difficult to interpret because of the degree of within group variability, it appears that the addition of the more difficult and costly intensive component (i.e., trained therapists providing separate instruction and coaching) was somewhat effective in improving the social behavior of the lower functioning children to the degree that they were indistinguishable from their peers (who were also improving due to intervention). Our results also suggest, however, that such intensive intervention is not enough to ensure more durable gains that are noticeable to caregivers. In a future investigation, whether following the intensive component with the continued implementation of the universal component would facilitate greater maintenance should be explored. Further, given the results of this study, it is worth speculating as to whether the Carpenter (2002) intervention also resulted in improvements in targeted skills that failed to impact the peer and teacher ratings.

## Summary, Conclusions, and Future Directions

In this chapter, we have described many of the challenges faced in attempting to transport evidence based intervention procedures into an applied setting. Among the obstacles we encountered were limited resources (i.e., money, time, and personnel), competing demands on teacher time and student schedules, variability across sites (e.g., class size, student composition, classroom environment, and teacher experience), methodological difficulties (e.g., conducting behavioral observations, attrition and continual changes in student composition impacting assessment and intervention), and the acceptability of intervention procedures to teachers and parents. Of course, such challenges are not unique to our efforts. In fact, the degree to which the available *efficacy* (i.e., the potency of an intervention delivered in ideal, well controlled conditions) findings translate into actual *effectiveness* (i.e., the potency of an intervention delivered in less controlled, real world conditions) has become a central question in the current treatment literature (e.g., Chorpita, 2003).

We offer the following conclusions for consideration. First, at the most basic level, our adherence to the laboratory approach led us to follow up on our clinical observations with a more objective analysis of the mental health referral flow, a format that facilitated collaboration with the coordinating community agency. Second, the use of standardized assessment measures (e.g., teacher ratings, behavioral observations) allowed us to monitor the effects (or absence of) of the implemented intervention procedures and make needed modifications along the way. Pointing to the need for data-based assessments in every day practice, our control group (study one) and baseline (study two) assessments failed to show any systematic social skills related improvements amongst the students as a result of already-in-place Head Start interventions. Third, one such measure, behavioral observation, appears to be necessary for adequate intervention evaluation, but is rather costly to implement in terms of time and personnel. Fourth, interventions capable of producing behavior change may not necessarily result in improved peer status or teacher perceptions. To do so may require increasing the "dose" of intervention in terms of amount and/or duration and both of these options are costly. For instance, we were able to use teachers to deliver the universal intervention component during already scheduled activities, but the delivery of the intensive component required added personnel and the separation of some students from the classroom.

**Table 1. Preliminary Pre/Post Outcomes for the COMPASS Program.**

| Measures | Mean Pre-treatment Scores | Mean Post-treatment Scores | Significance Level |
|---|---|---|---|
| Social Skills Rating Scale, Parent Form: Social Skills Subscale | 78 | 90 | *$p$<.01 |
| Social Skills Rating Scale, Parent Form: Problem Behaviors Subscale | 123 | 112 | **$p$<.01 |
| Quality of Play Questionnaire: Conflict Score | 6.8 | 2 | ***$p$<.01 |

Note. Preliminary sample size of 23 participants.
*t(22)=-3.97, p<.01
**t(22)=3.07, p<.01
***t(18)=4.07, p<.01

As far as directions for future research, we, of course, first need to more fully analyze the data from our second effectiveness study. As noted, higher than expected degrees of within child variability is likely to impact our ability to detect reliable changes as a function of the different intervention components. Given the apparent effectiveness of the easier to implement universal component, we need to determine whether the intensive component led to added improvement. Regardless of these findings, however, it is clear that even the combination of these components was not sufficient to ensure durable behavioral improvement that impacted teacher perception. Perhaps we could determine whether extending the universal component after the termination of the intensive component helps with maintenance and generalization. Another option might be to "boost the dose of instruction" in other ways (e.g., lengthen the course of intervention, include more instruction modules).

Closing on an optimistic note, we provide an update on the efforts of the second author (EMC) to adapt the COMPASS curriculum to an outpatient setting at the UCLA Neuropsychiatric Institute. In collaboration with Fred Frankel and incorporating some of the elements of his successful parent-assisted friendship intervention program for elementary-aged children (Frankel & Myatt, 2003), she developed a revised COMPASS curriculum targeting a wide range of children aged 4 to 6 with social-skills deficits. Similar to the original curriculum, children are taught how to share, take turns, obey game rules, join in with fun ideas and questions, talk nicely, and to listen. In a new component, parents learn how to manage child behavior on play dates, as well as other techniques for facilitating their children's friendships, such as how to network with other parents, supervise play dates, and coach their child in outdoor games. Two group leaders deliver the training in 12 one-hour sessions that are attended by both children and parents. Preliminary outcome data is very promising. Thus far, pre/post comparisons for the 23 outpatient children (40% with a primary diagnosis of Autism Spectrum Disorder, 36% Attention-Deficit/Hyperactivity Disorder) completing the COMPASS program show significant improvements on parent ratings of social skills and related behavior problems (Social Skills Rating Scale, Parent Form; see Table 1). In addition, the ntervention has also resulted in significant decreases in conflict during scheduled play dates (Quality of Play Questionnaire; see Table 1). Notably, the parent-rated improvements in social skills are also clinically significant, moving the typical child into the normative range on the standardized measure.

## REFERENCES


Altmann, J. (1974). Observational study of behavior: Sampling methods. *Behaviour, 49,* 227-267

Asher, S. R., & Parker, J. G. (1989). The significance of peer relationship problems in childhood. In B. H. Schenider, G. Attili, J. Nadel, & R. P. Weissberg (Eds.), *Social competence in developmental perspective* (pp. 5-23). Amsterdam: Kluwer Academic Publishing.

Barkley, R. A., Shelton, T. L., Crosswait, C., Moorehouse, M., Fletcher, K., Barrett, S., Jenkins, L., & Metevia, L. (2000). Multi-method psycho-educational intervention for preschool children with disruptive behavior: Preliminary results at post-treatment. *Journal of Child Psychology and Psychiatry, 41*, 319-332.

Bierman, K. L. (2004). *Peer rejection: Developmental processes and intervention strategies.* New York: The Guilford Press.

Bierman, K. L., Miller, C. L., & Stabb, S. D. (1987). Improving the social behavior and peer acceptance of rejected boys: Effects of social skill training with instructions and prohibitions. *Journal of Consulting and Clinical Psychology, 55*, 194-200.

Bierman, K. L., & Montminy, H. P. (1993). Developmental issues in social-skills assessment and intervention with children and adolescents. *Behavior Modification, 17*, 229-254.

Carpenter, E.M. (2002). A curriculum-based approach for social-cognitive skills training: An intervention targeting aggression in Head Start preschoolers. *Dissertation Abstracts International: Section B: The Sciences and Engineering, 63*, 3001.

Carpenter, E.M., & Nangle, D.W. (1999). *Mental health referrals in Maine Head Start preschoolers.* Unpublished technical report, Psychological Services Center, University of Maine, Orono.

Carpenter, E. M., & Nangle, D. W. (2002). Effects of brief verbal instructions on aggression: A replication in a Head Start setting. *Child and Family Behavior Therapy, 24,* 21-38.

Cartledge, G., & Kleefield, J. (1990). *Taking Part Curriculum.* Circle Pines, MN: American Guidance Service.

Chandler, L. K., Lubeck, R. C., & Fowler, S. A. (1992). Generalization and maintenance of preschool children's social skills: A critical review and analysis. *Journal of Applied Behavior Analysis, 25,* 415-428.

Chorpita, B.F. (2003). The frontier of evidence-based practice. In A.E. Kazdin & J.R. Weisz (Eds.), *Evidence-based psychotherapies for children and adolescents* (pp. 42-59). New York, NY: Guilford Press.

Eisenberg, N., Guthrie, I. K., Murphy, B. C., Shepard, S. A., Cumberland, A., & Carlo, G. (1999). Consistency and development of prosocial dispositions: A longitudinal study. *Child Development, 70*, 1360-1372.

Elliott, S. N., & Gresham, F. M. (1993). Social skills interventions for children. *Behavior Modification, 17*, 287-313.

Factor, D. C., & Schilmoeller, G. L. (1983). Social skill training of preschool children. *Child Study Journal, 13*, 41-56.

Fox, J. J., & McEvoy, M. A. (1993). Assessing and enhancing generalization and social validity of social-skills interventions with children and adolescents. *Behavior Modification, 17*, 339-366.

Frankel, F. & Myatt, R. (2003). *Children's friendship training.* New York: Brunner-Routledge.

Gresham, F.M. & Elliott, S.N. (1990). *Social Skills Rating System: Manual.* Circle Pines, MN: American Guidance Service.

Guglielmo, H. M., & Tryon, G. S. (2001). Social skill training in an integrated preschool program. *School Psychology Quarterly, 16*, 158-175.

Kelly, J. A. (1980). The simultaneous replication design: The use of a multiple baseline to establish experimental control in single group social skills treatment studies. *Journal of Behavior Therapy and Experimental Psychiatry, 11*, 203-207.

Kupersmidt, J. B., Coie, J. D., & Dodge, K. A. (1990). The role of poor peer relationships in the development of disorder. In S. R. Asher & J. D. Coie (Eds.), *Peer rejection in childhood* (pp. 274-308). New York: Cambridge University Press.

Ladd, G. W., & Mize, J. (1983a). A cognitive-social learning model of social skill training. *Psychological Review, 90*, 127-157.

Ladd, G.W., & Mize, J. (1983b). Social skills training and assessment with children: A cognitive-social learning approach. *Child and Youth Services, 5*, 61-74.

Lee, V. E., Brooks-Gunn, J., Schnur, E., & Liaw, F. (1990). Are Head Start effects sustained? A longitudinal follow-up comparison of disadvantaged children attending Head Start, no preschool, and other preschool programs. *Child Development, 61*, 495-507.

Locurto, C. (1991). Beyond IQ in preschool programs? *Intelligence, 15*, 295-312.

Lumpkin, P. W., Silverman, W. K., Weems, C. F., Markham, M. R., & Kurtines, W. M. (2002). Treating a heterogeneous set of anxiety disorders in youths with group cognitive behavioral therapy: A partially nonconcurrent multiple-baseline evaluation. *Behavior Therapy, 33*, 163-177.

McConnell, S. R., Sisson, L. A., Cort, C. A., & Strain, P. S. (1991). Effects of social skills training and contingency management on reciprocal interaction of preschool children with behavioral handicaps. *Journal of Special Education, 24*, 473-495.

McFadyen-Ketchum, S. A., & Dodge, K. A. (1998). Problems in social relationships. In E. J. Mash & R. A. Barkley (Eds.), *Treatment of childhood disorders* (2nd ed., pp. 338-365). New York: Guilford Press.

McKinney, E. P., & Rust, J. O. (1998). Enhancing preschool African American children's social skills. *Journal of Instructional Psychology, 25*, 235-241.

Mize, J., & Ladd. G. W. (1990). A cognitive-social learning approach to social skills training with low-status preschool children. *Developmental Psychology, 26*, 388-397.

Nangle, D. W., Erdley, C. A., Carpenter, E. M., & Newman, J. E. (2002). Social skills training as a treatment for aggressive children and adolescents: A developmental-clinical integration. *Aggression and Violent Behavior, 7*, 169-199.

Oden, S. L., & Asher, S. R. (1977). Coaching children in social skills for friendship making. *Child Development, 48*, 495-506.

Parker, J. G., & Asher, S. R. (1987). Peer relations and later personal adjustment: Are low-accepted children at risk? *Psychological Bulletin, 102*, 357-389.

Parker, J. G., Rubin, K. H., Price, J. M., & DeRosier, M. E. (1995). Peer relationships, child development, and adjustment: A developmental psychopathology perspective. In D. J. Cohen & D. Cicchetti (Eds), *Developmental psychopathology: Vol 2. Risk, disorder, and adaptation* (pp 96-161). Oxford: John Wiley & Sons.

Price, J. M., & Ladd, G. W. (1986). Assessment of children's friendships: Implications for social competence and social adjustment. In R. J. Prinz (Ed.), *Advances in behavioral assessment of children and families* (Vol. 2, pp. 121-149). Greenwich, CT: JAI Press.

Raudenbush, S. W., & Bryk, A. S. (2002). *Hierarchical linear models: Applications and data analysis methods*. Thousand Oaks, CA: Sage Publications.

Ravler, C.C. & Zigler, E.F. (1997). Social competence: An untapped dimension in evaluating Head Start's success. *Early Childhood Research Quarterly, 12*, 363-385.

Rickel, A. U., Eshelman, A. K., & Loigman, G. A. (1983). Social problem solving training: A follow-up study of cognitive and behavioral effects. *Journal of Abnormal Child Psychology, 11*, 15-28.

Ripple, C. H., Gilliam, W. S., Chanana, N., & Zigler, E. (1999). Will fifty cooks spoil the broth? The debate over entrusting Head Start to the states. *American Psychologist, 54*, 327-343.

Schneider, B. H., & Byrne, B. M. (1987). Individualizing social skills training for behavior disordered children. *Journal of Consulting and Clinical Psychology, 55*, 444-445.

Sharp, K. C. (1981). Impact of interpersonal problem-solving training on preschoolers' social competency. *Journal of Applied Developmental Psychology, 2*, 129-143.

Shepherd, E. J. (2007). *Intervening to promote social skill usage in Head Start preschoolers: A single-group design evaluation of effectiveness*. Unpublished doctoral dissertation, University of Maine, Orono.

Shepherd, E. J., Nangle, D. W., Rivera, M. S., Erdley, C. A., & Hecker, J. E. (2003, November). *Parents as facilitators of their children's social development: Piloting a minimal therapist contact intervention in a Head Start setting*. Paper presented at the annual meeting of the Association for Advancement of Behavior Therapy, Boston, MA.

Shure, M. B., & Spivack, G. (1982). Interpersonal problem-solving in young children: A cognitive approach to prevention. *American Journal of Community Psychology, 10*, 341-356.

Spivack, G., & Shure, M.B. (1974). *Social adjustment of young children: A cognitive approach to solving real-life problems*. Oxford, England: Jossey-Bass.

Stokes, T. F., & Osnes, P. G. (1989). An operant pursuit of generalization. *Behavior Therapy, 20*, 337-355.

Tremblay, R. E., Masse, L. C., Pagani, L., & Vitaro, F. (1996). From childhood physical aggression to adolescent maladjustment: The Montreal prevention experiment. In R. D. Peters & R. J. McMahon (Eds.), *Preventing childhood disorders, substance abuse, and delinquency* (pp. 268-298). Thousand Oaks, CA: Sage.

Vaughn, S. R., Ridley, C. A., & Bullock, D. D. (1984). Interpersonal problem-solving skills training with aggressive young children. *Journal of Applied Developmental Psychology, 5*, 213-223.

Webster-Stratton, C. (1992). Individually administered videotape parent training: "Who benefits?" *Cognitive Therapy and Research, 16*, 31-52.

Webster-Stratton, C., & Hammond, M. (1997). Treating children with early-onset conduct problems: A comparison of child and parent training interventions. *Journal of Consulting and Clinical Psychology, 65*, 93-109.

Webster-Stratton, C., & Hammond, M. (1998). Conduct problems and level of social competence in Head Start children: Prevalence, pervasiveness, and associated risk factors. *Clinical Child and Family Psychology Review, 1*, 101-124.

Webster-Stratton, C., Reid, J., & Hammond, M. (2001). Preventing conduct problems, promoting social competence: A parent and teacher training partnership in Head Start. *Journal of Clinical Child Psychology, 30*, 283-302.

Zahavi, S., & Asher, S. R. (1978). The effect of verbal instructions on preschool children's aggressive behavior. *Journal of School Psychology, 16,* 146-153.

In: Toward a Science of Clinical Psychology
Editor: Luciano L'Abate, pp. 101-116
ISBN: 978-1-60456-062-6


*Chapter V*

# TEACHING SAFETY SKILLS TO CHILDREN: ISSUES IN TRAINING AND GENERALIZATION

***Raymond G. Miltenberger***[1]

## ABSTRACT

Children may encounter a variety of threats to personal safety in their interaction with the physical and social environment. These safety threats could result in injury or death if appropriate action is not taken by the child or responsible adults. One type of safety threat involves activities or situations that the child encounters on a frequent, even daily basis. In these situations the child has repeated opportunities to practice safe behavior. Examples include wearing a seatbelt when traveling in a car, wearing a helmet when riding a bike, or staying in the yard or on the sidewalk when in close proximity to a street. Another type of safety threat involves low incidence but potentially life threatening situations (e.g., Miltenberger & Gross, in press). Examples include an abduction attempt, finding an unattended firearm, or experiencing a home fire. Although most children will never encounter such safety threats, if faced with such a threat, the child has one opportunity to engage in safe behavior. Failure to do so may result in serious injury or death (e.g., Eber, Annest, Mercy, & Ryan, 2004).

It is the responsibility of parents and other adults to eliminate safety threats to the extent possible from the environment and/or to teach their children to engage in safe behavior at the appropriate time (Dowd, Sege, Smith, & Wright, 2004; Miltenberger & Gross, in press; Miltenberger & Himle, 2004). For frequently occurring safety threats that cannot be eliminated (e.g., riding in a car, riding a bike, being near or having to cross a street), parents must be sure their children learn to engage in safe behavior on a consistent basis. Children have repeated opportunities to wear seat belts or use car seats, to wear bike helmets, and to stop and look both ways before crossing a street. With appropriate training and contingencies

[1] FMHI, MHC 2113A, Tampa, FL 33612, (813) 974 5079, rmiltenberger@fmhi.usf.edu
Applied Behavior Analysis Masters Program, Department of Child and Family Studies, University of South Florida

from parents, children can learn to engage in such behaviors consistently. Parents also have the responsibility to eliminate or minimize children's exposure to low incidence safety threats. By keeping their children in sight in a public place, parents minimize the chance of abduction. By keeping guns stored safely (locked, unloaded, with a safety device), parents minimize the chance their children will find and be injured by a loaded weapon. By keeping a house free of combustibles and ignition sources parents minimize the chance of a house fire. In addition to their efforts to eliminate serious, low incidence safety threats however, parents also have a responsibility to teach their children safety skills that could prevent injury or death in the event that the safety threat should occur (e.g., Miltenberger & Himle, 2004).

The focus of this chapter is on teaching safety skills to children to respond to low incidence, life threatening situations. Following a review of important safety skills and methods for assessing those skills, the chapter focuses on evidenced-based practices for teaching safety skills and promoting the generalized use of the safety skills. Recent research on teaching safety skills to prevent firearm injuries is highlighted in the chapter. Before proceeding however, a caveat is in order. Even though this chapter is about teaching safety skills to children, the intent of the chapter is not to suggest that children are responsible for ensuring their own safety. First and foremost, it is always the parents' responsibility to remove important safety threats from the environment in an attempt to ensure their children's safety. Teaching safety skills to children should be seen as secondary to the parents' responsibility to remove safety threats from the environment. For example, teaching children abduction-prevention skills does not absolve parents of the responsibility for closely supervising their children in a public place. Likewise, teaching children skills to respond safely upon finding an unattended firearm does not absolve parents of the responsibility for storing their guns safely. Nevertheless, because safety threats will continue to occur in spite of parents' best efforts to keep their children's environments safe, it is important for children to learn safety skills and the appropriate situations in which to use these skills. Furthermore, it is important for parents to arrange the appropriate contingencies to promote the use of the skills.

## TYPES OF SAFETY SKILLS

Although the specific safety skills will vary depending on the nature of the safety threat, three safety skills are common to most threat situations. The first skill is to discriminate the presence of the safety threat. The second skill is to engage in behavior that functions to escape from the threat situation. The third is to inform a supervising adult (e. g., parent or teacher) about the threat so the threat can be removed (e. g., Himle, Miltenberger, Flessner, & Gatheridge, 2004; Johnson et al., 2005: 2006; Lumley, Miltenberger, Long, Rapp, & Roberts, 1998).

### Discriminate the Presence of the Threat

The child must discriminate the presence of the safety threat so that the remaining safety skills can be executed at the right time. Through training, a simulated safety threat becomes a discriminative stimulus in the presence of which the safety skills are executed and reinforced. As a result, the safety skills are more likely to occur in the future when a similar safety threat is present in the child's natural environment (Miltenberger, 2004). For example, a child must learn to engage in the appropriate safety skills when an abduction lure is provided by an adult to entice the child to leave; when finding a firearm either alone or with a peer; or when hearing a smoke detector. Learning to discriminate the presence of the safety threat is critical so that the child can immediately engage in behavior to escape from the threat. In most safety threat situations an immediate response is critical as the longer the child is exposed to the safety threat without taking action, the more likely the child will be harmed (Poche, Yoder, & Miltenberger, 1988).

In the case of abduction prevention skills training, children are taught to engage in the safety skills immediately (say "no", run away, and tell an adult) in response to four possible abduction lures from an adult. These include a simple lure in which the adult simply asks the child to leave; an incentive lure in which the adult offers the child something tangible to leave (e.g., a toy or candy); an assistance lure in which the adult asks the child for help (e.g., to help find a lost puppy); and an authority lure in which the adult tells the child that a parent said it was okay to leave with him (e.g., Miltenberger & Olson, 1996). When training is successful, the child will discriminate the presence of any of these lures and engage in the safety skills.

## Escape from the Threat Situation

Once the child discriminates the presence of the threat, the second essential skill is to escape from the situation. Escaping the situation means putting physical distance between the child and the threat, most often by running away. Once the child is no longer in the physical presence of the safety threat, the likelihood of harm is eliminated or greatly diminished. For example, when faced with an abduction lure or when finding a firearm the child escapes from the situation by running to a parent or supervising adult (e.g., teacher, babysitter). Once the child is away from the potential abductor, the child cannot be taken by force. Once the child is away from the firearm, the child cannot be harmed by the gun if it were to be handled and discharged by a peer. It is not enough for the child to say "no" or otherwise verbally refuse an abduction lure or to simply refuse to touch a found firearm. Getting away from the safety threat is critical for ensuring safety. By running to a parent or supervising adult, the child is then in a position to report the safety threat, the final safety skill.

Although immediately escaping from the situation is the most important response to the safety threat, researchers also teach the child to provide a verbal refusal prior to running away when the safety threat comes from another individual (e. g., an abduction lure). For example, in research on teaching sexual abuse prevention skills or abduction prevention skills, the child is taught to say "no" when presented with an abduction or sexual abuse lure and immediately run away and report the incident (Johnson et al., 2005; 2006; Lumley et al., 1998; Miltenberger et al., 1999).

## Report the Safety Threat

After the child gets away from the safety threat, the child is no longer at immediate risk, but the safety threat may continue to exist for other children or for the child at a later time.

Therefore, the third safety skill is to report the threat to a parent or other responsible adult who can then take the appropriate action to eliminate the threat. For example, the adult can remove the unattended firearm or call the police about the potential abductor.

The three safety skills described in this section have been evaluated in recent research on teaching abduction prevention skills to children and teaching skills to prevent firearm injury (Gatheridge et al., 2004; Gross, Miltenberger, Knudson, Bosch, & Brower-Breitwieser, in press; Himle, Miltenberger, Flessner, et al., 2004; Himle, Miltenberger, Gatheridge, & Flessner, 2004; Johnson et al., 2005; 2006; Miltenberger et al., 2004; 2005). However, the same three skills would have generality to any of a number of other safety threats as well. These may include for example:

- finding an unattended bottle of medicine or poison,
- finding an open gate to a swimming pool,
- finding a lighter or matches,
- being asked by an adult to engage in sexual activity or other inappropriate touch,
- being asked by an older child to consume alcohol or drugs, or
- being asked by another person to engage in any dangerous behavior.

Whether the safety threat comes from contact with a danger in the physical environment or from an action of another person, the child's safety is best assured by his or her ability to a) discriminate the presence of the threat, b) get away from the threat, and c) report the threat to a responsible adult.

## Assessment of Safety Skills

Assessment of safety skills appropriate for low incidence safety threats can be a challenge because the opportunity to engage in the behavior in a natural context is infrequent (or nonexistent for many children) and because, by their very nature, these safety threats occur when an adult is not present. To address these assessment challenges, researchers have devised three strategies for assessing safety skills; knowledge assessment, skills assessment, and in situ assessment (e.g., Carroll, Miltenberger, & O'Neill, 1992; Gatheridge et al., 2004; Himle, Miltenberger, Gatheridge, et al., 2004; Lumley et al., 1998; Roberts & Miltenberger, 1999). These strategies vary in terms of their ecological validity and ease of implementation.

### Knowledge Assessment

Assessing a child's knowledge of safety skills typically is conducted by describing a scenario involving a safety threat and asking the child how he/she would respond to the situation. For example, in assessing knowledge of abduction prevention skills, the trainer might ask, "What would you do if you were on the playground after school and a man walked up and asked you to come with him to help him look for his lost puppy?" (e.g., Olson-Woods, Miltenberger, & Foreman, 1998). For assessing safety skills related to firearm injury, the trainer would describe a scenario in which a child found a gun while alone and ask the child what he or she would do in that situation (Himle Miltenberger, Gatheridge, et al., 2004).

In assessing knowledge of safety skills, you are assessing the child's verbal repertoire, in particular the child's ability to verbalize the correct behaviors for the situation. Knowledge assessment is easy to conduct and has been the primary mode of assessment in a number of studies evaluating safety skills training programs (Carroll et al., 1992). However knowledge assessment may have limited validity as numerous research studies have shown poor correspondence between what children say they would do in a given situation and what they actually do in the situation (e.g., Caroll-Rowan & Miltenberger, 1994; Himle, Miltenberger, Gatheridge et al., 2004; Miltenberger & Thiesse-Duffy, 1988; Olson-Woods et al., 1998). Given the poor correspondence between saying and doing, it is important to assess actual safety skills as well as knowledge of safety skills.

## Skills Assessment

Safety skills assessment typically is conducted in the context of a role play simulating the safety threat. To conduct a skills assessment the trainer tells the child that he/she will act out a situation and ask the child to "show me what you would do in this situation?" (e.g., Gatheridge et al., 2004; Miltenberger & Olson, 1996). The trainer then creates the scenario and assesses the child's skills as the child responds to the simulated safety threat. To assess safety skills related to finding a gun, the trainer might say the following, "Pretend you walk into your parents' bedroom and see this gun sitting on the bed," as the trainer puts a realistic replica of a handgun (or a disabled handgun) on a table. "Pretend you are alone and your parents are in the next room. I'll pretend to be your parent." As the trainer walks toward the adjacent room the trainer says, "Now show me what you would do if you found this gun on your parents' bed."

By conducting a skills assessment, you are assessing the child's actual safety skills, not the child's verbal description of the behavior. An advantage of a skills assessment is that you can determine whether the skills are in the child's repertoire. A limitation of a skills assessment is that you are asking the child to exhibit the skills in your presence and, therefore, the behavior is under the stimulus control of your presence. You cannot assess whether the child would use the skills in a naturalistic threat situation when an adult is not present. Recent research has demonstrated that children may exhibit safety skills during a skills assessment in the presence of the trainer but then fail to use the skills during a naturalistic assessment in which they do know they are being assessed (Gatheridge et al., 2004; Himle, Miltenberger, Gatherideg et al., 2004; Kelso, Miltenberger, Waters, Egemo-Helm, & Bagne, in press).

## In Situ Assessment

The third and most ecologically valid assessment of safety skills is called in situ assessment (e. g., Himle, Miltenberger, Flessner, et al., 2004; Johnson et al., 2005; 2006). An in situ assessment measures the use of the skills when a simulated safety threat is presented in the natural environment while the child is unaware that an assessment is occurring. Because the child is not in the presence of an adult and is not aware an assessment is occurring, the child's behavior during an in situ assessment is not under the stimulus control of the trainer, another adult, or the training context. Rather, the child's use of the safety skills is under the stimulus control of the threat situation. Although a skills assessment measures the acquisition of the skills, an in situ assessment measures the generalized use of the skills. To determine whether the skills generalized to the natural environment where exposure to an actual safety threat would occur, an in situ assessment is necessary.

To conduct an in situ assessment, the parent (or teacher) arranges a situation where the child will be alone while exposed to the simulated safety threat. The child is not cued in any way to the safety threat during an in situ assessment. Therefore, from the child's perspective the safety threat is real. To assess abduction prevention skills, the child is left alone briefly (e.g., in the yard, on the playground) while the parent observes surreptitiously. Once the child is alone, a confederate approaches the child and presents the abduction lure. The confederate (and possibly another observer) records the child's response to the lure (e.g., Johnson et al., 2005; 2006). To assess a child's safety skills when finding a firearm, a replica of a firearm (or a disabled firearm) is placed in another room where the child would find it if the child entered the room. The child is then sent to the room for another purpose and the child's behavior upon finding the gun is recorded by a hidden video camera. For example, a parent might place the gun on a kitchen counter near a snack, turn on a video camera placed out of sight on a shelf, and then send the child to the kitchen for the snack (e.g., Himle, Miltenberger, Flessner, et al., 2004; Miltenberger et al., 2004; 2005). It is important to note that the firearm used in an assessment must be a replica, or be disabled if it is a real gun. A working gun should never be used in an assessment or in a training session as a mistake could be made (failure to unload it completely) that might result in unintentional injury.

Whether using knowledge assessment, skills assessment, or in situ assessment, the safety skills exhibited by the child are scored numerically. For example, Johnson et al. (2005) used a 0 to 4 point scale to measure abduction prevention skills as follows:

0 = agreed to leave when presented with an abduction lure
1 = did not agree to leave but did not engage in any other safety skills
2 = said "no," but failed to run away or tell an adult
3 = said "no,", and ran away but did not tell
4 = said "no," ran away, and told an adult.

Himle, Miltenberger, Gatheridge, et al. (2004) used a 0 to 3 point scale to assess safety skills when a child found a firearm:

0 = touched the gun
1 = did not touch the gun but stayed near
2 = did not touch the gun and immediately left the room
3 = did not touch the gun, immediately left the room, and told an adult

## TRAINING STRATEGIES

Research on teaching safety skills to children illustrates two basic approaches to instruction; an informational approach and an active learning approach.

### Informational Approach

In an informational approach to teaching safety skills, information about safety threats and safety skills is presented in a number of ways such as lectures, movies, animation, readings, coloring books, skits, or plays (Carroll et al., 1992). The children watch and listen to the information and sometimes respond verbally, but do not engage in overt practice or rehearsal of the safety skills. The Eddie Eagle GunSafe Program is an example of an informational program to teach safety skills to prevent gun play (Gatheridge et al., 2004; Himle, Miltenberger, Gatheridge et al., 2004). In the Eddie Eagle program, small groups of children (4 to 7 year olds) participate in five 10 minute training sessions conducted daily over five days. In this program, the children receive instructions from a trainer, color in coloring books, watch a video, and look at a poster to learn the Eddie Eagle message (Stop, Don't Touch, Get Away, Tell an Adult). The children also respond verbally with the Eddie Eagle message when the trainer describes scenarios in which children find a gun. Although the children rehearse the safety message, they do not engage in any actual rehearsal or practice of the safety skills in role plays simulating a situation in which they find a gun.

An informational approach can be an efficient method of training as the materials can be made available on video, in books or manuals, and on the internet so that they are easily accessible. In addition, the use of such materials may not require the time and cost of a trainer. With the Eddie Eagle program for example, the materials can be purchased online along with an Instructor's Guide that provides directions for using the materials to teach safety skills (The National Rifle Association, 2007). However, there is very little research evaluating informational approaches to teaching safety skills, and the research that has been done is not promising (e.g., Hardy, 2002; Hardy, Armstrong, Martin, & Strawn, 1996; Miltenberger & Thiesse-Duffy, 1988; Poche et al., 1988; Wurtele, Saslawsky, Miller, Marrs, & Britcher, 1986).

In recent years, researchers have evaluated the effectiveness of the Eddie Eagle GunSafe program for teaching safety skills to prevent gun play to children ages 4-7 years old (Gatheridge et al., 2004; Himle Miltenberger, Gatheridge, et al., 2004). These researchers used knowledge assessments, skills assessments, and in situ assessments to measure the effects of the Eddie Eagle program. The results showed that, following training, most children could describe the safety skills, but few could demonstrate the skills in role play or in situ assessments. In other words, the Eddie Eagle program taught children to recite the safety message but did not teach children the safety skills or promote the generalized use of the skills. It was noteworthy that most children could say what to do when finding a gun (don't touch it, run away, tell an adult) but most could not actually execute the behavior they had just described when asked to "show me what to do" in a role play.

The provision of information on safety threats and safety skills through instructions or modeling can occur in person or through various media (e.g., workbooks, video). However, research has yet to substantiate the effectiveness of such an approach to training safety skills. Rather, researchers have shown that an active learning approach is superior to an informational approach for teaching various safety skills to children including firearm injury prevention (Gatheridge et al., 2004; Himle, Miltenberger, Gatheridge et al., 2004), abduction prevention (Poche et al., 1988), and sexual abuse prevention (Miltenberger & Thiesse-Duffy, 1988; Wurtele et al. 1986).

## Active Learning Approach

In an active learning approach children not only receive instructions and modeling, but also have repeated opportunities to rehearse the safety skills with praise and corrective feedback in role plays simulating the safety threat. An active learning approach to teaching safety skills typically is referred to as behavioral skills training (e.g., Himle & Miltenberger, 2004). Behavioral skills training (BST), consisting of the combination of instructions, modeling, rehearsal, and feedback, has been shown to be effective in teaching a variety of safety skills including pedestrian safety skills (e. g., Yeaton & Bailey, 1978), fire safety skills (e. g., Jones, Kazdin, & Haney, 1981; Jones, Ollendick, McLaughlin, & Williams, 1989), sexual abuse prevention skills (e. g., Lumley et al., 1998; Miltenberger et al., 1999; Miltenberger & Thiesse-Duffy, 1988; Miltenberger, Thiesse-Duffy, Suda, Kozak, & Bruellman, 1990; Stillwell, Lutzker, & Green, 1988), abduction prevention skills (e. g., Johnson et al., 2005; 2006; Marchand-Martella, Huber, Martella, & Wood, 1996; Miltenberger & Olson, 1996; Poche, Brower, & Swearingen, 1981; Poche et al., 1988), and firearm injury prevention skills (e. g., Himle, Miltenberger, Flessner, et al., 2004; Miltenberger et al., 2004; 2005). Recent research evaluating BST for teaching skills to prevent gun play illustrates the application of BST and procedures for enhancing generalization following the use of BST.

*BST to prevent gun play*. In spite of efforts to promote safe storage practices by gun owning parents, loaded firearms continue to be accessible to children (Azrael, Miller, & Hemmenway, 2000; Grossman, Reay, & Baker, 1999). Compounding this problem, research by Hardy (2002), Hardy et al. (1996), and Jackman, Kellerman, Farah, and Simon (2001) shows that when children find firearms, they are likely to play with them. Sadly, playing with firearms found in the home resulted in a yearly average of 143 deaths and 1222 injuries to children in the years 1993 to 2001 (Eber et al., 2004). Clearly, children need to learn the skills to prevent gun play in order to prevent firearm injury and death. Fortunately, BST has been evaluated in a number of studies for teaching safety skills to prevent gun play.

The first study to evaluate BST for teaching safety skills to prevent gun play compared BST with the Eddie Eagle GunSafe Program implemented in a small group format with 4 to 5 year old children (Himle, Miltenberger, Gatheridge, et al., 2004). Children in the Eddie Eagle group were trained in five 15-min sessions in a manner consistent with the Instructors Guide provided with the Eddie Eagle training materials. Children in the BST program received instructions and modeling and then rehearsed the skills across a variety of scenarios in which they found a gun in each of the five, 15-min sessions. Following each rehearsal, the children received praise and correction as necessary. The researchers used a real (but disabled) gun in training and created simulations in which the child found a gun in different situations in the home to promote generalization. The results showed that following training, children in the Eddie Eagle and BST groups could describe the safety skills, but that only children trained with BST could demonstrate the safety skills in a role play assessment. Unfortunately, although BST produced acquisition of the skills, most of the BST children failed to use the skills during an in situ assessment. Because the skills failed to generalize following BST, subsequent research evaluated strategies for promoting generalization.

In an attempt to promote the generalized use of the safety skills researchers evaluated individual BST with booster sessions as needed with 4 and 5 year olds (Himle, Miltenberger, Flessner, et al., 2004) and 6 and 7 year olds (Miltenberger et al., 2004). Children were trained individually in two, 30-min BST sessions. In each session, the child rehearsed the safety skills with praise and feedback until exhibiting the skills correctly 5 times in a row upon finding a gun in a variety of scenarios. Children then were assessed (with in situ assessments) and were given up to 3 booster sessions if not performing correctly. Booster sessions included instructions, modeling, rehearsal, and feedback similar to the initial training sessions. In situ training was implemented if the child still did not perform correctly during the assessment that followed the third booster session. During in situ training, the trainer entered the assessment situation, caught the child failing to exhibit the safety skills correctly, and provided a short training session in which the child was required to rehearse the safety skills correctly five consecutive times.

The results showed that three of the eight 4 and 5 year olds demonstrated the skills following BST, but that five needed in situ training before they demonstrated the skills consistently during in situ assessments (Himle, Miltenberger, Flessner, et al., 2004). Similarly three of the six 6 and 7 year olds demonstrated the skills following BST while the other three needed in situ training before demonstrating the skills (Miltenberger et al. 2004). In both studies, the children continued to exhibit the safety skills when assessed from 2 weeks to 5 months following training. The results from these studies suggest that 4 to 7 year old children can learn the safety skills and use them during in situ assessments following individual BST and in situ training.

In a replication of Himle, Miltenberger, Gatheridge, et al. (2004) comparing BST and Eddie Eagle with 4 and 5 year olds, Gatheridge et al. (2004) compared BST and Eddie Eagle implemented in a small group format with 6 and 7 year olds. Gatheridge et al. (2004) found that children trained with Eddie Eagle performed well on the knowledge assessment, but that most failed to exhibit the skills during the skills assessment or the in situ assessment. However, children trained with BST performed well during the knowledge assessment and the skills assessment. In addition, most of the 6 and 7 year olds trained with BST exhibited the safety skills during the in situ assessment as well. For the BST and Eddie Eagle children who did not exhibit the safety skills following training, one in situ training session was implemented. Following in situ training, all the BST children exhibited the skills and the majority of Eddie Eagle children also exhibited the skills.

## In situ training

The results of Himle, Miltenberger, Flessner et al. (2004), Miltenberger et al. (2004), and Gatheridge et al. (2004) demonstrated the importance of in situ training for teaching safety skills to children. Although BST was effective for some children, in situ training resulted in successful performance for all children who did not perform the safety skills following BST. In each of these studies evaluating in situ training, the procedure was implemented following the failure of BST to promote the generalized use of the safety skills. To determine whether BST would be more effective if in situ training were implemented as part of BST and to determine whether training could be streamlined, Miltenberger et al. (2005) evaluated in situ training incorporated into the BST procedure.

In this study, ten 4 and 5 year olds received two 30-min BST sessions followed by an in situ assessment and in situ training session 30 min after the second session. If the child did not exhibit the safety skills during the assessment, a trainer entered the assessment situation, caught the child in the presence of the gun, and had the child rehearse the skills five times. If the child engaged in the safety skills correctly and reported the gun during the in situ assessment, the child received substantial praise. Further in situ training sessions were conducted if needed until the children used the safety skills in subsequent assessments. Miltenberger et al. (2005) found that all ten children learned the skills in just a few training sessions and that the skills generalized and maintained over a three-month follow-up. Furthermore, five of the participants participated in a dyad assessment in which they found the gun while with a peer, and all five engaged in the safety skills successfully. These results suggest that the inclusion of in situ training may make BST more effective and efficient. Similar results have been found evaluating in situ training for teaching abduction prevention skills to young children (Johnson et al., 2005) and for teaching sexual abuse prevention skills to women with mental retardation (Egemo-Helm et al., 2007).

## Increasing Training Efficiency

Although the studies by Miltenberger et al. (2005) and Johnson et al. (2005) showed that BST could be more effective and efficient when in situ training is incorporated into the procedure, trained staff are required to carry out the training procedures, thus limiting the efficiency and possible widespread adoption of the training approach. Two potential solutions to this challenge would be the development of a training package that could be carried out effectively by parents and the demonstration that peers could be effective trainers of safety skills (Jostad & Miltenberger, 2004).

In a recent study, Jostad, Miltenberger, Kelso, and Knudson (in press) evaluated the effectiveness of peer training for teaching safety skills to prevent gun play. The researchers used BST to train four 6 and 7 year olds how to conduct BST to teach safety skills to six 4 and 5 year olds. Once they were trained by the researchers, the 6 and 7 year olds conducted BST sessions without any assistance from the researchers. The 6 and 7 year olds also conducted in situ training when needed. The results showed that all of the 4 and 5 year olds exhibited the safety skills during in situ assessments following training by their peers. Similar to the results of Himle, Miltenberger, Flessner, et al. (2004) and Miltenberger et al. (2004), half of the children engaged in the safety skills following BST and half needed in situ training before engaging in the safety skills during in situ assessments. The results of Jostad et al. (in press) also showed that the children continued to engage in the safety skills when assessed many months after training.

In another recent investigation, Gross et al. (in press) developed and evaluated training materials for parents to use to teach safety skills to their own children. In this study, four parents of 4 to 7 year old children received a training manual with step by step instructions how to conduct BST and in situ training sessions with their child and a video showing two initial BST sessions and in situ training sessions. The parents read the manual and watched the video and then, without any input or training from the researchers, conducted two BST sessions with their child on consecutive days. Within 30 min following the second session, they conducted an in situ training session as well. The results showed that three of the four children trained by their parents used the safety skills during three consecutive in situ assessments conducted in their home and in a day care setting. The one child who did not exhibit the skills engaged in noncompliant behavior during the training sessions conducted by her father. Video recording of the training sessions showed that her father was unable to complete all of the training components due to her noncompliance.

The results of studies by Jostad et al. (in press) and Gross et al. (in press) provide preliminary evidence that peer training and parent training of safety skills to prevent gun play may be successful. If further research substantiates these findings, these strategies may be viable ways to increase training efficiency and make training accessible to more children. If peer training were shown to be successful in further research, researchers could train a number of peer trainers who could then provide training for many children. Likewise, if the effectiveness of the training package for parents is substantiated in further research, the materials could be made widely available for parents, making training accessible to many children.

## Promoting Generalization

The issue of generalization is critical to child safety skills training. Generalization refers to the use of the skills by the child in an actual safety threat situation. Skill acquisition without the generalized use of the skills does not benefit the child. The child must use the skills in a real safety threat situation for safety skills training to be deemed successful. Considering the importance of generalization, any study evaluating procedures for teaching safety skills must assess generalization of the skills. In situ assessment is the only strategy that can adequately assess generalization because it simulates the threat situation in a manner that makes it indistinguishable from an actual threat situation.

Research in safety skills training shows that BST and in situ training are the most effective strategies for promoting generalization of safety skills. Although the use of BST has resulted in generalization of safety skills for some children, the use of in situ training has been required for others (Himle, Miltenberger, Flessner, et al., 2004; Miltenberger et al., 2004). Unfortunately, it is not possible to determine in advance whether in situ training will be necessary for promoting generalization for any particular child. For this reason, in situ assessment must be conducted following training to determine whether further in situ training is necessary and how many sessions are necessary. In some cases, one in situ training session was effective and in other cases up to three in situ training sessions were necessary before a child used the safety skills (Himle, Miltenberger, Flessner, et al., 2004; Jostad et al., in press; Miltenberger et al., 2004; 2005).

Although it is not clear why BST produces generalized responding for some children and not others, BST does incorporate two known generalization strategies (e.g., Stokes & Baer, 1977). First, during BST, the trainer uses multiple exemplars when having the child role play the safety skills in response to a variety of different scenarios. For example, a child will practice responding to a variety of abduction lures or practice the safety skills when finding a firearm in a variety of different locations. Second, common stimuli often are used during training. A variety of disabled firearms or replicas of firearms is used when training skills to prevent gun play (Himle, Miltenberger, Flessner, et al., 2004; Miltenberger et al., 2004; 2005). Likewise, abduction prevention training sometimes occurs in locations where an actual abduction attempt might occur, such as outside the school or on the playground (e. g., Poche et al., 1981).

In situ training incorporates still other strategies to promote generalization. When the child is caught near the gun failing to engage in the safety skills in the natural environment, contingencies are delivered for the behavior in that environment. If getting caught near the gun or getting caught touching the gun is an aversive event (because the child receives a disapproving statement or expression of disapproval from the researcher), the child is less likely to approach or touch a found gun in the future as a result of a positive punishment process (Miltenberger et al., 2005). In addition, running away and telling when finding a gun in the future would be negatively reinforced by avoiding the aversive event (getting caught again) (Miltenberger et al., 2005). In addition, having to rehearse the safety skills five times during in situ training may serve two functions as well; positive punishment for approaching or touching the gun and negative reinforcement as the future use of the safety skills functions to avoid such rehearsal in the future.

## SUMMARY

A number of conclusions can be drawn from the research on teaching safety skills to children.

1. A behavioral skills training approach, in which the child receives instructions and modeling and then rehearses the skills with feedback in response to a variety of simulated situations, is more effective than an informational approach that does not have the active learning component (e. g., Gatheridge et al., 2004; Himle, Miltenberger, Gatheridge, et al., 2004; Miltenberger & Thiesse-Duffy, 1988; Poche et al., 1988; Wurtele et al., 1986).
2. Although BST consistently results in skill acquisition, the skills do not always generalize to the natural environment when in situ assessments are conducted (e. g., Himle, Miltenberger, Flessner et al., 2004; Miltenberger et al., 2004).
3. In situ training is the most reliable method for producing the generalized use of safety skills across a number of skill domains (e. g., Egemo-Helm et al., 2007; Johnson et al., 2005; 2006; Miltenberger et al., 1999; 2004; 2005).
4. The efficiency of BST and in situ training can be increased when training is delivered by peers (Jostad et al., in press) or by parents in the home (Gross et al., in press).

5. In situ assessment is the only way to conduct a valid assessment of the generalized use of the skills in response to a seemingly real safety threat following safety skills training (e. g., Gatheridge et al., 2004; Himle, Miltenberger, Gatheridge et al., 2004; Poche et al., 1981).

Future research in the area of safety skills training should proceed in a number of ways. First, research should seek to replicate the effects of peer training with a variety of safety skills. Second, research should continue to evaluate training materials that can be used by parents to teach their children safety skills in a variety of domains. Both of these areas of research could help make training more efficient. Third, research should evaluate ways to use technology (e. g., interactive video or computer simulations) to increase the effectiveness and efficiency of training. Finally, research should seek to better understand the child or family factors that might help predict the success of training procedures. By making safety skills training as effective, efficient, and accessible as possible, more children will benefit from training with the eventual reduction of accidental childhood injuries and deaths.

## REFERENCES

Azrael, D., Miller, M., & Hemenway, D. (2000). Are household firearms stored safely? It depends whom you ask. *Pediatrics, 106*, e31-e36.

Carroll-Rowan, L., & Miltenberger, R. (1994). A comparison of procedures for teaching abduction prevention to preschoolers. *Education & Treatment of Children*, 17, 113-128.

Carroll, L., Miltenberger, R., & O'Neill, K. (1992). A review and critique of research evaluating child sexual abuse prevention programs. *Education & Treatment of Children*, 15, 335-354.

Dowd, M. D., Sege, R., Smith, G. A., & Wright, H. (2004). Firearm injury prevention; failure of gun safety education (letter). *Pediatrics*, 113, 1847.

Eber, G. B., Annest, J. L., Mercy, J. A., & Ryan, G. W. (2004). Nonfatal and fatal firearm-related injuries among children aged 14 years and younger: United States, 1993-2000. *Pediatrics, 113(6),* 1686-1692.

Egemo-Helm, K.R., Miltenberger, R. G., Knudson, P., Finstrom, N., Jostad, C., & Johnson, B. (2007). An evaluation of in situ training to teach sexual abuse prevention skills to women with mental retardation. *Behavioral Interventions, 22*, 99-119.

Gatheridge, B. J., Miltenberger, R. G., Huneke, D. F., Satterlund, M. J., Mattern, A. R., Johnson, B. M., & Flessner, C. A. (2004). Comparison of two programs to teach firearm injury prevention skills to 6- and 7- year-old children. *Pediatrics, 114(3),* 294-299.

Grossman, D. C., Reay, D. T., & Baker, S. A. (1999). Self-inflicted and unintentional firearm injuries among children and adolescents; the source of the firearm. *Archives of Pediatrics & Adolescent Medicine, 153 (8),* 875-882.

Hardy, M. S. (2002). Teaching firearm safety to children: failure of a program. *Developmental and Behavioral Pediatrics, 23(2),* 71-76.

Hardy, M. S., Armstrong, F. D., Martin, B. L., & Strawn, K. N. (1996). A firearm safety program for children: they just can't say no. *Developmental and Behavioral Pediatrics, 17(4),* 216-221.

Himle, M., & Miltenberger, R. (2004). Preventing unintentional firearm injury in children: The need for behavioral skills training. *Education & Treatment of Children, 27,* 161-177

Himle, M. B., Miltenberger, R. G., Flessner, C., & Gatheridge, B. (2004). Teaching safety skills to children to prevent gun play. *Journal of Applied Behavior Analysis, 37,* 1-9.

Himle, M. B., Miltenberger, R. G., Gatheridge, B., & Flessner, C. (2004). An evaluation of two procedures for training skills to prevent gun play in children. *Pediatrics, 113(1),* 70-77.

Gross, A., Miltenberger, R., Knudson, P., Bosch, A., & Brower-Breitwieser, C. (in press). Preliminary evaluation of a parent training program to prevent gun play. *Journal of Applied Behavior Analysis.*

Jackman, G. A., Simon, H. K., Farah, M. M., & Kellerman, A. L. (2001). Seeing is believing: what do boys do when they find a real gun? *Pediatrics, 107(6),* 1247-1250.

Johnson, B. M., Miltenberger, R. G., Egemo-Helm, K., Jostad, C. J., Flessner, C., & Gatheridge, B. (2005). Evaluation of behavioral skills training for teaching abduction-prevention skills to young children. *Journal of Applied Behavior Analysis, 38,* 67-78.

Johnson, B. M., Miltenberger, R. G., Knudson, P., Egemo-Helm, K, Kelso, P., Jostad, C. & Langley, L. (2006). A preliminary evaluation of two behavioral skills training procedures for teaching abduction prevention skills to school-age children. *Journal of Applied Behavior Analysis, 39*, 25-34.

Jones, R. T., Kazdin, A. E., & Haney, J. I. (1981). Social validation and training of emergency fire safety skills for potential injury prevention and life saving. *Journal of Applied Behavior Analysis, 14*, 249-260.

Jones, R. T., Ollendick, T. H., McLaughlin, K. J., & Williams, C. E. (1989). Elaborative and behavioral rehearsal in the acquisition of fire emergency skills and the reduction of fear of fire. *Behavior Therapy, 20,* 93-101.

Jostad, C. M., & Miltenberger, R. G. (2004). Firearm injury prevention skills: Increasing the efficiency of training with peer tutoring. *Child & Family Behavior Therapy, 26(3*), 21-35.

Jostad, C. M., Miltenberger, R. G., Kelso, P., & Knudson, P. (in press). Peer tutoring to prevent gun play: Acquisition, generalization, and maintenance of safety skills. *Journal of Applied Behavior Analysis.*

Kelso, P., Miltenberger, R., Waters, M., Egemo-Helm, K., & Bagne, A. (in press). Teaching skills to second and third grade children to prevent gun play: A comparison of procedures. *Education and Treatment of Children.*

Lumley, V. A., Miltenberger, R. G., Long, E. S., Rapp, J. T., & Roberts, J. A. (1998). Evaluation of a sexual abuse prevention program for adults with mental retardation. *Journal of Applied Behavior Analysis, 31,* 91-101.

Marchand-Martella, N., & Huber, G., Martella, R. C., & Wood, W. S. (1996). Assessing the long-term maintenance of abduction prevention skills by disadvantaged preschoolers. *Education & Treatment of Children, 19(1),* 55-58.

Miltenberger, R. G., (2004). *Behavior modification: Principles and procedures* (3rd ed.). Pacific Grove, CA: Wadsworth.

Miltenberger, R. G., Flessner, C., Gatheridge, B., Johnson, B., Satterlund, M., & Egemo, K. (2004). Evaluation of behavioral skills training procedures to prevent gun play in children. *Journal of Applied Behavior Analysis, 37,* 513-516.

Miltenberger, R. G., Gatheridge, B. J., Satterlund, M., Egemo-Helm, K. R., Johnson, B. M., Jostad, C., Kelso, P., & Flessner, C. A. (2005). Teaching safety skills to prevent gun play: an evaluation of in situ training. *Journal of Applied Behavior Analysis, 38,* 395-398.

Miltenberger, R. G., & Gross, A. (in press). Teaching safety skills to children. In W. Fisher, C. Piazza, & H. Roane (Eds.), *Handbook of applied behavior analysis.* New York: Guilford.

Miltenberger, R. G., & Himle, M. B. (2004). Firearm injury prevention: Failure of gun safety education. (letter). *Pediatrics*, 113, 1847-1848.

Miltenberger, R., & Olsen, L. (1996). Abduction prevention training: A review of findings and issues for future research. *Education & Treatment of Children*, 19, 69-82.

Miltenberger, R. G., Roberts, J. A., Ellingson, S., Galensky, T., Rapp, J. T., Long, E. S., & Lumley, V. A. (1999). Training and generalization of sexual abuse prevention skills for women with mental retardation. *Journal of Applied Behavior Analysis, 32,* 385-388.

Miltenberger, R., & Thiesse-Duffy, E. (1988). Evaluation of home-based programs for teaching personal safety skills to children. *Journal of Applied Behavior Analysis*, 21, 81-88.

Miltenberger, R. G., Thiesse-Duffy, E., Suda, K. T., Kozak, C., & Bruellman, J. (1990). Teaching prevention skills to children: the use of multiple measures to evaluate parent versus expert instruction. *Child & Family Behavior Therapy, 12(4),* 65-87.

Olsen-Woods, L. A., Miltenberger, R. G., & Forman, G. (1998). Effects of correspondence training in an abduction prevention training program. *Child & Family Behavior Therapy, 20(1),* 15-34.

Poche, C., Brouwer, R., & Swearingen, M. (1981). Teaching self-protection to young children. *Journal of Applied Behavior Analysis, 14,* 169-176.

Poche, C., Yoder, P., & Miltenberger, R. (1988). Teaching self-protection to children using television techniques. *Journal of Applied Behavior Analysis, 21,* 253-261.

Roberts, J., & Miltenberger, R. (1999). Emerging issues in the research on child sexual abuse prevention. *Education & Treatment of Children*, 22, 84-102.

Stillwell, S. L., Lutzker, J. R., & Greene, B. F. (1988). Evaluation of a sexual abuse prevention program for preschoolers. *Journal of Family Violence, 3*, 269-281.

Stokes T. F., & Baer, D. M. (1977). An implicit technology of generalization. *Journal of Applied Behavior Analysis, 10*, 349-367.

The National Rifle Association (2007). Eddie Eagle Program Materials. Retrieved June 11, 2007 from http://www.nrahq.org/safety/eddie/materials.asp.

Yeaton W. H., & Bailey, J. S. (1978). Teaching pedestrian safety skills to young children: an analysis and one-year follow up. *Journal of Applied Behavior Analysis, 11,* 315-329.

Wurtele, S.K., Saslawsky, D.A., Miller, C.L., Marrs, S.R., & Britcher, J.C. (1986). Teaching personal safety skills for potential prevention of sexual abuse: A comparison of treatments. *Journal of Consulting and Clinical Psychology*, 54, 688-692.

In: Toward a Science of Clinical Psychology
Editor: Luciano L'Abate, pp. 117-131
ISBN: 978-1-60456-062-6


*Chapter VI*

# A Clinical Laboratory Approach to Reducing Bullying and Aggression In Schools and Families

***Arthur M. Horne, Katherine Raczynski and Pamela Orpinas***

## Abstract

Children have the right to attend schools where they have a sense of belonging and security; thus, allowing them to maximize their academic, emotional, behavioral, and personal development. The availability of a safe, inviting, and engaging school should be the right of every child, and yet thousands of students often do not experience this positive environment. Instead, students regularly encounter various forms of aggression and coercion as they attempt to attend to the academic focus of their school. Unfortunately, the problem of aggression challenges students repeatedly, often with painful consequences. For example, recent reports on the Youth Risk Behavior Survey (Eaton et al., 2006) provide very disturbing results. In 2005, 43% of boys and 28% of girls reported they were in a physical fight, and one-third of those fights occurred in school. Almost a third of all students had property stolen or deliberately damaged on school property, and 6% of boys and girls avoided school because they felt unsafe.

High school students also reported high rates of dating violence, with more than 9% of adolescents being hit, slapped, or otherwise physically hurt by a dating partner, and more than 10% of girls and 4% of boys reported being forced to have sexual intercourse. Weapon carrying among high school students has been steadily decreasing since 1991, but the downward trend has not continued in the past two surveys. Even during the best of reporting years, as many as 6% of students reported carrying a gun, knife, or club to school (Eaton et al., 2006). These are serious levels of violence with damaging consequences for all students: for those individuals who are the targets of aggression, for the perpetrators, and for the bystanders or witnesses.

While the focus of the Youth Risk Behavior Survey is on high school students, the prevalence of aggression and bullying in the lower grades is also high. In fact, from the beginning of school in kindergarten bullying occurs, and the frequency increases by grade level up to middle school, at which time it levels off and actually begins to decrease in high school. The extent of bullying in elementary and middle school may vary by school depending on educational policies, characteristics of students and educators, and enforcement of school rules. The prevalence of bullying is also influenced by how the behavior is defined and which time frame is used for data collection. In spite of these differences, the prevalence remains high in most studies, with a third to a half of students reporting victimization (see Orpinas & Horne, 2006, for a review of the prevalence of perpetration and victimization). Clearly, bullying is a public health problem that calls for prevention and intervention.

## Defining the Aggressive Behavior

The World Health Organization defines violence as: "the intentional use of physical force or power, threatened or actual, against oneself, another person, or against a group or community that either results in or has a high likelihood of resulting in injury, death, psychological harm, maldevelopment or deprivation" (Krug, Mercy, Dahlberg, & Zwi, 2002, p. 1084). While violence—or extreme forms of aggression, such as homicide, assault, and rape—is a major concern to all school personnel, it does not occur frequently and, when it does occur in schools, it is most often the result of escalating problems related to verbal or relational aggression and bullying.

Aggression refers to intentional behaviors that may cause psychological or physical harm to others. Aggression includes physical (e.g., hitting, pushing, or scratching), verbal (e.g., name-calling, teasing or threatening), and relational (e.g., isolating a peer on purpose or passing negative or untruthful rumors) behaviors. A relatively new form of aggression is cyberbullying, in which students use the Internet, phones, emails and other electronic means to attack peers. Many acts of violence and physical aggression result as an escalation of milder forms of aggression, such as name-calling, verbal abuse, and threats of intimidation. Thus, steps to reduce initial acts of verbal and relational aggression are likely to reduce the overall level of aggression.

Bullying and aggression are often used interchangeably, although some researchers define bullying behaviors as a subset of aggression (Olweus, 1993; Orpinas & Horne, 2006). Bullying is defined as intentional acts intended to hurt others, inflicted repeatedly and over time on someone who has less power (Olweus & Limber, 2002). Thus, the main difference between aggression and bullying is that the latter one involves an imbalance of strength and power between the bully and the target and that the behavior is repetitive. Many people experience isolated incidents of aggression, but children who are bullied live with the ongoing fear of the recurring abuse from the bully, which is usually more damaging than an isolated and unpredicted event. As with aggression, bullying can be physical, verbal, or relational.

Unfortunately, bullying in school is not unusual (Batsche & Porter, 2006). The reported prevalence of bullying in the United States varies considerably among studies, with rates ranging from a low of 10% for "extreme victims" of bullying (Perry, Kusel, & Perry, 1988) to a high of 75% of school-aged children who reported being bullied at least one time during their school years (Hoover, Oliver, & Hazler, 1992). Nansel et al. (2001), in examining reports of bullying in grades 6-10 in a large representative sample in the United States, cited that 17% of students had been bullied with some regularity (i.e., several times or more within the semester) and 19% had bullied others. Clearly, bullying is a major problem for schools and one warranting attention and treatment, for if medical diseases (measles, mumps, E-coli) were occurring at these rates, they would justify a major public health intervention.

Programs to address the problem have been developed and evaluated to examine the most effective manner to reduce the problem of bullying. A number of authors have examined the problem of bullying and have summarized the prevalence, theoretical explanations for the problem, and the various approaches to understanding the problem and methods for reducing the incidence of bullying (Olweus & Limber, 2003; Orpinas & Horne, 2006; Ross, 2003). The remainder of this chapter describes approaches established to prevent and reduce the problem of aggression, followed by recommendations for effectively implementing the prevention programs.

## Development of Interventions

Since bullying and aggression have been a part of the school environment from historical times, educators and researchers have attempted a number of different responses to prevent the problem. Some adults view bullying and aggression in school as a normal, if unpleasant, part of growing up. They argue that all children need to learn to manage the problem on their own; it is a developmental learning process. While it is true that all children need to learn to manage conflict, it is not true that bullying is "normal." Rather it is learned behavior that is maintained in environments where it is tolerated or ignored by the adults of the school system. Based on the well-documented negative outcomes of bullying (e.g., Baldry, 2004; Bond, Carlin, Thomas, Rubin, & Patton, 2001; Kim, Leventhal, Koh, Hubbard, & Boyce, 2003; Nishina, & Juvonen, 2005), many researchers, parents, and school officials have rejected the idea that ignoring bullying is best.

Many schools make an effort to identify victims and perpetrators of aggression and provide counseling to them. While some efforts in this direction have been effective (Hazler, 1996), overall large-scale studies of relying upon counseling to reduce aggression have resulted in poor outcomes (Gottfredson & Gottfredson, 2002). Because of the relatively disappointing outcomes of programs that target specific students, the remainder of this chapter will focus on school-wide approaches.

Two different levels of manualized school-wide interventions are available: the first approach provides a manualized process, and the second approach provides a manualized curriculum. A manualized process will offer guidelines for improving school climate based on a theoretical framework, such as social cognitive theory. These programs may include a general description of steps or goals, but implementation at each school may vary. The second approach refers to a specific curriculum, in addition to a theoretically based process for reducing bullying. The curriculum guides each step of the program, and implementation should be standard across schools.

## Process-based Prevention

Some examples of programs that include a manualized process without a specific curriculum are BreakAway (Lofquist, 1983; Lynn & Lofquist, 2002), Bullying Prevention: Creating a Positive School Climate and Developing Social Competence (Orpinas, Horne 2006), the Olweus Bully Prevention Program (Olweus, 1993), Positive Behavior Support (Lewis, Powers, Kelk, & Newcomer, 2002), Bullying Prevention Handbook (Hoover and Oliver, 2008) and the Protective School Model (Bosworth, 2000). Each of the programs shares many of the same characteristics, suggesting that researchers generally agree on how bullying prevention programs should be implemented. These steps include: 1) having a strong commitment to evaluate and reduce bullying, 2) a preliminary assessment of the school to identify problems and goals, 3) assembling a team of stakeholders who will provide leadership for the program; 4) developing a written action plan which is articulated to the school community; 5) providing appropriate training to involved parties; 6) implementing the steps of the action plan; and 7) collecting and analyzing data to evaluate the process.

The BreakAway model targets school improvement by empowering student leaders to actively identify problems and develop solutions (Lofquist, 1983; Lynn & Lofquist, 2002). The initial step of the BreakAway model is to educate teachers and school personnel about organizational change, needs assessment, action planning, and the principles of prevention. Faculty also build collaboration and leadership skills for working with groups of students. After this initial training, adults in the school select a group of youth leaders that constitute the core action team. This team selects an area for school improvement, such as reducing bullying, and creates an action plan for addressing the problem. The core team also identifies and recruits other students and school personnel to help implement the action plan. Case studies suggest that the BreakAway model increases school engagement and connectedness and reduces discipline referrals (Lynn & Lofquist, 2002).

The Orpinas and Horne Bullying Prevention Program (2006) provide guidelines for teachers, counselors, parents, and school administrators to foster a positive school climate and develop social competence in adolescents. They suggest an eight-step evaluation process, based on principles of program evaluation, to guide the development, implementation, and evaluation of bullying prevention programs. The initial steps include developing a team of stakeholders who are committed to change, defining the problem of bullying, and identifying clear and measurable objectives. Using this input, the stakeholders identify the best-suited intervention for the school, create a plan for evaluation, and actually implement that program. Finally, stakeholders collect the evaluation data, analyze it, and refine the process for future implementation.

The Olweus Bully Prevention Program (Olweus, 1993; Olweus & Limber, 2002) focuses on increasing awareness among students, teachers, and parents, highlighting the need for clear and consistent guidelines or rules against bullying. The Olweus Program is divided into several steps. Preliminary steps include administering a student questionnaire to determine the extent of the problem, reporting the findings to teachers, administrators, and parents, and developing a long-term plan of action. Olweus also encourages teachers to create teacher support groups in which 10 to 12 teachers meet regularly to discuss efforts and challenges. At the classroom level, teachers and students collaboratively generate rules about bullying. The

Olweus Program calls for implementing individual interventions for bullies, victims, and their parents. This takes the form of talks with bullies and victims, which occur quickly after incidents. Parents of bullies are encouraged to create family rules at home against bullying, as well as sanctions when these rules are broken.

The Positive Behavior Support (PBS) approach is designed to reduce disruptive and aggressive behaviors at school by modeling and rewarding pro-social alternatives (Lewis, Powers, Kelk, & Newcomer, 2002). PBS is based on social cognitive theory and emphasizes creating consistent rules, procedures, and expectations. School faculty members agree on three to five positively stated rules that encompass the values and goals of the school, such as "Be Kind." A smaller group of stakeholders takes the rules and decides how they will be applied in different locations around the school, such as the lunchroom and the library. This group also determines an appropriate reward system, like redeemable tokens or points, which will reinforce following the rules. Teachers and administrators work with students to ensure that they understand the rules and rewards. Stakeholders meet regularly during the year to monitor implementation and make adjustments as needed.

The Protective School Model (Bosworth, 2000) identifies 10 dimensions of a "protective" school environment, meaning a school that fosters students' social and academic development. The dimensions are: a vision of success, school culture that promotes student bonding, effective school leaders, a strong academic program, an effective prevention program, use of varied strategies to meet the needs of students and parents, professional development, funding and resources, community support, and appropriate data used in decision-making. The model provides suggestions for promoting these goals using a step-by-step process. First, educators identify a core group of stakeholders. This group arranges for teachers and staff to assess the school on the 10 dimensions, using the Protective Schools Assessment. Once the data are collected, the core team determines the areas that need improvement and develop a written action plan. The core team identifies other important players to assist in implementing the action plan, such as parents, students and school staff. The core team monitors the progress of the program throughout the year.

Each of the programs highlighted above are presented as a general intervention that relies upon implementation of specific steps for restructuring the social environment. The advantage of these process-based approaches is that they promote ownership of the program and the development of interventions catered to the specific needs of the school. These approaches leave considerable latitude to individual school, administrator, teacher, and parent interpretation. On the other hand, programs that provide a more systematic and structured approach to clinical problems may also be desirable, even to the point of establishing written protocols for each step of the intervention. This idea is supported by Gottfredson and Gottfredson (2002), who reported that the programs resulting in the most positive change for reducing aggression in schools were those with specific curricula that implemented a psychoeducational approach, thus providing less variation for implementation.

## Aggression Prevention Curricula

To address the call for more structured or manualized curriculum based approaches to prevent bullying, several curricula have been developed. A common characteristic of these programs is that they have specific modules or lesson plans for each topic of concern.

### *Steps to Respect: A Bullying Prevention Program*

Steps to Respect: A Bullying Prevention Program was developed by the Committee for Children (www.cfchildren.org) and has demonstrated promising results (Hodges, Boivin, Vitaro, & Bukowskii, 1999). The program has three levels: Grades 3-4, grades 4-5, and grades 5-6 and focuses on establishing a safe, caring, and respectful culture. Similar to the process-based programs, Steps to Respect starts by developing a school-wide framework that establishes the role of the administrator as a supportive leader of the implementation and of the program evaluation. In addition, a steering committee which includes teachers, administrators, and others who encounter students during the school day (e.g., bus drivers, nurses, secretaries) is formed to implement the program. Worksheets are available to guide the steering committee in their planning to increase the efficacy and sustainability of the program. For example, specific worksheets address challenges such as obtaining school buy-in, developing an anti-bullying policy, examining the school's physical characteristics, carrying out staff training, and beginning the curriculum.

The second phase of Steps to Respect involves training of all staff, conducting a curriculum orientation for classroom teachers, and then booster training for staff and faculty. The training follows specific written scripts to facilitate fidelity to the program. The third phase is to implement the curriculum in classrooms. During this phase, bully prevention lessons are incorporated into academic lessons so that the learning of subject matter, the prevention of bullying, and the development social skills complement each other. In addition to the classroom training, all staff participate in a school-wide anti-bullying campaign.

The Steps to Respect program has demonstrated some impressive gains in reducing the problem of aggression in the schools. For example, a fairly minimal intervention promoted by the program includes specific training and skills development for having peers step in to tell bullies to stop the bullying. The project reports that over half of the time the bullying stopped within a few seconds when peers spoke up and that there were reductions in bullying and argumentative behavior on the playground after the intervention (Frey et al., 2005).

### *Bullying Intervention Program (BIP)*

Unlike other universal programs—those that focus on changing the entire school and are designed for all students regardless of the level of risk—BIP is an individual cognitive-behavioral intervention for students who bully others (Swearer & Givens, 2006). BIP posits that the perceptions of students involved in bullying are as critical as their aggressive behaviors. Perceptions and cognitions of the bullies serve to stimulate, perpetuate, and escalate bullying interactions (Doll & Swearer, 2005; Swearer & Cary, 2003). The program is applied one-on-one with students who engage in bullying behavior, rather than with whole classrooms. This individual approach is, in part, a function of research that suggests homogenous group interventions are less effective for severely aggressive youth and, in fact, group interventions with aggressive youth may result in increasing rather than decreasing aggression (Dishion, McCord, & Poulin, 1999). Thus, the program was developed for school counselors and school psychologists to work directly with students who bully others.

BIP offers an alternative to in-school suspension for bullying behaviors. In schools using this program, parents of students who bully others can choose whether their child be suspended or participate in BIP; if parents elect BIP, active parental consent and student assent are obtained. BIP participants, then, adhere to the same policies, procedures, and scheduling that the school uses for in-school suspension.

BIP is a 3-hour, one-on-one cognitive behavioral intervention session with three components: (a) assessment, (b) psychoeducation, and (c) feedback. In the assessment, which takes approximately 1 hour, the child completes widely-used measures developed to evaluate experiences with bullying, depression, anxiety, cognitive distortions, school climate, and self-concept. In the psychoeducation component, which lasts about two hours, a masters-level student-therapist under the supervision of a licensed psychologist or counselor presents written structured material about bullying, followed by a short quiz to assess the student's understanding. Next, the student completes several worksheet activities about bullying behavior from Bully Busters (Newman et al., 2000). The program finishes with the student-therapist and the referred student watching a video about bullying produced by MTV. Finally, in the feedback phase the referred student talks about his or her experiences with bullying and impressions of BIP. The student-therapist then prepares a written bullying intervention report based on the assessment data and the interactions with the referred student. This report is reviewed by the parents, student, and school personnel during a face-to-face solution-oriented meeting.

To date the BIP intervention has been implemented in a limited number of schools, and the results are promising (Swearer & Givens, 2006). In addition, this program fulfils many of the expectations for implementing a clinical laboratory method for reducing bullying: 1) it is theoretically based, 2) it has been manualized to standardize delivery and to evaluate fidelity of implementation, and 3) it uses standardized assessment protocols. BIP could be implemented by less than doctoral level practitioners, with adequate training.

### *Bully Busters: A Teacher's Manual For Helping Bullies, Victims, And Bystanders*

In the schools where we have worked, counselors, psychologists, and teachers have requested a program that is both affordable and that has a focused curriculum. Teachers have also expressed a desire to have a program that may be implemented in an individual classroom, by a particular teaching team, a specific grade level, or universally throughout the entire school. The program we have been using is Bully Busters (Horne, Bartolomucci, & Newman-Carlson, 2003; Horne, Stoddard, & Bell, 2008; Newman, Horne, & Bartolomucci, 2000) which addresses a number of bullying topics. The Bully Busters program is theoretically developed following an ecological model for understanding the problem of bullying and the steps to reduce the problem. The manual provides written direction for teachers, activities to conduct in the classrooms with students, specific processing questions to assist students in examining the impact of each activity, and evaluation instruments for each module and for overall program accomplishments.

Bully Busters begins with two levels of assessment. First, teachers complete a survey to evaluate the extent of their self-efficacy for working with problems of bullying and their classroom management skills and practices. Second, students and teachers complete a survey to examine the extent of bullying and aggression that occurs in the schools and to describe where the bullying problems occur. The results are then used to provide feedback to school personnel (teachers, administrators, support staff), to parents, and to other interested stakeholders (community agencies, religious/spiritual leaders).

Bully Busters includes seven modules, and every module is composed of several sections: 1) the theoretical background for the topic discussed; 2) relevant research related to the topic; 3) guidelines for implementing activities with students; 4) a teacher goal form, in which the teacher defines her or his goals related to the module and identifies specific students in special need; 5) a final review of the content so that teachers may evaluate their knowledge of the topic and, following the implementation of the module, review their teacher goal form to assess the success of the implementation; 6) written guidelines for directing discussions related to the topic of the module; and 7) written activities for students; each activity is followed by questions that facilitate processing each of the activities with students.

Module One is designed to increase awareness of bullying. Teachers receive standard definitions of bullying but then, collaboratively with students, develop a "working definition" of bullying to use in their classrooms. Written guidelines facilitate a conversation among students about who is a bully, what is bullying, and where bullying happens. Students then participate in several activities to recognize how their words and actions can be hurtful. Students role-play constructive ways of interacting following scripts and scenarios provided in Module One, specifically focused on increasing awareness of the problem of bullying.

Module Two examines how bullying develops and the variety of forms it can take. Teachers lead students in discussions of aggressive and passive forms of bullying, and possible differences between male and female bullying. Activities in this module include viewing movies in which characters are victims or bullies. This module ends with a guided discussion on common misconceptions about bullying.

Module Three focuses on recognizing the victim of bulling. Students discuss the effects of victimization, and teachers challenge myths about victims. Students learn to differentiate among types of victims, including individuals who are passive, provocative, and bystanders. Incorporating bystanders into the process of stopping bullying receives considerable attention and is a major focus of the Bully Busters intervention. Teachers encourage students to break the "code of silence" that causes some students to withdraw from involvement. Involving bystanders helps create a safer climate for all students. The majority of students are not actively engaged in bullying episodes but their reluctance to intervene in a bully incident can further promote this behavior by having bullies believe their aggression is supported. Students learn that bystanders are either part of the problem or part of the solution.

Module Four provides specific strategies to create a bully-free classroom. Teachers receive written materials detailing strategies (e.g., setting rules, acting quickly). Most importantly, teachers also receive training in empathy skills education, social skills training, and anger control skills.

Module Five expands on students' skills development by providing specific strategies to work with students who are victimized by bullies. Activities assist victims to become aware of their strengths, to view themselves in a positive manner, and to build skills and confidence in joining groups.

Module Six examines the role of prevention, for it is better to establish a classroom environment that prevents problems than to have to solve problems after they develop. Teachers are encouraged to identify how their attitudes and behaviors, as well as characteristics of the school, influence student behavior. Student activities focus on skills to prevent conflict from developing, such as problem solving, decision making, and social interaction skills. These skills build upon material from previous modules.

The final module focuses on relaxation training, stress coping, and management of personal emotions. Teachers first learn to apply the skills to themselves and then teach them to their students. The program finishes with a follow-up assessment of teachers' knowledge and self-efficacy, as well as a student and teacher survey of bullying in the school. Teachers receiving the Bully Buster training reported significantly higher levels of self efficacy for managing bullying behavior, demonstrated greater knowledge of classroom behavior management, and had fewer classroom behavior problems and office referrals than comparison teachers (Bell, 2007; Browning, Cooker & Sullivan, 2005; Howard, Horne, & Jolliff, 2002; Newman & Horne, 2004; Orpinas, Horne & Staniszewski, 2003).

### *The Good Behavior Game*

The Good Behavior Game is an approach to improving classroom management and reducing disruptive behavior that has shown far-reaching effects in and out of the classroom, particularly among elementary school students. Researchers developed the game in the 1960s as a way to incorporate principles of behavioral psychology into classroom management (Barrish, Sauders, & Wolf, 1969). The two-fold aim of the approach is to reduce peer reinforcement of disruptive behavior and to reward students for inhibiting inappropriate behavior.

The team-based game is played in short time intervals in the classroom. The teacher divides the class into two or more teams, and teams receive marks for violating classroom rules during game play. The team(s) that fall below the pre-determined number of marks for the game interval receive a reward, such as special activity time or a small treat (sticker, candy).

A manual describes the rules and step-by-step procedures for the game, including how to prepare to use the game, how to work with noncompliant students, and how to keep students interested in the game over time (Embry & Straatemeier, 2001). Although the nature of the game allows for some flexibility on the part of the teacher (such as the length of each game interval and the type of reward given), the manual designates the procedures that are essential to the game's efficacy. Critical procedures include clear and repeated explanation of the game rules, consistency in giving marks, and awarding a desirable consequence to the winning team.

The Good Behavior Game has been extensively researched with very positive results. (For a detailed review of these studies, see Embry, 2002.) Numerous multiple baseline studies resulted in considerable reductions of disruptive behaviors during game intervals as measured by direct classroom observation by trained observers (Barrish, Sauders, & Wolf, 1969; Medland & Stachnik, 1972). A large randomized trial (Dolan, et al. 1993) found improvement in on-task classroom behavior and suggested that the game effectively reduces aggressive behavior, especially in highly aggressive students. These outcomes were from teacher ratings, peer ratings, and direct observation of aggressive behavior.

The Good Behavior Game is praised by teachers for being simple to learn and implement. It also has the advantage of being appropriate for use within a single classroom or across an entire school system. It is easily generalizable; once students are familiar with the game, it can be used outside of the classroom, such as in the cafeteria or library. Further, it can be included as a component in other bullying reduction programs.

## Key Components of Successful Implementation of Bullying Prevention Programs in Schools

When school administrators, teachers, staff, and stakeholders adopt a bullying prevention curriculum, they must be willing to commit the time and effort required to achieve proper implementation. In this section, we outline two major challenges to attaining success: providing high quality implementation, and overcoming student, family and community factors which run counter to bullying prevention efforts (Gottfredson & Gottfredson, 2002; Greenberg et al., 2003).

To provide quality implementation, administrators and teachers must be sincerely committed to decreasing bullying using the program. This internalization of program goals is colloquially known as "buy-in" or "ownership." Ideally, buy-in should pervade all levels of the school (administrators, teachers, support staff, students), and extend to the community at large (parents, coaches and other youth services workers).

Buy-in and leadership at the administrative level is crucial to enact positive change. Administrators and other school leaders have a specific role in ensuring that rules, policies and procedures within school cultivate a positive school climate. Initially, administrators should carefully select the curriculum, provide adequate training for teachers or implementers, and allocate sufficient time to implement the program components. Administrators should also develop a plan to monitor the progress of the program. Other steps that ensure success include enforcing a clearly communicated school-wide anti-bullying discipline plan and providing support to personnel who need assistance in program implementation. Additionally, administrators should lead by example by refraining from coercive interaction with employees and students, and work to eliminate bullying by adults in the school (e.g., teacher-teacher, teacher-student, administrator-teacher). The Steps to Respect program described earlier offers advice to administrators about how to plan and prepare for program implementation.

Administrative buy-in, while fundamental, cannot be assumed, even in schools where administrators seek out a bullying-prevention curriculum to implement. Manualized programs may be attractive to administrators who wish to address school bullying "on paper" but not in practice. School officials may believe that implementing a program is as easy as putting a manual in the hands of teachers with no other support or guidance. The reasons for lack of buy-in are numerous. Administrators may not believe that bullying is a problem within the school. In this case, a school-wide evaluation would be appropriate to assess the extent of bullying. Administrators may have misconceptions about the nature of bullying, such as that it is "just a part of growing up." or that "kids need to learn to stick up for themselves." To remedy these types of fallacies, administrators should be educated about the consequences of bullying, such as psychological distress and decreased academic achievement.

Similar ideas that hinder buy-in may be shared by teachers, counselors or other school personnel who are asked to implement a bullying-prevention curriculum. It is essential that these program implementers receive adequate training and possess a high level of commitment to the program goals. The attitudes of these adults will dramatically impact student receptiveness to the program. When students hear a strong and consistent message about the unacceptability of bullying in school, they are more likely to internalize the message. Alternatively, students will not enact positive change if they do not think that adults in the school will support their decision to alter their behavior, whether they are bullies, victims or bystanders.

In addition to the beliefs outlined above, program implementers may also lack buy-in because they already feel overwhelmed and overworked. They may feel that their jobs encompass solely in-class academic instruction, not monitoring positive social interaction in and out of the classroom. Teachers may also resent being asked to use instruction time to teach social skills, especially in the age of high-stakes testing. We can easily sympathize with these objections; however, the time invested in implementing bullying prevention program may pay rich dividends. Program implementers should be instructed about the positive outcomes that accompany a drop in bullying at school: better attendance, increased student engagement, and better academic success. Prevention, in the end, saves class time. Teachers who are skilled at intervening in student interpersonal disputes—bullying or otherwise—have a repertoire of solutions that can be quickly implemented when problems arise. In serious cases, it may be necessary to address teacher burnout and stress before embarking on a bullying prevention curriculum.

Adults implementing the bullying prevention curriculum may also express concerns about the impact of a program where community, family, and student factors may work against the program goals. A number of out-of-school risk factors contribute to the prevalence of bullying in schools, such as living in a community where aggressive behavior is glorified, family dysfunction is typical, and student expectations for success are low. Teachers may wonder, "is it possible for me to get Callie to stop bullying at school when I can see that her brother victimizes her every day at home?" or "How can I ask Deon to not fight with the bullies at school when I know he will fight them in his neighborhood?" These are wrenching questions that may discourage even the most committed program implementer. While school personnel may not be able to overcome every external impediment, they should focus on the factors that can be changed within the school. Administrators, teachers, and counselors do have control over school rules and values. Implementers need to set attainable goals, such as "I can help Callie learn to control her anger at school, even if I cannot change her life at home." Children and adolescents exhibit a remarkable ability to adapt to different sets of acceptable behaviors. Just as students understand that rules for the classroom and the playground differ, they will learn that conventions at the school may be different than those practiced at home and in the community.

In addition to counteracting negative external influences, schools ideally will work to extend the impact of the bullying prevention curriculum outside the classroom walls. That is, students will generalize the positive social skills learned at school in their lives at home and in the community. School personnel may work outside of the school (e.g., churches, libraries, after school groups) to mobilize community resources. For specific recommendations about enhancing students' ability to generalize social skills learned in class, see McGinnis and Goldstein (2003).

## Recommendations for Further Refinement of Clinical Laboratory Implementation

The field of applied psychology has been criticized for relying upon face-to-face, talk based interventions which may be based upon unproven, unverified, and undocumented methods for alleviating problems in the field of mental health (L'Abate, this volume). Psychologists have been called upon to adopt a clinical laboratory method that is theoretically based and that will address not only the shortcomings of previous attempts at solving the mental health problems of our society, but that will do it more economically and more effectively. Researchers who wish to test the efficacy of violence prevention programs in schools must take into consideration different individual, school, and community factors that may impact the outcome of the programs they implement. Some of these factors may be difficult to measure; therefore, we recommend that studies include a strong process evaluation component. First, the level of community, administration, and classroom commitment to the program should be measured and taken into account when analyzing program outcomes. Stronger buy-in should result in better outcomes. What is less clear is whether a minimum level of commitment is necessary to achieve desired results. Data on school commitment can also be used to differentiate between programs that fail because they are not effective or because of a lack of commitment. The relation between buy-in and quality and intensity of implementation needs further research. Second, program evaluators and researchers need to further investigate the qualities of most successful program implementers. Schools would benefit by knowing which personal characteristics of program facilitators are critical to successful implementation. Finally, researchers need to investigate which programs work best for schools with different student populations. We cannot expect that one ideal "one-size-fits-all" program does exist.

## References

Baldry, A. C. (2004). The impact of direct and indirect bullying on the mental and physical health of Italian youngsters. *Aggressive Behavior, 30*(5), 343-355.

Barrish, H., Saunders, M., & Wolf, M. M. (1969). Good Behavior Game: Effects of individual contingencies for group consequences on disruptive behavior in a classroom. *Journal of Applied Behavior Analysis*, *2,* 119–124.

Batsche, G.M., & Porter, L.J. (2006). Bullying. In Bear, G.G., & Minke, K.M. (Eds*),*

*Children's needs III: Development, prevention, and intervention* (pp. 135-148). Washington, DC, US: National Association of School Psychologists.

Bell, C. (2007). *Evaluation of an implementation of an abbreviated bully prevention program for reducing aggression in middle school*. Unpublished doctoral dissertation, University of Georgia.

Bond, L., Carlin, J. B., Thomas, L., Rubin, K., & Patton, G. (2001). Does bullying cause emotional problems? A prospective study of young teenagers. *British Medical Journal, 323*(7311), 480-484.

Browning, C. M., Cooker, P. g., & Sullivan, K. (2005). Help for the bully/peer abuse problem: Is bully busters in-service training effective? In G. R. Walz & R. K Yep (Eds.), *Vistas: Compelling perspectives on counseling* (pp. 231-234). Alexandria, VA: American Counseling Association.

Bosworth, K. (2000). *Protective schools: Linking drug abuse prevention with student success*. Tucson, AZ: University of Arizona, College of Education.

Dishion, T. J., McCord, J., & Poulin, F. (1999). When Interventions Harm: Peer Groups and Problem Behavior. *American Psychologist, 54*, 755-764.

Doll, B., & Swearer, S. M., (2005). Cognitive behavior interventions for participants in bullying and coercion. In R. B. Mennuti, A. Freeman, & R. Christner (Eds.), *Cognitive Behavioral Interventions in Educational Settings*. New York: Brunner-Routledge.

Eaton, D. K., Kann, L., Kinchen, S., Ross, J., Hawkins, J., Harris, W. A. et al. (2006). Youth risk behavior surveillance - United States, 2005. *Journal of School Health, 76,* 353-372.

Embry, D.D. (2002). The good behavior game: A best practice candidate as a universal behavioral vaccine. *Clinical Child and Family Psychology Review*, 5(4), 273–297.

Embry, D. D., & Straatemeier, G. (2001). *The PAX Acts Game Manual: How to apply the Good Behavior Game*. Tucson, AZ: PAXIS Institute.

Frey, K. S., Hirschstein, M. K., Snell, J. L., Edstrom, L.V., MacKenzie, E. P., & Broderick, C. J. (2005). Reducing Playground Bullying and Supporting Beliefs: An Experimental Trial of the *Steps to Respect* Program. *Developmental Psychology. 41*(3), 479–491.

Greenberg, M. T., Weissberg, R. P., O'Brien, M. U., Zins, J. E., Fredericks, L., Resnick, H., et al (2003). Enhancing school-based prevention and youth development through coordinated social, emotional, and academic learning. *American Psychologist, 58,* 466-474.

Gottfredson, D. C. & Gottfredson, G. D. (2002). Quality of school-based prevention programs: Results from a national survey. *Journal of Research in Crime and Delinquency, 39,* 3-35.

Hazler, R. J. (1996). *Breaking the cycle of violence: Interventions for bullying and victimization*. Washington, DC: Accelerated Development: A member of the Taylor and Francis Group.

Hodges, E. V. E., Boivin, M., Vitaro, F., & Bukowski, W. M. (1999). The power of friendship: protection against an escalating cycle of peer victimization. *Developmental Psychology, 35,* 94–101

Horne A. M., Bartolomucci C. L., & Newman-Carlson D. A. (2003). *Bully Busters: A teacher's manual for helping bullies, victims, and bystanders (Grades K-5)*. Champaign, IL: Research Press.

Horne, A., Stoddard, J., & Bell, C. (2008). *A parent's guide to understanding and responding to bullying: The bully busters approach*. Champaign, IL: Research Press.

Hoover, J. & Oliver, R. (2008). *Bullying Prevention Handbook.* Bloomington, IN: Solution Tree.

Hoover, J., Oliver, R., & Hazler, R. (1992). *Causal attributions: From cognitive processes to collective beliefs.* Oxford, UK: Basil Blackwell.

Howard, N., Horne, A., & Jolliff, D. (2002). Self-efficacy in a new training model for the prevention of bullying in schools. In R. Geffner, M. Loring, & C. Young (Eds.), *Bully behavior: Current issues, research, and interventions* (pp. 181-192). New York: Haworth Press.

Kim Y.S., Leventhal B.L., Koh Y.J., Hubbard A., & Boyce W.T (2006). School bullying and youth violence - Causes or consequences of psychopathologic behavior? *Archives of General Psychiatry,63*(9),1035- 1041.

Krug, E. G., Mercy, J. A., Dahlberg, L. L., & Zwi, A. B. (2002). The world report on violence and health. *Lancet, 360,* 1083-1088.

Lewis, T. J., Powers, L. J., Kelk, M. J., & Newcomer, L. (2002). Reducing problem behaviors on the playground: An investigation of the application of school-wide positive behavior supports. *Psychology in the Schools, 39,* 181-190.

Lofquist, W. A. (1983). *Discovering the meaning of prevention: A practical approach to positive change* Tucson, AZ: Associates for Youth Development.

Lynn, D. D. & Lofquist, W. A. (2002). *Breakaway: A framework for creating positive school communities. A leadership team workbook.* Tucson, AZ: Development Publications.

McGinnis, E., & Goldstein, A. P., (2003) *Skillstreaming in early childhood: New strategies and perspectives for teaching prosocial skills.* Champaign, IL: Research Press.

Medland, M. B., & Stachnik, T. J. (1972). Good Behavior Game: A replication and systematic analysis. *Journal of Applied Behavior Analysis, 5,* 45–51.

Nansel, T. R., Overpeck, M., Pilla, R. S., Ruan, W. J., Simons-Morton, B., & Scheidt, P. (2001). Bullying behaviors among U.S. youth: Prevalence and association with psychosocial adjustment. *JAMA, 285*, 2094-2100.

Newman, D. A., Horne, A. M., & Bartolomucci, C. L. (2000). *Bully busters: A teacher's manual for helping bullies, victims, and bystanders*. Champaign, IL: Research Press.

Newman-Carlson, D. & Horne, A. (2004). Bully Busters: A psychoeducational intervention for reducing bullying behavior in middle school students. *Journal of Counseling and Developmen*t, *82*, 259–267.

Nishina, A., & Juvonen, J. (2005). Daily reports of witnessing and experiencing peer harassment in middle school. *Child Development, 76*(2), 435-450.

Olweus, D. (1993). *Bullying at school: What we know and what we can do*. Cambridge, MA: Blackwell Publishers.

Olweus, D. (2001). Peer harassment: a critical analysis and some important issues. In S. Graham & J. Juvonen (Eds.), *Peer Harassment in School: The Plight of the Vulnerable and Victimized* (pp. 3-20). New York: Guilford Press.

Olweus, D. & Limber, S. (2002). *Bullying prevention program* (Rep. No. Book nine). Boulder, CO: Center for the Study and Prevention of Violence, Institute of Behavioral Science, University of Colorado at Boulder.

Orpinas, P., & Horne, A. (2006). *Bully prevention: Creating a positive school climate and developing social competence.* Washington, DC: American Psychological Association.

Orpinas, P., Horne, A. M., & Staniszewski, D. (2003). School bullying: Changing the problem by changing the school. *School Psychology Review, 32*, 431-444.

Perry, D.G., Kusel, S. J., & Perry, C., L. (1988). Victims of peer aggression. *Developmental Psychology, 24,* 807-814.

Ross, D. M. (2003). *Childhood bullying, teasing, and violence: What school personnel, other professionals, and parents can do.* (2nd ed.) Alexandria, VA: American Counseling Association.

Swearer, S. M., & Cary, P. T. (2003). Perceptions and attitudes toward bullying in middle school youth: A developmental examination across the bully/victim continuum. *Journal of Applied School Psychology, 19*, 63-79.

Swearer, S. M., & Givens, J. E. (March, 2006). *Designing an alternative to suspension for middle school bullies.* Paper presented at the annual convention of the National Association of School Psychologists, Anaheim, CA.

In: Toward a Science of Clinical Psychology
Editor: Luciano L'Abate, pp. 133-146
ISBN: 978-1-60456-062-6


*Chapter VII*

# Empirically Supported Interventions in School Settings: Fostering Children's Social and Emotional Competence

***Douglas C. Smith***

## Abstract

School-based mental health services for children and adolescents have expanded significantly in recent years with increasing numbers of clinical and counseling psychologists now supplementing services provided by school personnel. School-based services mental health services include both universal (schoolwide) prevention strategies as well as more targeted interventions designed to address the psychological and emotional needs of students and their families. Empirically supported interventions falling under the rubric of social and emotional learning have been found to enhance both the emotional and academic well being of students while, at the same time, reducing risk for a wide range of negative behaviors including substance abuse, aggression, school dropout, pregnancy, and suicide. This chapter reviews empirically supported treatments for children and adolescents in the areas of emotional literacy, conflict resolution, and anger management.

## Introduction

The purpose of this chapter is to provide an overview of empirically supported treatments for working with children and families in school settings. Other contributors to this volume have discussed the utility of evidence-based psychological interventions in a wide range of treatment settings. Nowhere is the need more evident than in the public school system. With the advent of the *No Child Left Behind Act of 2001* (NCLB), public schools are now held accountable, not only for the success of academic programs, but also for support practices and policies, including mental health services, that presumably contribute to the overall development and well being of children and adolescents.

This chapter will begin with an overview of mental health services delivered by clinical psychologists and others in school settings. A focus on primary prevention and positive youth development characterizes the evolution of these services. The major thrust of this chapter will be on empirically supported treatments that further the social and emotional development of children and youth in school settings. I will focus specifically on three areas of social-emotional learning that have gained the most empirical support. These include: 1) emotional literacy, 2) conflict resolution and 3) anger management.

## School-Based Mental Health Services

Both the philosophy and delivery of school-based mental health services have changed dramatically over the last decade. Clinical and counseling psychologists are now working in school settings in increasing numbers (Pluymert, 2002; Waxman & Weist, 1999). In part, this may be attributable to the advent of managed health care with subsequent reductions in allotments for private mental health services (Short & Talley, 1997). On the other hand, many clinicians now recognize some of the advantages of working in the school environment, which include: 1) relatively easy access to children and those families in need of services, 2) the opportunity to provide treatment in an ecologically valid and real life setting, and 3) the opportunity to develop comprehensive treatment plans in collaboration with other professionals including teachers, counselors, administrators, and other educational and related services specialists (Adelman & Taylor, 2006; Dryfoos, 1994; Weist, 1999).

School-based mental health services often include a continuum of services, which may range from universal, school wide prevention efforts to more targeted treatment approaches (Adelman & Taylor, 2000; Dwyer, Osher, & Warger, 1998). For example, at the school wide level, a universal prevention approach for all students might include working with the teacher to create an engaging and supportive classroom environment in the interest of maximizing students' interest and motivation and thereby preventing behavior problems. At a secondary level of intervention, there are likely to be some students at risk for more challenging behavioral and emotional concerns who may require additional assistance in the form of group or individual skill building, e.g., social skills training, academic tutoring, etc. At the tertiary level, there may be a few students who require more intensive and individualized services to overcome chronic and severe behavior problems that have not been responsive to primary or secondary level interventions. Empirically supported treatments in school settings may include interventions at any or all of the levels mentioned here.

Exemplary school-based treatment strategies also employ a coordinated and integrated service delivery system. It is widely recognized, for example, that problem behaviors and attitudes observed in the school setting are very likely the product of a myriad of personal, social, ecological and cultural factors including family and peer influences, community and cultural norms and expectations, and even the impact of more distal influences such as television and other types of multimedia (Bronfenbrenner, 1979; Howard, Flora, & Griffin, 1999; Sameroff, Peck, & Eccles, 2004). Thus, the most powerful and effective interventions are comprehensive and systemic in their efforts to address the multiplicity of factors that contribute to the perceived problem.

## A Positive Approach to Prevention and Intervention

For most of its history, clinical psychology has focused on the treatment of mental "disorders". A positive approach to the prevention of mental illness focuses on building a set of social and emotional strengths that are incompatible with mental distress. These include developing emotional literacy skills, such as empathy and respect for the rights of others; boosting resiliency factors, such as self-esteem and academic success; and establishing a high degree of "connectedness" between students and their families, peers, schools, and communities (Cowen, Wyman, Work, & Iker, 1995; Elias et al., 1994; Weissberg & Greenberg, 1998). Unlike traditional problem-focused approaches, the positive approach to mental health in schools is preventive, solution-driven, and systemic in its efforts. Its goal is to enhance the overall well being of students and others in the context of schooling.

The impetus for a positive approach to mental health in schools draws upon a model of human functioning that, rather than attempting to repair psychological disease and dysfunction, attempts to promote optimal levels of development (see Seligman & Csikszentmihalyi, 2000, for a more detailed discussion of a positive approach to psychological treatment). In short, a positive approach is primarily concerned with the facilitation of psychological health and well-being. Regarding prevention of mental distress, a positive approach engenders development of prosocial interpersonal skills and such noble personal qualities as wisdom, courage, altruism, civility, and tolerance for the views of others.

## Promoting Social and Emotional Learning in Schools

The positive approach to mental health described above is compatible with a growing national movement toward comprehensive (kindergarten through Grade 12) psychosocial education that (a) emphasizes personal and social skills training; (b) promotes positive social values and health attitudes; and (c) provides honest, relevant information about public health issues including societal violence, substance abuse, gang involvement and other issues of concern to parents and educators (National Center for Health Education, 1997). The Collaborative for Academic, Social and Emotional Learning (CASEL) serves as a clearinghouse for research and practice in the area of social and emotional learning (SEL) in schools. This collaborative of distinguished scholars and practitioners publishes and disseminates information on how schools can establish comprehensive efforts to foster social and emotional learning, what specific strategies are most effective for which populations, and the impact of social and emotional learning on academic success (CASEL; www.casel.org). Social and emotional learning is defined as "the process of acquiring the skills to recognize and manage emotions, set and achieve positive goals, appreciate the perspectives of others, establish and maintain positive relationships, make responsible decisions, and handle interpersonal situations effectively" (CASEL, 2005). In a comprehensive review of prevention strategies designed to enhance social and emotional competence, Weissberg and Greenberg (1998) discussed a range of competence-enhancement strategies for elementary age students. The major goal of such programs is "to teach children to make use of both personal and environmental resources to achieve prosocial goals" (p. 890). Because specific acts of misbehavior are viewed primarily as learned behaviors, they can be unlearned and thus prevented by acquisition of more prosocial and positive behaviors. Hawkins, Catalano, Kosterman, Abbot, and Hill (1999) suggested that healthy bonding of children to adults, peers, and institutions that promote healthy beliefs and prosocial attitudes is likely to result in adoption of similar beliefs and attitudes.

In a recent meta-analysis of some 263 social and emotional learning programs for kindergarten through high school students, Weissberg et al. (in press) found convincing support for the notion that social and emotional learning programs, delivered in the context of schools, can not only modify disruptive and antisocial behaviors but also contribute to enhanced academic functioning. Specifically, when compared to control group students who did not receive social and emotional skills training across studies, students who received training demonstrated more positive social interactions, an enhanced degree of self-esteem, and a greater sense of connectedness with regard to school. These students manifested significant decreases in antisocial behaviors including disruptiveness in the classroom, aggressive behavior, and substance use. Students also showed reductions in internalizing symptoms, including depression and anxiety. Perhaps of most interest to educators in the NCLB era, students who participated in social and emotional training programs produced a consistent pattern of improved school performance as indicated by standardized achievement test scores. Even more impressively, for the 44 studies that collected follow-up data at a minimum of six months following the intervention, significant gains remained for the treatment groups in terms of social skills and attitudes, prosocial behaviors, and academic performance, as well as significant reductions in disruptive externalizing behaviors, internalizing symptoms, and substance abuse.

Given the positive impact of social and emotional learning programs in general, this review will focus on some of the key components of those programs that have received the most empirical support within school settings. These include: 1) strategies designed to foster emotional literacy, 2) social problem-solving and conflict resolution training, and 3) programs focused on anger management. Within each area, I will provide a brief overview and rationale for the targeted skills and a more detailed review of exemplary programs.

## Empirically Supported Treatments that Facillitate Emotional Literacy

### Overview

Daniel Goleman's (1995) book Emotional Intelligence: Why It Can Matter More Than IQ popularized the notion that one's emotional reasoning may be equal to or more important than cognitive intelligence as a predictor of life success. There is now compelling evidence that emotional competence is indeed related to a range of positive outcomes both at school and in the larger community, including friendships, social status, and achievement (Elias et al., 1994; Weissberg & Greenberg, 1998).

Goleman (1995) and others (e.g., Salovey & Mayer, 1990) have identified at least five domains of emotional competence important to overall functioning and success. The first and most basic, self-awareness, refers to the ability to recognize and identify internal feeling states such as anger, disappointment, fear, and exhilaration. Closely related, but at a higher developmental level, is awareness of others, including such skills as empathy, or understanding others' feelings, and role taking, or understanding others' points of view. Both self-awareness and awareness of others are critical to positive interactions with peers, resolving interpersonal conflicts, and, ultimately, preventing and reducing the likelihood of aggression and other misbehaviors at school.

The third domain, managing one's emotions, refers to the ability to regulate and control potentially troublesome emotions, such as frustration, resentment, guilt, and despair. One such emotion that has been the subject of numerous school-based intervention projects is anger. Anger management and regulation is an important skill in terms of social and emotional competence.

The fourth domain, motivating oneself, has particular relevance for school. Students who have the ability and skill to motivate themselves academically, both extrinsically and intrinsically, are likely to view school as a positive experience, are less likely to engage in problematic or antisocial behaviors, and generally perform at higher levels than their counterparts (Resnick et al., 1997).

Finally, negotiating/resolving conflicts, the fifth domain, is a critical skill for enhancing interpersonal success (Johnson & Johnson, 1996; Tolan & Guerra, 1994). If disagreements, grievances, and other relatively minor conflicts can be resolved effectively, it is unlikely that these events will lead to aggressive/violent confrontations. Negotiation/conflict resolution builds upon a number of more fundamental interpersonal skills including cooperation, problem solving, and empathy.

## Programs Fostering Emotional Literacy in Schools

A number of programs have emerged in recent years that are designed to help students acquire and utilize emotional literacy skills. These programs are broad-based in the sense that they target a wide range of social and emotional skills and are usually applied in the context of the classroom or the larger school environment. To be truly effective, efforts to enhance emotional literacy must become an integral part of the school's educational mission. What is required is a concerted, school wide effort to foster these skills and to establish a climate of respect and tolerance.

One highly regarded program that includes a formal curriculum and daily lessons to develop and refine emotional literacy skills is *The Incredible Years* (www.incredible years.com), an early prevention/intervention program designed for children ages 2 – 10. The program was identified as a model program by the University of Colorado's Center for the Study and Prevention of Violence (Webster-Stratton et al., 2001). Like most empirically supported treatment packages in the area of emotional literacy, the program actually targets multiple risk factors across settings. Thus, The Incredible Years Series includes three comprehensive, multi-faceted, and developmentally-based curriculums for parents, teachers, ad children. As a whole, the programs are designed to promote social and emotional competence in young children at risk for or presenting with conduct problems in home or school settings.

In all three of the training programs, trained facilitators use videotape scenes to encourage group discussion, problem-solving, and sharing of ideas. The program for parents emphasizes parenting skills known to promote social competence and reduce problem behaviors, such as how to play with children, helping children learn, effective praise and use of incentives, effective limit-setting and strategies to handle misbehavior. Additional parent training components focus on parent interpersonal skills, such as effective communication, anger management, problem-solving between adults, and ways to give and receive support. In addition, the parent module assists parents in fostering reading skills in their children, setting up predictable homework routines, and building collaborative relationships with teachers.

The teacher training module emphasizes effective classroom management skills including effective use of teacher attention, praise and encouragement, proactive teaching strategies, the importance of building positive relationships with students, managing inappropriate classroom behaviors, and how to teach empathy, social skills and problem-solving in the classroom.

The child module is designed as either a "pull out" program for small groups of children at school or as a classroom wide curriculum. It emphasizes training children in a wide range of emotional literacy skills, such as empathy and perspective taking, friendship skills, anger management, interpersonal problem-solving, school rules and how to be successful at school.

Webster-Stratton et al. (2001) document multiple randomized control group evaluations of the parenting, teacher, and child training modules that attest to the utility of *The Incredible Years* series. Studies in the United States, England, Wales, Norway and Canada demonstrate increases in children's appropriate use of problem-solving strategies and prosocial conflict management with peers. Participating parents manifested increased levels of positive affect and more effective use of limit-setting as opposed to use of criticism, negative commands, and physical punishment in interactions with their children. Parents also expressed higher levels of self-confidence and reduced feelings of depression as well as improved positive family communication and problem-solving. Teachers who participated in the training also showed increases in their use of praise and encouragement and reductions in criticism and harsher forms of discipline in their interactions with students. Their students were perceived as being more engaged in school activities and less aggressive in their interactions with peers.

Overall, *The Incredible Years* is an excellent example of a comprehensive, multi-faceted prevention and intervention program delivered within the school setting but focusing on a wide range of social and emotional skills, not only targeting children, but teachers and parents as well.

# EMPIRICALLY SUPPORTED TREATMENTS THAT FACILLITATE CONFLICT RESOLUTION AND SOCIAL PROBLEM-SOLVING

## Overview

Social problem-solving training is designed to help students recognize interpersonal conflict situations, increase their repertoire of problem-solving strategies, analyze and evaluate the consequences of various actions, and select and implement socially appropriate solutions (Goldstein, 1999). Most programs use modeling, role-playing, and didactic teaching methods to promote problem-solving skills. The goal of such programs is to build positive peer relations by helping children learn to avoid interpersonal conflict and to handle those conflicts that are unavoidable in nonviolent, socially appropriate ways.

Johnson and Johnson (1995) make the case that effective conflict resolution training occurs within a school environment that purposely structures constructive conflict. This begins by creating a cooperative context in which long-term mutual interests outweigh the possible benefits of short-term individual gains. Use of cooperative learning procedures in the classroom establishes the context necessary for positive social interaction and mutual resolution of conflicts.

Effective conflict resolution also involves teaching students how to negotiate and mediate disputes with others, as well as regulating their own behavior. Negotiation involves the more basic skills of communicating one's needs as well as being able to invoke a range of strategies for maximizing joint positive outcomes. Social problem-solving and conflict resolution, like many other social-emotional skills, involves multiple components including the ability to listen to others, to understand others' thoughts and feelings, to communicate effectively, to develop a wide range of problem-solving alternatives, and to carefully consider the consequences of one's actions prior to actually responding.

## Programs Fostering Social Problem-Solving and Conflict Resolution in Schools

The PATHS (Promoting Alternative THinking Strategies) Curriculum is another model program for promoting emotional and social competencies and reducing aggression and behavior problems identified by the University of Colorado's Center for the Study and Prevention of Violence (Greenberg, Kusche, & Mihalic, 1998). This innovative curriculum is designed to be used by educators and counselors in a multi-year, universal prevention model. Although primarily focused on the school and classroom settings, information and activities are also included for use with parents.

The PATHS Curriculum was developed for use in the classroom setting with elementary school aged-children in grades K-5. Lessons are taught three times per week for a minimum of 20-30 minutes per day and include instruction in identifying and labeling feelings, expressing feelings, assessing the intensity of feelings, managing feelings, understanding the difference between feelings and behaviors, delaying gratification, controlling impulses, reducing stress, self-talk, reading and interpreting social cues, understanding the perspectives of others, using steps for problem-solving and decision-making, having a positive attitude toward life, self-awareness, nonverbal communication skills, and verbal communication skills. A key objective of promoting these developmental skills is to prevent or reduce behavioral and emotional problems. PATHS lessons teachers receive training in a two- to three-day workshop and in bi-weekly meetings with the curriculum consultant.

In their review of a number of controlled studies evaluating the PATHS curriculum, Greenberg, Kusche, & Mihalic (1998) report consistent data indicating improved protective factors and reduced behavioral risk factors in students exposed to PATHS. Evaluations have demonstrated significant improvements for program youth (regular education, special needs, and deaf) compared to control youth across a number of domains including self-control, understanding and recognition of emotions, ability to tolerate frustration, use of more effective conflict-resolution strategies, and thinking and planning skills. Significant decreases were also noted in such areas as anxiety and depression and conduct problems.

Another example of an ecological approach to conflict resolution incorporating a classroom and school wide value system of nonviolence is the Resolving Conflict Creatively Program (RCCP, DeJong, 1994). RCCP is a comprehensive, school-based, program designed for use with children in kindergarten through eighth grade and was designated as one of the "promising" violence prevention programs by the Promising Practices Network on Children, Families, and Communities (www.promisingpractices.net). The 51-lesson program curriculum and accompanying activities are tailored to be developmentally appropriate for specific age groups. Through promoting positive conflict resolution and understanding of different cultures, the program strives to create a more caring and peaceful school environment. RCCP now serves over 400 schools in 16 urban, suburban, and rural districts across the country. The primary goal of the program is to increase children's knowledge of ways to approach conflict situations and to resolve conflicts effectively in an effort to enhance children's positive interpersonal and intergroup relations. In addition, RCCP attempts to combat prejudice and stereotypes and the various types of conflict and violence that may arise as a result of these issues by teaching children how to recognize and oppose prejudice and by increasing their respect for and understanding of diversity. Finally, RCCP aims to transform the overall school culture into one that exemplifies nonviolent conflict resolution and a respect for and openness to diversity. In addition to in class lessons by trained teachers, the program includes the recruitment, training, and supervision of children to act as peer mediators. These mediators help facilitate the resolution of conflicts among children both in the classroom and elsewhere in school.

The RCCP curriculum has been evaluated in a number of quasi-experimental studies by Aber and colleagues (Aber, Brown, & Henrich, 1999; Aber, Brown, & Jones, 2003) in public schools in New York City. Results suggest that students who participated in the program were evaluated more positively by teachers in terms of their social behavior and emotional control. In addition, both suspension and dropout rates decreased significantly in those schools implementing the program and 90% of parents of participants reported increases in their own communication and problem-solving skills. These findings suggest that the impact of comprehensive programs like this one may stretch beyond the students who participated directly.

# Empirically Supported Treatments that Facillitate Anger Management

## Overview

School- and clinic-based anger management programs for children have proliferated in recent years (Smith, Larson, & Nuckles, 2006). Because anger is conceptualized as a multidimensional construct that includes affective, cognitive, and behavioral dimensions, most of these programs have multiple prevention and treatment components. In their review of anger management programs for youth, Smith et al. (2000) found that the most successful programs included emotion-focused strategies such as relaxation, increased self-awareness, and awareness of the feelings of others; cognitive strategies, such as problem solving and self-regulation; and behavioral strategies, such as developing specific skills in communication and assertiveness. In addition, successful interventions included clear efforts to encourage maintenance and generalization of skills outside the classroom or training setting. As a group, school- and clinic-based anger management programs for youth appeared to exert a strong influence on the control and regulation of aggressive and antisocial behaviors (Smith et al., 2000).

In a more recent review, Smith, Larson, and Nuckles (2006) examined a total of 28 school-based anger management interventions for treatment content and fidelity. Given its centrality in the clinical literature since the mid-1970's and their limitation to short-term, school-based treatment environments, it was not surprising to find that virtually all of the studies examined employed cognitive-behavioral techniques as a primary focus of the treatment package. Whereas there were variations in the preponderance of one clinical technique over another among the studies, three major divisions of cognitive-behavioral therapies dominated the anger management literature. These were: (a) coping skills therapies; (b) problem-solving therapies, and; (c) cognitive restructuring methods. Many of the interventions also referenced operant components, such as point systems, self-monitoring, or behavioral rehearsal.

Coping skills therapy involves the use of education, therapist modeling, skills rehearsal, and *in vivo* trials so that the student acquires a repertoire of adaptive responses to use in potentially volatile situations. Coping skills are not constrained by any established boundaries and subsume a variety of trainable behaviors. Common to most training programs are skills associated with anger regulation and alternatives to aggressive behavior. A sampling of coping skills included in the studies reviewed by Smith et al., (2006) include teaching adolescents coping skills for anger recognition and regulation, alternatives to aggression through assertiveness skills, social skills training, use of self-instruction phrases (e.g., "Cool it. Calm down.") to regulate levels of anger arousal, and skills to avoid victimization and in how to seek social support through friendships.

Problem-solving procedures generally follow a model that initially trains the student to recognize a problem when it is encountered and then to apply a prescriptive set of problem-solving skills leading toward an effective solution (D'Zurilla & Nezu, 2001). These problem-solving "steps" are typically trained as self-interrogatories:

1. What is the problem?
2. What are my choices?
3. What are the possible consequences?
4. Which one should I choose?
5. Now do it!
6. How did it work?

Problem-solving training is a substantial component in many anger management interventions with both elementary and secondary level students.

Cognitive-restructuring methods presuppose that anger is, in part, a function of maladaptive thought processes, and interventions focus on challenging and replacing those thoughts with more adaptive cognitions (Dobson & Dozois, 2001). This methodology requires that clients be developmentally able to reflect upon their own cognitions, thus it is typically reserved for older students. Cognitive-behavioral techniques were employed in the overwhelming number of intervention studies reviewed by Smith et al., (2006).

## Programs Fostering Anger Management in Schools

The Anger Coping Program (Lochman, 1992: Lochman & Wells, 1996) is on the best practices list compiled by the Hamilton Fish National Institute on School and Community Violence (www.hamfish.org). It is a school-based group intervention effort designed to reduce conduct problems, delinquency and substance abuse among 9-12 year-old students already identified as manifesting problem behaviors related to anger and aggression. Based on a social-cognitive model of anger arousal and consistent with social information processing models of social competence, the intervention focuses on the cognitive distortions and cognitive deficiencies often found in aggressive children. Group lessons, which take place over 12-18 sessions, promote self-instruction and awareness and serve to build social cognitive skills.

Research conducted by Lochman and colleagues provides empirical support for the notion that anger coping training utilizing social cognitive treatment methods can reduce the disruptive behaviors of students previously identified as manifesting externalizing problems at school. Both parents and teachers of students who participated in the training report less aggressive behavior after completion of training.

On the basis of the same contextual sociocognitive model, Lochman and colleagues (Lochman, 2004; Lochman & Wells, 2002) expanded the Anger Coping Program to include a parent training component. The new program, called the Coping Power Program, designed for boys, takes place over a 15 month intervention period. The child component includes eight intervention sessions in the 1st intervention year and 25 in the 2nd intervention year. Each group session lasts 40–60 minutes. The sessions include four to six boys and are co-led by a program specialist with a master's or doctoral degree in psychology or social work and by a school guidance counselor. Like the aforementioned Anger Coping Program, the Coping Power child component sessions emphasize the following: behavioral and personal goal-setting, awareness of feelings and associated physiological arousal, use of coping self-statements, distraction techniques and relaxation methods when provoked and made angry, organizational and study skills, perspective taking and attribution retraining, social problem–solving skills, and dealing with peer pressure and neighborhood-based problems by using refusal skills.

The parent component consists of 16 group sessions over the same 15-month intervention period. It is delivered in groups of four to six single parents or couples. Groups usually meet at the boys' schools and are led by two staff persons. Assertive attempts are made to promote parent attendance and to include both mothers and fathers in parent groups. The content of the parent component was derived from social-learning-theory–based parent training programs. Parents learn skills for identifying prosocial and disruptive behavioral targets in their children, rewarding appropriate child behaviors, giving effective instructions, establishing age-appropriate rules and expectations for children, applying effective consequences to negative child behavior, and establishing ongoing family communication through weekly family meetings. In addition, parents learn to support the sociocognitive skills that children learn in the Coping Power child component and to use stress-management skills to remain calm and in control during stressful or irritating disciplinary interactions with their children.

Evaluation of the Coping Power Program demonstrated significant impacts on several follow-up outcomes (Lochman, 2004). Specifically, boys who had participated in the program along with their parents had lower rates of self-reported covert delinquent behavior (theft, fraud, property damage) at 1-year follow-up. The program also had significant follow-up effects on teachers' ratings of children's improvements in school behavioral problems during the academic year after the program was completed. Boys who had been in the program demonstrated increasing behavioral improvements in school throughout the follow-up year, suggesting that intervention-produced changes in children's abilities to cope effectively with difficult peer and adult conflicts had continued to grow in the year following intervention.

Finally, both the parent and child components appear to have important roles in influencing boys' functioning at a 1-year follow-up. While the child component influenced improvements in boys' behavior at school, the parent component appeared to be the most critical intervention influence on boys' covert delinquency and substance use at follow-up. In addition, there was evidence that Coping Power had clearer effects on white boys' parent-rated substance use and school behavior functioning than was the case for minority children, most of whom were African-American.

Overall, these results suggest that social cognitive interventions, and particularly those that include a parent component in addition to the typical child training, can have a substantial effect on students' ability to regulate their anger and to develop more effective and socially desirable coping strategies when faced with stressful situations.

## Conclusions and Future Considerations

Given that greater numbers of clinicians are now finding schools to be an interesting and often inviting context for the delivery of mental health services, it is important to understand some of the parameters of effective service delivery in this particular setting. School-based empirically supported treatments in school settings share a number of key characteristics. For one, they are comprehensive and multisystemic in their approach, often targeting multiple agents including families, teachers, the school ecology, and even the community, in addition to the identified "problem" child. Secondly, effective strategies tend to be preventative in nature and are often delivered on a universal or school wide basis. Thirdly, many of these strategies tend to be "solution driven"; that is they are focused on enhancing overall well-being and competence rather than ameliorating a specific deficit. Finally, effective school-based therapeutic interventions tend to involve a collaborative service delivery model, whereby a variety of stakeholders are involved in establishing and reaching treatment goals.

This chapter reviewed a number of empirically supported treatment programs under the general umbrella of social and emotional learning. These programs face the somewhat daunting challenge of not only enhancing students' repertoire of prosocial attitudes and skills while simultaneously reducing problematic, disruptive, and antagonistic behaviors but also must contribute to students academic performance if they are to be taken seriously by parents and educators. Although it is still very early in the overall evaluation scheme, initial results suggest that programs designed to promote emotional literacy, problem-solving and conflict resolution skills, and effective anger management in schools may go a long way in producing not only academically capable students but those who contribute to the fabric of our society by way of being caring and respectful human beings.

## REFERENCES

Aber, L.J., Brown, J.L., & Henrich, CC. (1999). *Teaching conflict resolution: An effective school-based approach to violence prevention.* New York: National Center for Children in Poverty.

Aber, L.J., Brown, J.L., & Jones, S.M. (2003). Developmental trajectories toward violence in middle childhood: Course, demographic differences, and response to school-based intervention. *Developmental Psychology, 39,* 324-348.

Adelman, H.S., & Taylor, L. (2000). Shaping the future of mental health in schools. *Psychology in the Schools, 37,* 49-60.

Adelman, H.S., & Taylor, L. (2006). *The school leader's guide to student learning supports.* Thousand Oaks, CA: Corwin Press.

Bronfenbrenner, U. (1979). *The ecology of human development.* Cambridge, MA: Harvard University Press.

Collaborative for Academic, Social, and Emotional Learning [CASEL]. (2005). *Safe and sound: An educational leader's guide to evidence-based social and emotional learning programs – Illinois edition.* Retrieved October 26, 2007, from *http://www.casel.org.*

Cowen, E. L., Wyman, P. A., Work, W. C., & Iker, M. R. (1995). A preventive intervention for enhancing resilience among highly stressed urban children. *The Journal of Primary Prevention, 15,* 247–260.

DeJong, W. (1994). *Building the peace: The resolving conflict creatively program.* Washington, DC: U.S. Department of Justice, National Institute of Justice.

Dobson, K.S., & Dozois, D.J.A. (2001). Historical and philosophical bases of the cognitive therapies. In K.S. Dobson (Ed.), *The handbook of cognitive-behavioral therapies* (2nd ed., pp 3-39). New York: Wiley.

Dryfoos, J. (1994). *Full service schools: A revolution in health and social services for children, youth and families.* San Francisco: Jossey-Bass.

Dwyer, K., Osher, D., & Warger, C. (1998). *Early warning, timely response: A guide to safe schools.* Washington, DC: U.S. Department of Education. Available at: *http://www.ed.gov/offices/OSERS/OSEP/earlywrn.html.*

D'Zurilla, T.J., & Nezu, A.M. (2001). Problem-solving therapies. In K.S. Dobson (Ed.), *The handbook of cognitive-behavioral therapies* (2nd ed., pp 211-245). New York: Wiley.

Elias, M. J., Weissberg, R. P., Hawkins, J. D., Perry, C. L., Zins, J. E., Dodge, K. A., et al. (1994). The school-based promotion of social competence: Theory, research, practice, and policy. In R. J. Haggerty, N. Garmezy, M. Rutter, & L. Sherrod (Eds.), *Stress, risk and resilience in children and adolescence: Processes, mechanisms, and interventions* (pp. 269–315). New York: Cambridge University Press.

Goldstein, A.P. (1999). Aggression reduction strategies: Effective and ineffective. *School Psychology Quarterly, 14,* 40-58.

Goleman, D. (1995). *Emotional intelligence: Why it can matter more than IQ.* New York: Bantam Books.

Greenberg, M.T., Kusche, C., & Mihalic, S.F. (1998). *Promoting Alternative Thinking Strategies (PATHS): Blueprints for Violence Prevention, Book Ten.* Blueprints for Violence Prevention Series (D.S. Elliott, Series Editor). Boulder, CO: Center for the Study and Prevention of Violence, Institute of Behavioral Science, University of Colorado.

Hawkins, J. D., Catalano, R. F., Kosterman, R., Abbot, R., & Hill, K. G. (1999). Preventing adolescent health-risk behaviors by strengthening protection during childhood. *Archives of Pediatrics and Adolescent Medicine, 153,* 225–234.

Howard, K.A., Flora, J., & Griffin, M. (1999). Violence-prevention programs in schools: State of the science and implications for future research. *Applied & Preventive Psychology, 8,* 197-215.

Johnson, D.W., & Johnson, R.T. (1995). *Teaching students to be peacemakers* (3rd ed.). Edina, MN: Interaction Book Company.

Lochman, J.E. (2004). The Coping Power Program for preadolescent aggressive boys and their parents: Outcome effects at the 1–year follow-up. *Journal of Consulting and Clinical Psychology 4,* 571–578.

Lochman, John E., and Karen C. Wells (2002). Contextual social–cognitive mediators and child outcome: A test of the theoretical model in the coping power program. *Development and Psychopathology, 14,* 971–93.

National Center for Health Education. (1997). *Growing healthy: An examination of comprehensive school health education's role in healthy lifestyles for youth.* Waco, TX: WRS Group.

Pluymert, K. (2002). Best practices in developing exemplary mental health programs in schools. In A. Thomas & J. Grimes (Eds.), *Best Practices in School Psychology IV* (Vol. 2, pp. 963-975). Bethesda, MD: National Association of School Psychologists.

Resnick, M. D., Bearman, P. S., Blum, R. W., Bauman, K. E., Harris, K. M., Jones, J., et al. (1997). Protecting adolescents from harm: Findings from the National Longitudinal Study on Adolescent Health. *Journal of the American Medical Association, 278,* 823–832.

Salovey, P., & Mayer, J. D. (1990). Emotional intelligence. *Imagination, Cognition and Personality, 9,* 185–211.

Sameroff, A.J., Peck, S.C., & Eccles, J.L. (2004). Changing ecological determinants of conduct problems from early adolescence to early adulthood. *Development and Psychopathology, 16,* 873-896.

Seligman, M. E. P., & Csikszentmihalyi, M. (2000). Positive psychology: An introduction. *American Psychologist, 55,* 5–14.

Short, R.J., & Talley, R.C. (1997). Rethinking psychology and the schools: Implications of recent national policy. *American Psychologist, 52,* 234-240.

Smith, D.C., Larson, J.D., DeBaryshe, B., & Salzman, M. (2000). Anger management for youth: What works and for whom? In D.S. Sandhu & C.B.Aspy (Eds.), *Violence in American schools: A practical guide for counselors* (pp. 217-230). Alexandria, VA: American Counseling Association.

Smith, D.C., Larson, J. & Nuckles, D.R. (2006). A critical analysis of school-based anger management programs for youth. In S.R. Jimerson and M.J. Furlong (Eds.), *Handbook of school violence and school safety: From research to practice* (pp. 365-382). Mahwah, NJ: Lawrence Erlbaum Associates.

U.S. Department of Education (1998). *Early warning, timely response: A guide to safe schools.* Available at: *http://cecp.air.org/guide/guide.pdf*

Waxman, R., & Weist, M. (1999). Toward collaboration in the growing education-mental health interface. *Clinical Psychology Review,* 19, 239-253.

Webster-Stratton, C., Mihalic, S., Fagan, A., Arnold, D., Taylor, T., & Tingley, C. (2001). *The Incredible Years: Parent, Teacher and Child Training Series: Blueprints for Violence Prevention, Book Eleven.* Blueprints for Violence Prevention Series (D.S. Elliott, Series Editor). Boulder, CO: Center for the Study and Prevention of Violence, Institute of Behavioral Science, University of Colorado.

Weissberg, R.P., Durlak, J.A., Taylor, R.D., Dymnicki, A.B., I O'Brien, M.U. (in press). Promoting social and emotional learning enhances school success: Implications of a meta-analysis. *American Psychologist, 62.*

Weissberg, R. P., & Greenberg, M. T. (1998). School and community competence-enhancement and prevention programs. In I. E. Sigel & K. A. Renninger (Eds.), *Handbook of child psychology* (Vol. 4, pp. 877–954). New York: Wiley.

Weist, M. (Ed.), (1999). Challenges and opportunities in expanded school mental health [Special issue]. *Clinical Psychology Review,* 19(2).

# Section III. The Laboratory Method in Psychotherapy: Manualized and Structured Treatments

In: Toward a Science of Clinical Psychology
Editor: Luciano L'Abate, pp. 149-159

ISBN: 978-1-60456-062-6


*Chapter VIII*

# MANUALIZED TREATMENTS IN PSYCHOTHERAPY

***Katherine L. Muller, Simon A. Rego and William C. Sanderson***

## ABSTRACT

Treatment manuals represent the standardization of a particular psychotherapeutic intervention and are at the heart of the application of the scientific method in psychotherapy. Over the last thirty years, treatment manuals have moved from their original birthplace in the realm of outcome research to the shelves of clinicians in practice settings. Along the way, treatment manuals and the so-called "manualized treatments" they represent have been the subject of praise, criticism, and controversy. In this chapter, we review the history and development of treatment manuals and describe their role in psychotherapy research and practice. We also consider the advantages and disadvantages of manualized treatments. We conclude with speculation about the future of treatment manuals in the field of psychotherapy.

## DEFINITION OF "TREATMENT MANUAL"

A treatment manual may be thought of as an "instruction book" for providing a psychotherapeutic intervention. Though their content and format vary widely, treatment manuals are typically defined as materials that present the essential components of a particular psychotherapy (Kazdin, 1998). These components include ideas (e.g., the goal of the treatment is to change illogical thinking), techniques (e.g., in order to accomplish this, use logical analysis which is defined as... ) , and procedures (e.g., in order to perform logical analysis complete a thought record with the patient by following these steps *......).* Manuals may take many material forms, especially with the technology available today. Originally presented in a text format, manual formats now include audio and video recordings, as well as digital media and Internet-based interactive websites.

Treatment manuals vary in their level of specificity. Some manuals are very specific; essentially, they serve as "scripts" designed to be used in a strict, stepwise manner. More frequently, manuals present essential components and timelines but allow for some flexibility in style of presentation and individualization to patient needs (Kendall, Chu, Gifford, Hayes, & Nauta, 1998). Yet other manuals are far less specific about required therapy content and procedures. These manuals are often deemed "principle-based" because they provide a framework for treatment formulation but do not specify timeframes or techniques (Hayes, 2002).

## PURPOSE OF TREATMENT MANUALS

Treatment manuals are distinguished from other books or writings about psychotherapy in that they provide a general framework and elaborate on the specific steps a therapist must take in conducting a therapy (Kendall et al., 1998). In addition, manuals present components and procedures that are considered essential to the therapy (Luborsky & DeRubeis, 1984). Manuals may serve many purposes depending on the context in which they are used, however, there appears to be some level of consensus in the field about their primary purposes (Carroll & Nuro, 2002; Luborksy & DeRubeis, 1984).

First, treatment manuals are used in the context of psychotherapy research. Manuals operationalize the procedures of psychotherapy, which increases uniformity and makes treatments testable and replicable (Weissman & Sanderson, 2002). They also allow for evaluation of outcome across studies utilizing the same treatment manuals. Manuals are also particularly useful in comparative studies of psychotherapy approaches (Luborsky & DeRubeis, 1984). In this context, the manual provides a way to develop measurement systems that may highlight the differences and similarities in treatment approaches. Treatment manuals are a major staple of identifying empirically-supported treatments in that they allow for replication of interventions in additional studies, aid in practitioner accountability for procedures utilized, and allow for outcome evaluation (Addis, 2002; Weissman & Sanderson, 2002).

Another primary purpose of treatment manuals is to assess therapist adherence to treatment protocol. In other words, treatment manuals assist in determining whether a given therapist "adhered to" or complied with the treatment protocol. Therapist adherence rating scales are often developed based on the content of a treatment manual (Addis & Waltz, 2002; Luborksy & DeRubeis, 1984). This is an essential part of the scientific method in that it allows investigators to assess the internal validity of the study or, in other words, confirm that in fact the treatment was delivered as specified.

Training of therapists is another important purpose of a treatment manual (Luborksy & DeRubeis, 1984; Wilson, 1998). The recommendations contained in a treatment manual may serve as a workbook for therapists learning a particular treatment in either clinical or research settings. Since manuals contain the essential components of a treatment intervention, they can be used for training with many different therapist audiences. Manuals also serve a role in supervision of therapists learning the procedures in the manuals. Supervisors can refer to the manual to assess therapist adherence and progress in learning how to apply the treatment.

Psychotherapy treatment manuals have also come to serve a significant clinical purpose in the last several years. Manuals have become the primary vehicle through which treatments are disseminated and shared in the field of psychotherapy (Addis & Waltz, 2002). Treatment manuals are the conduits that allow investigators to convey information from the research context to the clinical frontlines. Manuals are efficient packages that contain information found to be efficacious in research settings. In some cases, clinicians are applying these interventions as written and assessing their outcomes in "real-world" settings (e.g.,Sanderson, Raue, & Wetzler, 1998; Wade, Treat, & Stuart, 1998).

## The History of Treatment Manuals

Initially, treatment manuals were designed to outline treatments for research pursuits and to provide training materials for therapists (Kazdin, 1998). In the last thirty years, however, manuals have not only become *de rigueur* for research studies but they have also become a centerpiece of clinical practice. The history of the treatment manual is a reflection of the evolution of the field of psychotherapy itself over the last three decades.

The nascence of the treatment manual can be traced back to behavior therapists in the late 1960's (e.g., Wolpe, 1969). These early "manuals" were sets of procedures with a prescribed system of implementation (Luborsky & DeRubeis, 1984). It is logical that behavior therapists were the first to create manuals, as the therapies used therein tended to be structured and prescriptive and more easily committed to text. Much as the behavior therapist would specify certain patient behaviors in the treatment, the manual was a specification of therapist behavior and procedure in session (Luborsky & DeRubeis, 1984). However, over the course of the last thirty years, all schools of thought in the field of psychotherapy have contributed their form of manual.

Many authors cite a growing advocacy for psychotherapy research in the late 1970's and early 1980's as the impetus for creation of formal treatment manuals as we know them today (Luborsky & DeRubeis, 1984; Moras, 2002). As psychotherapy outcome studies were pursued during the 1980's, concern about treatment methodology within the studies grew. Researchers committed to sound research designs advocated for more "systematic" treatment manuals to guide the implementation of the therapies being considered in these outcome studies (Luborksy & DeRubeis, 1984). Other advocates for this more scientific approach to psychotherapy research included congressional committees during President Jimmy Carter's administration, third-party insurance payers, and many research psychologists and psychiatrists. One of these psychiatrists was Gerald Klerman, then director of the Alcohol, Drug Abuse and Mental Health Administration (ADAMHA) and a pioneer in the scientific evaluation of psychotherapeutic interventions (Luborsky & DeRubeis, 1984; Weissman, 2007). Klerman and others argued that the field should employ the same rigorous methods and measures in psychotherapy outcome research that had been successfully utilized in pharmacological research.

With the support and influence of these various camps of advocates, funding for psychotherapy outcome studies soon followed. Other interested parties, such as the American Psychological Association and the American Psychiatric Association, worked with the Senate Finance Health Subcommittee to establish clinical trials of psychotherapy. This push for research continued throughout President Reagan's administration in the 1980's. Though some of the funds initially committed to these research efforts were cut, the level of enthusiasm for this scientific approach to psychotherapy research remained high (Luborsky & DeRubeis, 1984).

Work in the area of psychotherapy research in the 1980's set the standard for years to come. During this decade, the field witnessed the landmark Treatment of Depression Collaborative Research Program (TDCRP). This multi-site study, initiated by the National Institute of Mental Health, utilized manualized treatment protocols to investigate the effectiveness of two forms of psychotherapy for depression. In the study, investigators compared cognitive behavior therapy and interpersonal psychotherapy to pharmacotherapy interventions. Since the study involved three treatment sites and multiple study therapists, all three treatment interventions had to be standardized and treatment manuals were the logical choice to accomplish this goal. This study established a standard for the use of treatment manuals in future psychotherapy comparison studies and is often cited as a marker of the paradigm shift in psychotherapy research (Elkin, Parloff, Hadley, & Autry, 1985; Luborsky & DeRubeis, 1984).

After this "small revolution" (Luborsky & DeRubeis, 1984) within the field in the 1980's, treatment manuals became standard equipment in the research of psychotherapy outcome. Indeed, some have deemed them as essential for the receipt of study funding (Carroll & Nuro, 2002; Kazdin, 1998). Treatment manuals have since become almost synonymous with empirical approaches in psychotherapy. In fact, the term "evidence-based treatment" (EBT) has been coined to describe a psychotherapy that has been defined *in a manual* and tested for efficacy in a controlled clinical trial (Chambless, et al., 1996). Treatment manuals have also been developed outside the research domain by clinicians in practice settings. Originally the territory of the behavior therapist, practitioners of many different types of psychotherapy have created manuals for their treatment approaches.

In 1995, Division 12 (Clinical Psychology) of the American Psychological Association provided their recommendations for training in and dissemination of empirically-supported treatments (Task Force on the Promotion and Dissemination of Psychological Procedures, 1995). This report's support of the use of empirically-supported treatments- and, by association, treatment manuals- in practice settings was both praised and criticized. Despite this polarization in response, this report increased the notoriety of treatment manuals (e.g., Woody & Sanderson, 1998). Throughout the 1990's and until the present, psychotherapy research has continued, both in the traditional "efficacy" research setting and in the "effectiveness" setting of regular clinical practice. In 1999, the National Institute of Mental Health spearheaded a "public health" research agenda that includes the goal of increasing the effectiveness and use of empirically-supported treatments in practice settings (Moras, 2002). This initiative bodes well for the continued use of treatment manuals, as they are a typical component of the application of an empirically-supported psychotherapeutic treatment.

## "Manual-Based" Treatments

Treatments that have been described in a manual are sometimes referred to as "manual-based" treatments or "manualized" treatments (Wilson, 1998). The term "manualized treatment" has become associated with, and is at times used interchangeably with, the terms "empirically-supported treatment" and/or "evidence-based treatment". This reflects the connection to research in the origin of treatment manuals. Most of the extant manuals have been used in research studies evaluating the efficacy of a certain psychotherapeutic treatment. If efficacy is indeed demonstrated for a certain treatment, it is deemed an "empirically-supported" treatment. Treatments developed as part of these studies- or treatments developed based on these studies- are said to be "evidence-based treatments" (see Chambless et al., 1996 for a comprehensive definition of an evidence-based treatment). It is worth noting that today there exist treatment manuals that are not empirically-supported. In fact, some treatment manuals are written and published without the methods having been tested for efficacy (Addis & Waltz, 2002) or are "supported" by the use of "pseudoscientific" evidence (cf. Lilienfeld, Lynn, & Lohr , 2002). For our purposes, we will use the term "manualized treatment" to refer to treatment interventions that have an associated manual and have peer-reviewed empirical support.

## Treatment Manual Development

The development of the first treatment manuals was more practical than purposeful. They were developed to assist in the conduct or replication of a psychotherapy intervention. Since that time, however, the roles of treatment manuals have expanded to include those of instructional guide, assessment instrument, and clinical practice guideline. These changing roles have required increased attention to the development and composition of treatment manuals. The original, at times overly simplistic, model of readily transporting a treatment found to be efficacious in a research trial to the clinical frontline has proven unrealistic. The obstacles have included funding for manual development, getting completed manuals into the hands of clinicians, manuals not being "clinician-friendly", and the criticism of manuals being too general to apply to a diverse array of clients (Carroll & Nuro, 2002). As a result, rather than being an aid to a scientific investigation, the development of a treatment manual itself has become the subject of research.

There are many opinions about the optimal way to develop a treatment manual (e.g., Carroll & Nuro, 2002; Chorpita, 2002; Westen, 2002 ). Some believe that treatment manuals should be developed *prior* to the initiation of a study to test an intervention. Others see value in studying certain procedures first and then creating treatment manuals based on the findings of these studies. New theories abound on ways to bridge the gap that has traditionally existed between research and practice through involving both camps in the design of treatment manuals. One of the most recent models of treatment manual development is the "stage model" (Carroll & Nuro, 2002). This model is based on extant stage approaches in psychotherapy research and suggests that treatment manuals progress through three stages that map relatively closely onto the stages of psychotherapy research. Stage I manuals provide initial specification of treatment goals, format, and techniques and are typically used in pilot trials and feasibility studies. Stage II treatment manuals are typically those used in randomized efficacy trials and provide standards for training and supervision of therapists, allow for discrimination from both control and other approaches, and aid in the evaluation of treatment process. Stage III manuals are utilized primarily for dissemination to the clinical community and are used as part of effectiveness trials.

## CURRENT STATUS OF TREATMENT MANUALS

Treatment manuals have allowed researchers- and now clinicians- to better communicate the nature of a treatment intervention. They have also aided in our understanding of the active ingredients in a psychotherapeutic treatment because they define interventions and allow for measurement of adherence to procedures (Luborsky & DeRubeis, 1984). Today, treatment manuals retain their place in the realm of research and are increasingly used in non-research, clinical practice settings. Despite their growing presence in the field, treatment manuals and manualized treatments continue to be a subject of debate among practitioners of psychotherapy. In fact, with the possible exception of the controversy over prescription privileges for psychologists, there is probably no issue more hotly debated among practicing psychologists today. Other topics that influence the status, acceptance, and use of treatment manuals today include dissemination efforts, new conceptualizations of manuals, and new applications of treatment manuals as training tools (Addis, 2002; Huppert, Fabbro, & Barlow, 2006).

### Acceptance of Treatment Manuals

While treatment manuals are generally accepted in research settings, their place in the clinical realm is a point of controversy. Many clinicians have embraced and praised the use of manualized treatments (Heimberg, 1998; Wilson, 1998), while others have been far less apt to accept this mode of treatment (Garfield, 1996). These reactions have ranged from cautious consideration to outright rejection (Kendall, 1998; Wilson, 1998). Though proponents of manualized treatments have not been able to address all of the concerns and complaints raised, they have attempted to respond to many of them, resulting in increasingly user-friendly and comprehensive manuals (Wilson, 1998). There has been an abundance of opinion papers on the topic of manualized treatments and their advantages and disadvantages. Herein, we provide a summary of the most frequently cited concerns and responses to them.

#### *Clinical Judgment and "Nonspecific" Factors*

A common criticism of manualized treatments is that they undermine or even remove the judgment of practitioners from the provision of the treatment (Kendall, 1998; Wilson, 1998). Additionally, some believe that manuals turn therapists into "robots", with no regard for therapeutic relationship and alliance. Supporters of manualized treatments respond to these criticisms with an emphasis on the "nonspecific" factors that are part of all psychotherapies, including manualized psychotherapies. These factors, which include but are not limited to, trust, alliance, listening, and collaboration, are also necessary in applying a manualized treatment. There are also some proponents who highlight the advantages of the "actuarial" approach of manuals, citing research that finds this approach to be more effective than interventions based on subjective clinical judgment over a broad range of therapists with varying competency (Wilson, 1998).

### *Comorbidity*

Critics of manual-based treatments also suggest that manuals do not address and account for comorbidity, the co-existence of symptoms and/or syndromes. They cite the typical treatment manual's focus on a certain diagnosis or set of symptoms as neglecting other co-occurring symptoms or diagnoses, and that this omission may detrimentally affect outcome. Proponents of manualized treatments cite findings of a number of studies that demonstrate that comorbidity does not negatively affect efficacy of the treatment (Kendall, 1998.) They also cite a handful of studies that find that manuals for a specific problem can actually reduce comorbid problems (Wilson, 1998). Supporters do note that this is an area for further research, as effectiveness studies of the treatments in community settings are needed to confirm these findings.

### *Innovation*

Another common criticism of manualized treatments is that, as they are widely used and recommended, they may restrict innovation in the field. Critics fear that use of these treatments will promote dogmatic adherence to certain treatment manuals and prevent further research and development of new psychotherapy approaches (Addis & Waltz, 2002). In response to these concerns, proponents recognize the fact that manualized treatments do not work for everyone, and this gap itself spurs further research and innovation (Wilson,1998). In addition, treatment manual advocates note that manualized treatments promote accountability and evaluation of use in diverse clinical settings. This evaluative process aids in connecting research and "real-life" clinical application. They suggest that this connection may then help identify gaps in knowledge and inspire further innovation and development (Wilson, 1998.)

### *Flexibility*

More than one clinician writing about treatment manuals has referred to them as "straitjackets" (Moras, 2002). Opponents cite a lack of flexibility as a significant drawback of manualized treatments. They believe that manuals limit the ability to tailor interventions as the therapist sees fit for an individual patient (Moras, 2002). Proponents of treatment manuals have refuted this claim by providing examples of manualized treatments being used in flexible ways by clinicians. They also emphasize the role of treatment manuals in guiding "what" is to be covered in the treatment but not the style in which it is delivered. Other users of treatment manuals report that it is common for clinicians to be very structured and vigilantly adherent at first, but that they experiment with flexibility and creativity as they become more comfortable with the manual (Kendall, 1998; Kendall et al., 1998). Flexibility in treatment manuals remains an issue to be further explored and, possibly, researched. Critics and supporters of manualized treatments appear to agree on this point.

For an illustration and pertinent discussion of the balance between adhering to a manual while being flexible enough to address the patient's individual psychopathology, interested readers should see the series describing the actual use of a manual in clinical practice published in the online journal *Pragmatic Case Studies in Psychotherapy* (http://pcsp.libraries.rutgers.edu/viewissue.php?id=14). The series includes a lead article on the challenges of utilizing a treatment manual for a patient with social phobia (Edwards &

Kannan, 2006) and features commentaries relevant to the issue of flexibility (Fishman, 2006; Sanderson, 2006; Turk, 2006).

## Dissemination

A logical "next step" in the process of manualized treatment development is the movement of these treatments from the research setting to the clinical setting. This process is typically referred to as "dissemination" (Addis, 2002). For the most part, dissemination has been conceived of as an effort to transport treatments with established empirical support to clinical settings. This transmission is typically accomplished through the vehicle of the treatment manual. In brief, once a treatment has demonstrated efficacy in a research trial, the manual used for the treatment intervention is then, ideally, made available to clinical practice settings.

Certain factors have affected the successful dissemination of manualized treatments. These factors include cost of dissemination, "clinician-friendliness" of treatment manuals, lack of training in and utilization of manualized treatments, and clinician's opinions of manualized treatments. While obstacles to successfully transmitting manualized treatments exist, dissemination efforts have been bolstered by a number of "benchmarking studies". "Benchmarking" is defined as "a method of measuring performance against established standards of best practice" (On-line Medical Dictionary, 2007). In the field of psychotherapy, benchmarking studies strive to apply an efficacious, empirically-supported treatment in a clinical setting to demonstrate its effectiveness in the "real world". A number of studies have demonstrated that manualized empirically-supported treatments maintain their effects when used in clinical practice. Examples of these benchmarking studies include the successful application of treatments for obsessive-compulsive disorder (Franklin, Abramowitz, Kozak, Levitt, and Foa, 2000), panic disorder (Sanderson, Raue, & Wetzler, 1998; Wade, Treat, & Stuart, 1998), and depression (Persons, Bostrom, & Bertagnolli, 1999). More studies like this are needed to confirm whether manualized treatments consistently enhance outcomes in clinical practice (Addis & Waltz, 2002).

## Treatment Manuals in Therapist Training

Recent assessments of patterns in clinical training suggest that the impact of manualized treatments has been modest at best (Weisz & Addis, 2006). Though it appears that doctoral psychology training programs are providing more information about these treatments, supervision in the application of manualized treatments has declined in recent years (Weisz & Addis, 2006). Some suggest that this absence of training in the academic setting is due the general lack of knowledge about manualized treatments in the field as a whole, preferences and biases of the instructors creating curricula, and a lack of consensus about which treatments should be provided. To remedy this, some proponents of manualized treatments are calling for training program accreditation guidelines to reflect a commitment to these treatments (Dobson & Hamilton, 2002; Moras, 2002). In contrast to the academic training situation, the private and public sectors have increased available training in manualized, empirically-supported treatments.

## Conclusions and Future Directions

Treatment manuals have indeed been the catalysts of a small revolution in psychotherapy research and practice (Luborsky & DeRubeis, 1984). This revolution began in the 1960's and 70's and continues to have an impact today. Despite continued controversy about the development and acceptance of manualized treatments, it is likely that they will remain a fixture in the future of psychotherapy.

Treatment manuals are likely to continue as a force in both the research and clinical realms of psychotherapy. These treatments fit well into the current general healthcare environment with its emphasis on evidence-based interventions (Strosahl, 1998) and therapist accountability (Carroll & Nuro, 2002). In addition, manualized treatments are particularly well suited to managed care approaches to healthcare, the preeminent healthcare system in the United States today.

It is likely that the movement to reconceptualize and dispel myths about manuals will continue. Efforts to encourage therapists to use treatment manuals appropriately with flexibility and sensitivity, while still adhering to the general principles outlined are supported by many in the field (Huppert et al, 2006). Many suggest creating manuals that are flexible, yet still structured enough to allow treatments to be distinguished from each other (Chorpita, 2002).

Both critics and proponents of manualized treatments have suggested that the field recognize the original purpose of psychotherapy research, which was to provide guidance for modification of actual clinical practices and, ultimately, improve clinical outcomes (Hayes, 2002). In keeping with this directive, attempts are being made to better bridge, and ultimately integrate, research and clinical perspectives and needs. Rather than viewing a treatment manual only as a product of a research study that is passed to the clinical realm, some suggest that clinicians be more involved in the initial development of the treatment and the resulting manual (Addis, 2002; Carroll & Nuro, 2002). This collaborative approach is likely to become more commonplace in treatment manual development and may aid in increasing the acceptance and use of manualized treatments by more clinicians.

## References

Addis, M.E. (2002). Methods for disseminating research products and increasing evidence-based practice:

Promises, obstacles and future directions. *Clinical psychology: Science and Practice, 9, 367-378.*

Addis, M.E., & Waltz, J. (2002). Implicit and untested assumptions about the role of psychotherapy treatment manuals in evidence-based mental health practice. *Clinical Psychology: Research and Practice, 9, 421-424.*

benchmarking. (n.d.). *On-line Medical Dictionary.* Retrieved April 15, 2007, from

Dictionary.com website: http://dictionary.reference.com/browse/benchmarking

Carroll, K.M., & Nuro, K.F. (2002). One size cannot fit all: A stage model for psychotherapy manual development. *Clinical Psychology: Research and Practice, 9, 396-406.*

Chambless, D.L., Sanderson, W.C., Shoham, V., Johnson, S.B., Pope, K., Crits-Christoph, P., Baker, M., Johnson,B., Woody, S.R., Sue, S., Beutler, L., Williams, D., & McCurry, S. (1996). Update on empirically validated therapies. *The Clinical Psychologist, 49(2), 5-15.*

Chorpita, B.F. (2002). Treatment manuals for the real world: Where do we build them? *Clinical Psychology: Research and Practice, 9, 431-433.*

Dobson, K.S. & Hamilton, K.E. (2002). The stage model for psychotherapy manual development: A valuable tool for promoting evidence-based practice. *Clinical Psychology: Science and Practice, 9, 407-409.*

Edwards, D. J.A., Kannan, S. (2006, February 17). Identifying and targeting idiosyncratic cognitive processes ingroup therapy for social phobia: The case of Vumile. *Pragmatic Case Studies in Psychotherapy,Vol. 2(1), Article 1.* Retrieved June 11, 2007 from http://pcsp.libraries.rutgers.edu/ include /getdoc.php?id =373&article=65&mode=pdf

Elkin, I., Parloff, M. B., Hadley, S. W., & Autry, J. H. (1985). NIMH Treatment of DepressionCollaborative Research Program: Background and research plan. *Archives of General Psychiatry, 42, 305-316.*

Fishman, S. T.. (2006, February 17). A yeoman's job in developing, refining, revising, and executing a manualized group version of the Clark and Wells (1995) model, although more remains to be done.

Pragmatic Case Studies in Psychotherapy,Vol. 2(1), Article 4. *Retrieved June 11, 2007 from http://pcsp.libraries.rutgers.edu/include/getdoc.php?id=389&article=68&mode=pdf*

Franklin, M.E., Abramowitz, J.S., Kozak, M.J., Levitt, J.T., & Foa, E.B. (2000). Effectiveness of exposure and ritual prevention for obsessive-compulsive disorder: Randomized compared with

nonrandomized samples. *Journal of Consulting and Clinical Psychology, 68, 594-602.*

Garfield, S.L., (1996). Some problems associated with "validated" forms of psychotherapy. *Clinical Psychology: Research and Practice, 3, 241-244.*

Hayes, S. C. (2002). Getting to dissemination. *Clinical Psychology: Science and Practice, 9, 410-415.*

Heimberg, R.G. (1998). Manual-based treatment: An essential ingredient of clinical practice in the 21st century. *Clinical Psychology: Research and Practice, 5, 387-390.*

Huppert, J.D., Fabbro, A. & Barlow, D.H. (2006). Evidence-based practice and psychological treatments.

In C. G. Goodheart, A.E.Kazdin, & R.J. Sternberg (Eds.), *Evidence-based Pscyhotherapy: Where Practice and Research Meet.* Washington, DC: American Psychological Association.

Kendall, P.C., Chu, B., Gifford, A., Hayes, C., & Nauta, M. (1998). Breathing life into a manual: Flexibility and creativity with manual-based treatments. *Cognitive and Behavioral Practice, 5, 177-198.*

Kazdin, A.E. (1998). Treatment manuals in clinical practice: Introduction to the series. *Clinical Psychology: Science and Practice, 5(3), 361-362.*

Lilienfeld, S.O., Lynn, S.J., & Lohr, J.M. (Eds.). (2002). *Science and Pseudoscience in Clinical Psychology*. New York: Guilford.

Luborsky, L. & DeRubeis, R. J. (1984). The use of psychotherapy treatment manuals: A small revolution in psychotherapy research style. *Clinical Psychology Review, 4, 5-14.*

Moras, K. (2002). A tool to advance the effectiveness and dissemination of empirically supported psychotherapies and the NIMH Public Health Research Agenda. *Clinical Psychology: Research and Practice, 9, 425-430.*

Persons, J.B., Bostrom, A., & Bertagnolli, A. (1999). Results of randomized controlled trials of cognitive therapy for depression generalize to private practice. *Cognitive Therapy and Research, 23, 535-548.*

Sanderson, W. C. (2006, February 17). Evaluating Adherence and Flexibility in the Use of a Manual in Clinical Practice. *Pragmatic Case Studies in Psychotherapy,Vol. 2(1), Article 3*. Retrieved June 11, 2007 from http://pcsp.libraries.rutgers.edu/include/getdoc.php?id=383&article=67&mode=pdf

Sanderson, W.C., Raue, P.J., & Wetzler, S. (1998). The generalizability of cognitive behavior therapy for panic disorder. *Journal of Cognitive Psychotherapy, 12, 323-330.*

Strosahl, K. (1998). The dissemination of manual-based psychotherapies in managed care: Promises, problems, and prospects. *Clinical Psycholog: Science and Practice, 5, 386.*

Turk, C. L. (2006, February 17). The case Of Vumile: Breathing life into a manual and model. *Pragmatic Case Studies in Psychotherapy,Vol. 2(1), Article 5*. Retrieved June 11, 2007 from http:// pcsp. libraries. rutgers.edu/include/getdoc.php?id=395& article=69&mode=pdf

Wade, W.A., Treat, T.A., & Stuart, G.L. (1998). Transporting an empirically supported treatment for panic disorder to a service clinic setting: A benchmarking strategy. *Journal of Consulting and Clinical Psychology, 66, 231-239.*

Weissman, M.M. (2007). Cognitive therapy and interpersonal psychotherapy: 30 years later. *American Journa of Psychiatry, 164, 693-696.l*

Weissman, M.M. & Sanderson, W.C. (2002). Promises and problems in modern psychotherapy: The need for increased training in evidence based therapies. In B. Hamburg (Ed.), *Modern Psychiatry:Challenges in Educating Health Professionals to Meet New Needs*. New York, Josiah Macy Foundation.

Weisz, J. R. & Addis, M.E. (2006). The research-practice tango and other choreographic challenges: Using and testing evidence-based psychotherapies in clinical care settings. In C. G. Goodheart,A.E.Kazdin, & R.J. Sternberg (Eds.), *Evidence-based Psyhotherapy: Where Practice and Research Meet*. Washington, DC: American Psychological Association.

Wilson, G.T. (1998). Manual-based treatment and clinical practice. *Clinical Psychology: Research and Practice, 5, 363-375.*

Wolpe, J. (1969). *The practice of behavior therapy*. New York, Pergamon.

Woody, S.R. & Sanderson, W.C. (1998). Manuals for empirically supported treatments: 1998 update from the task force on psychological interventions. *The Clinical Psychologist, 51(1), 17-21.*

In: Toward a Science of Clinical Psychology
Editor: Luciano L'Abate, pp. 161-176
ISBN: 978-1-60456-062-6


Chapter IX

# EVTs, EBPs, ESRs, and RIPs: Inspecting the Varieties of Research Based Practices

*T. Mark Harwood and Larry E. Beutler*

## Abstract

Research based practices have been investigated empirically, as organized initiatives, for only about 15 years (Paul, 2006). This is a relatively short period of time considering the complexity of psychotherapy outcome research. In the early years of psychotherapy, empirical investigation of psychotherapy process was essentially nonexistent. During the period between 1920 and 1940, clinicians began to publish results of uncontrolled case studies in an attempt to justify psychotherapy as a legitimate and effective treatment. Spurred in large part by the demands created during World War II, the mid to late 1940s and early 1950s experienced a surge in empiricism and its merger with psychotherapy finally resulting in a meaningful and useful scientific endeavor (Paul, 2006). Further, it wasn't until the 1960s that statistical and methodological sophistication had advanced to the point of rendering results that had clinical utility with respect to psychotherapy process and outcome research (Paul, 2006). Today, statistical and methodological sophistication has resulted in a growing body of psychotherapy process and outcome research convincing many that psychotherapy is more than a simplistic conglomeration of common relationship-oriented elements—in fact, there is a growing consensus that psychotherapy is a complex process involving manifold therapist x therapy x patient x phase interactions (Beutler et al, 2003, Harwood et al., 2006; Karno et al., 2004; Paul 2006). These therapist, therapy intervention, patient, and phase qualities must all be considered when attempting to disentangle the complexity of psychotherapy process.

This chapter briefly explores the major varieties of research based practices and introduces a model that integrates the various research based findings. Empirically validated treatments (EVTs or, perhaps more appropriately, empirically supported treatments, ESTs), empirically based practices (EBPs), empirically supported relationships (ESRs) and research informed principles (RIPs) comprise the varieties of research based practices that will be reviewed herein.

Empirically supported treatments are those well-defined (typically manualized) treatments that have received empirical support from several investigations, with at least one investigation being conducted independently from others. The methodology for this type of research is expected to be rigorous, well-planned, and able to rule out competing or alternative hypotheses. Of course, the foregoing can be said with respect to each of the research based practices discussed in this chapter. Treatment fidelity is a must, patient recruitment and selection should be conducted to enhance generalizability, and assessment should be ongoing, extensive, and psychometrically sound. Currently, there are approximately 150 different treatment manuals describing various models or approaches that have been demonstrated to be effective for specific types of patients (Chambless & Ollendick, 2001)

Empirically based practices stem from ESTs; that is, once a treatment has received sufficient support to be classified as an EST, it is often adopted by those in the treatment community. Benchmarking is often employed to explore the effectiveness of EBPs in treatment program evaluation (Weersing, 2005). Briefly, the method of benchmarking involves comparing the outcomes of a particular treatment applied to a specific sample and in a specific setting to the results obtained in two published clinical trials. The comparison is made more rigorous and meaningful by employing the same outcome measures and definitions of positive change utilized in the clinical trials. For detailed information on how to implement the benchmarking method, see Weersing (2005).

Empirically supported relationships (ESRs) or empirically supported therapeutic relationships (ESTRs) involve identifying the qualities of the therapist and qualities of the patient and their interaction that facilitate improvement. The Division 29 Task Force (Norcross, 2002) identified two types of relationship variables related to outcome: variables that predict the likelihood of growth or positive change and variables that moderate the effects of psychotherapy and, therefore; can be applied systematically in the process of tailoring treatments to fit patients. Examples of either of these types of variables include: coping style, resistance, functional impairment, stages of change and attachment style. Factors specific to the therapeutic relationship; i.e., qualities that interact between patient and therapist and involve the skill of the therapists were identified by the Division 29 Task Force as relationship factors, these include: therapeutic alliance, empathy, goal consensus and collaboration, positive regard, congruence/genuineness, feedback and the repair of alliance ruptures (Norcross, 2002).

Research informed principles may be conceptualized as the end product of each of the foregoing research practices. More specifically, RIPs represent the spectrum of generalizable statements that can be recognized to constitute principles of effective change (Castonguay & Beutler, 2006). Typically, these generalizations are derived from an inspection of the research from which ESTs, EBPs, and ESRs are derived. RIPs, by their very nature, allow for maximal flexibility in the application of technique because these principles relate to families of techniques. That is, these principles may call for practices that foster exposure or insight, or symptom change, or arousal modulation—any number of technique or interventions may be useful in meeting the patient's needs designated by the governing principle of change. Moreover, RIPs extend to the basic (i.e., common) necessary (but not necessarily sufficient) conditions that facilitate therapy. For example, these basic principles can include such elements as the establishment of trust, rapport, and the conditions of professionalism and positive regard.

## Systematic Treatment Selection and the Integration of Research Based Practices

One method of patient-treatment matching has been particularly noteworthy for its integration of RIPs. Based on decades of research, Systematic Treatment Selection (STS, Beutler & Clarkin, 1990, Beutler, Clarkin, & Bongar, 2000) and its practitioner-friendly variant, Prescriptive Psychotherapy (PT, Beutler & Harwood, 2000), has incorporated aspects of each of the foregoing research based practices in an effort to optimally tailor treatment to research based patient dimensions. These methods of treatment planning are probably most effective for patients suffering from complex/chronic problems such as depression and co-morbid substance abuse (Beutler, Clarkin, & Bongar, 2000; Beutler & Harwood, 2000).

STS guides the clinician in the assessment of presenting problems on the following six treatment relevant patient dimensions: 1) coping style, 2) functional impairment, 3) reactance level, 4) subjective distress, 5) social support, and 6) problem complexity/chronicity. In addition to thorough assessment, STS is an empirically-based method of treatment planning and a system designed to provide feedback to both the treating clinician and the patient. We will briefly discuss each of the foregoing patient dimensions and their relevance to treatment. There are at least three examples to standardize the application of principles, within the context of research-informed principles. Beutler, Clarkin, and Bongar (2000) applied the concepts broadly to conditions that were defined by or related to the presence of depression. In contrast, Beutler and Harwood (2000) exemplify a manualized application of principles to patients with co-morbid depression and substance abuse. Finally, Housley and Beutler (2007) is a step-by-step manual of a phase-based intervention for those who are victims of mass trauma or terrorism.

In each case, the manuals provide a foundation in empirically defined or extrapolated principles that have been judged to generalize across patients and treatments (Beutler, Clarkin, & Bongar, 2000; Beutler & Harwood, 2000; Beutler et al., 2003). Within the context of these principles, interventions are suggested that also are supported by a body of research. Thus, experiential, cognitive, relationship, and other types of interventions are identified as being consistent with the principles that are illustrated as an integrated intervention (Beutler, Clarkin, & Bongar, 2000; Beutler & Harwood, 2000; Beutler et al., 2003). The interested reader is directed to the foregoing volumes to obtain more detailed information on STS and PT and their application to the treatment of patients suffering from complex problems Moreover, a Joint Task Force of the Society for Clinical Psychology (Division 12 of the American Psychological Association) and the North American Society for Psychotherapy Research (Castonguay & Beutler, 2006a; Castonguay & Beutler, 2006b; Castonguay 2006c) has provided a further extension of these efforts by identifying principles that integrate participant, treatment, and relationship-based principles among patients with depressive, anxiety based, personality, and substance abuse disorders.

A recent empirical investigation on the efficacy of PT found strong empirical support for this method of patient-treatment matching. In this RCT investigation, patients were randomly assigned to one of three treatment conditions: PT (Beutler & Harwood, 2000; Beutler et al., 2003), a standard Cognitive Therapy for substance abuse (CT, Beck et al., 1993), or a contrasting Cognitive Narrative Therapy (NT, Gonçalves, 1995). As the careful reader will have already gathered, the PT condition selectively matched interventions in an aptitude by treatment interaction (ATI) model. A hierarchical multiple regression analysis was utilized and variables were entered to provide for the most stringent test of patient-treatment matching hypotheses. That is, patient variables were the first to be entered into the regression equation, followed by treatment variables and the strength of the therapeutic alliance. The final entry of variables involved the ATIs—the patient-treatment matching interaction variables. By entering our ATIs last, we were able to determine if our patient-treatment matching variables explained unique variance and contributed to the predictive power over and above what was accounted for by patient, therapy, and alliance variables. Further, residualized change scores were utilized in our analyses to eliminate regression to the mean effects.

The Prescriptive Psychotherapy model, based on ATIs was found to play a stronger predictive role than treatment interventions, alliance, or patient characteristics than treatment, patient, therapist, or relationship variables alone. More specifically, approximately 90% of the variance in scores on the Hamilton Rating Scale for Depression (HRSD; Endicott, Cohen, Nee, Fleiss, & Sarantakos, 1981) was accounted for by the four sets of predictors; however, the strongest predictors of sustained effectiveness were the Prescriptive Therapy Aptitude by Treatment Interaction matching variables (Beutler et al., 2003). The effect size for the finding on the HRSD translated to $r = 0.94$ ($p < 0.01$). The smallest effect size on the other major outcome measures in our investigation: the Beck Depression Inventory (BDI-II; Beck, Steer, & Brown, 1996), the Addiction Severity Index (ASI; McLellan, Luborsky, Woody, & O'Brien, 1980), and Time Line Follow Back (TLFB; Sobell & Sobell, 1992) was $r = 0.67$ ($p < 0.01$). Meaningful clinical change was indicated by all of the estimated effect sizes in each of the regression analyses.

As previously stated, the STS and PT manuals provide systematic procedures for the assessment of specific patient dimensions—the results of this assessment indicate which treatment principles or strategies are indicated. It is these principles or strategies that form the basis for a more fine-grained selection of specific and principle-consistent interventions. For example, if the principle of exposure is indicated, the clinician may select Systematic Desensitization, in any one of its variations, to accomplish this task. If arousal reduction is indicated, the imposition of structure and use of closed ended questions may be employed; however, other techniques are at the clinician's disposal. If patient resistance is an issue, therapists may select a more patient-driven method of treatment or simply become non-directive in their present stance. In each case, therapists have the flexibility to select from a variety of interventions to accomplish the goals indicated by the assessment-driven principles. Each of these patient dimensions are able to predict the likelihood of change or magnitude of change and are most applicable when dysphoria, anxiety, personality disorder, or substance abuse are prominent features of the presenting problem (Beutler et al., 2003; Castonguay & Beutler, 2006a; Castonguay & Beutler 2006b; Castonguay & Beutler 2006c).

The following discussion on patient dimensions includes a brief discussion of technique factors that correspond to each patient dimension. These technique factors or principles of change were extracted from specific treatment manuals by the Division 12 Task Force and identified as having empirical support for their patient-treatment matching effects (Castonguay & Beutler, 2006a).

## Coping Style

The assessment and determination of patient coping style (CS) is accomplished through a variety of methods. For example, a ratio of various internalizing and externalizing MMPI-2 scales (Butcher, 1990; Butcher et al., 1989) a careful assessment of patient history, a STS Clinician Rating Form (STS-CRF, Fisher, D., Beutler, L.E., & Williams, O.B. 1999), or a patient-driven computerized Systematic Treatment system can all provide the necessary information to identify a patient's dominant coping style, their Internalizing Ratio. The specific formula we have used is:

IR = Hy + Pd + Pa + Ma/Hs + D + Pt + Si

Coping style refers to a patient's dominant method of dealing with problems or people. Dominant coping styles are identified as either externalizing or internalizing and one's coping style informs the selection of treatment focus (symptom-focused or insight focused, respectively). An externalizing coping style is suggested when the IR is greater than 1.0 and an internalizing coping style is suggested when the IR is less than 1.0 (Beutler & Harwood, 2000). To briefly illustrate, an externalizer is characterized by excessive and disruptive behavior—they are likely to present as gregarious or extroverted, they have a tendency to act out and blame others for their problems, and they often have problems with authority. On the other hand, internalizers are characterized as inhibited—they tend to blame themselves for their problems, they are typically shy and ruminative, and they are usually compliant with authority figures. The STS principle that applies to an externalizing coping style is: "Extroverted/externalizing/impulsive coping styles indicate the use of interventions designed to directly affect symptoms and enhance skills.

Introverted/internalizing/restricted coping styles indicate the use of interventions designed to directly affect insight and awareness" (Beutler et al., 2000, pp. 203). Coping style was identified as a participant factor by the Division 29 Task Force and the foregoing STS principle may be considered an empirically based principle based on "a preponderance of the available evidence" (Castonguay & Beutler, 2006a, pp. 634) as evaluated by the Division 12 or Division 29 Task Force. Coping style is a patient factor that, when addressed properly in treatment, has the potential to increase the magnitude of positive change Beutler, Clarkin, & Bongar, 2000; Beutler et al., 2003). The guiding principle for this application states, "Therapeutic change is greatest when the relative balance of interventions either favors the use of skill building and symptom removal procedures among patients who externalize or favors the use of insight and relationship-focused procedures among patients who internalize." (Beutler, Clarkin, and Bongar, 2000, pp. 204).

Empirical support for the assessment of coping style and application of this information in treatment selection comes from at least 30 investigations involving both in-patient and out-patient populations (Beutler, Clarkin, & Bongar, 2000). The combined sample size for these investigations totals to more than 5,600 participants suffering from a variety of disorders. More specifically, these samples included primarily depressed individuals; however, co-morbidity was a prominent feature with substance abuse, anxiety disorders, personality disorders, and severe psychopathology well represented among the samples. Additionally, treatment formats included individual, group, and both married and cohabiting couples.

## Functional Impairment

A patient's level of functional impairment (FI) may be assessed with the Global Assessment of Functioning from the DSM-IV-TR (American Psychiatric Association, 2000) or a careful clinical assessment of current functioning. A consideration of FI results in a principle that impacts on the magnitude of change and it is also a prognostic indicator. More specifically, the STS principle on FI is "[b]enefit corresponds with treatment intensity among high functionally impaired patients" (Beutler & Harwood, 2000, pp. 149). In other words, as patient functional impairment increases, so should the number of treatment session per week, or the length of treatment sessions, or therapy may take on a multi-person treatment (group, family, couple, pharmacotherapy). This STS principle for FI may be characterized as a Level of Care Principle as well as a prognostic indicator. As with CS, FI has been identified by the division 29 Task Force as a Participant Factor (Castonguay & Beutler, 2006a, Beutler et al., 2006); however, it has also been identified by the dysphoria work group of the Task Force on Empirically Based Principles of Therapeutic Change (Castonguay & Beutler, 2006c).

Empirical support for the assessment of functional impairment and application of this information in treatment planning can be found in more than 45 investigations (Beutler, Clarkin, & Bongar, 2000). The combined sample size from these studies sums to more than 7,700 participants from both in-patient and out-patient settings. Almost all diagnostic categories were represented in the foregoing studies and myriad types of psychosocial treatments, including a variety of modes and formats, were administered.

## Reactance Level

A patient's level of reactance (or resistance) can be assessed with various MMPI-2 treatment indicator scales (e.g., Do, Cn, Aut, and TRT) or with the Dowd Trait Reactance Scale (Dowd TRS, 1991). Resistance or reactance is defined as the patient's perception of efforts on the part of the therapist to control his or her behavior—it may become activated when "...a patient's sense of freedom, image of self, safety, or psychological integrity, or power is threatened" (Beutler & Harwood, 2000, pp. 115). A high level of trait resistance is indicated by a number of behaviors including expressed resentment of others, often dominates in relationships, distrusts and is suspicious of others' motives, and enjoys competition. Low levels of trait resistance are indicated if patients tend to follow the advice of those in authority and avoid confrontation (Beutler & Harwood, 2000). Further, resistance has a state-like quality; that is, the clinician must remain vigilant to in-session cues that indicate when resistance has been activated; e.g., if the patient is often late or avoids appointments, has trouble following or understanding directions, holds a grudge, or becomes overly angry at the therapist (Beutler, Clarkin, & Bongar, 2000; Beutler & Harwood, 2000).

Resistance has been identified by the Division 29 Task Force as a participant factor (Castonguay & Beutler, 2006c). The STS principles related to resistance are "[t]herapeutic change is most likely when the therapeutic procedures do not evoke patient resistance" and [t]herapeutic change is greatest when the directiveness of the intervention is either inversely correspondent with the patient's current level of resistance or authoritatively prescribes a continuation of the symptomatic behavior" (Beutler & Harwood, 2000, pp. 116-117). As the careful reader may have noted, resistance has implications for both the likelihood of change and the magnitude of change (Beutler et al., 2003).

Empirical support for the assessment of reactance and the application of reactance level information in treatment planning can be found in more than 30 investigations (Beutler, Clarkin, & Bongar, 2000). The combined sample size from the aforementioned studies totals to more than 8,000 inpatient and outpatient participants. Psychosocial treatment formats included individual, family, group, and parent training with a variety of psychotherapies and pharmacological agents employed among myriad diagnostic categories.

## Subjective Distress

Although not specifically identified as a participant factor by Division 29, the therapeutic management of subjective distress (SD) has received empirical support (Beutler, Clarkin, & Bongar, 2000; Beutler & Harwood, 2000; Castonguay & Beutler, 2006c). The STS principles for managing SD (also referred to as one of the "Common Principles for Selecting Techniques and Interventions", Castonguay & Beutler 2006b) are [t]he likelihood of therapeutic change is greatest when the patient's level of emotional stress is moderate, neither being excessively high nor excessively low" and "[t]herapeutic change is greatest when a patient is stimulated to emotional arousal in a safe environment until problematic responses diminish or extinguish" (Beutler & Harwood, 2000, pp. 135-136). As with resistance, the principles governing the management of subjective distress have implications for both the likelihood and magnitude of positive growth (Beutler et al., 2003).

Subjective distress can be assessed via indexing cues (i.e., patient behaviors or reports and clinician ratings). For example, clinicians may identify high levels of SD when they note apathy, low energy levels, anxiety, and an unsteady or shaky voice in their patients. Patient reports may indicate the foregoing as well as frequently feeling like crying, difficulty making decisions, uncertainty about the future, and poor expectations with respect to the future (Beutler & Harwood, 2000). SD may also be assessed by the State-Trait Anxiety Inventory (STAI-State; Spielberger et al. 1983), the STS Clinician Rating Form, or the revised Client Emotional Arousal Scale (CEAS-R; Daldrup et al., 1988; Machado, Beutler, & Greenberg, 1999).

The patient-treatment matching dimension of Subjective Distress has not received as much empirical support as coping style, functional impairment, or reactance; however, at least eleven investigations have provided support for the use of this patient dimension in both pretreatment planning and the selection of specific interventions (Beutler, Clarkin, & Bongar, 2000). The combined sample size, comprised of both in-patients and out-patients, totaled to more than 1,250. A variety of diagnoses were represented in these eleven studies and several psychosocial and pharmacological treatments were delivered.

## Social Support

Perceived levels of social support is a positive prognostic indicator in the STS model (Beutler, Clarkin, & Bongar, 2000; Beutler & Harwood, 2000; Beutler et al. 2003). Treatment benefit is correspondent with social support suggesting that improvement in the quality of social support may also be a specific treatment factor (Castonguay & Beutler, 2006a). Social support was recently identified by the dysphoria work group of the Task Force on Empirically Based Principles of Therapeutic Change (Castonguay & Beutler, 2006b) as a patient prognostic indicator.

The STS principles associated with social support are "[a] certain level of experienced or felt support may be necessary to activate the power of interpersonal and relationship therapies" (Beutler, Clarkin, & Bongar, 2000, pp. 190), social support may be enhanced through multi-person treatment, and enhancing social support may result in greater likelihood and magnitude of positive change. Social support levels may be assessed through clinical interview or via self-report measures such as the Sarason Social Support Questionnaire (Sarason, Levine, Basham, & Sarason, 1983).

The patient-treatment matching dimension of social support has received empirically-based endorsement in at least 37 investigations involving a combined sample comprised of more than 7,700 in-patients and out-patients (Beutler, Clarkin, & Bongar, 2000). As with the aforementioned studies, a variety of diagnoses, formats, modalities, and psychosocial treatments were represented in the 37 investigations involving social support and its importance in psychosocial and pharmacological treatment.

## Problem Complexity/Chronicity

This patient dimension is often related to functional impairment; however, some patients are able to function adequately, in various aspects of their lives, even when dealing with complex/chronic problems (Beutler, L.E., Brookman, L., Harwood, T.M., Alimohamed, S. & Malik, M.M., 2002). For example, some alcoholics are functional and their disorder may actually operate as a coping mechanism for a period of time. In the present context, we are discussing complex/chronic problems that are causing distress for the patient and perhaps those who work or live with the patient. Problem complexity/chronicity (PCC) is a prognostic indicator, an indicator of treatment intensity, and suggests the need for multi-person treatment (Beutler, Clarkin, & Bongar, 2000; Beutler & Harwood, 2000). In other words, highly complex problems respond better to broad-band treatment; within the domain of psychotherapy, systemic and dynamic treatments should perform better than symptom-focused ones—among medical treatments, ECT would be favored over pharmacotherapy (Beutler, Clarkin, & Bongar, 2000; Gaw & Beutler, 1995).

Complexity and chronicity may be assessed clinically and identified by patterns or recurrence, persistence of problems, co-morbidity, and broadly generalized disturbances in interpersonal relationships (Beutler & Harwood, 2000). The STS Clinician Rating Form also provides for a clinician-derived assessment of PCC. In general, prognosis is attenuated by problem complexity/chronicity and by the absence of patient distress (Beutler, Clarkin, &

Bongar, 2000). Further, facilitating social support increases the likelihood of positive change among patients with complex/chronic problems (Harwood & Williams, 2003).

The treatment matching dimension of problem complexity and chronicity has received empirical support in at least 23 investigations (Beutler, Clarkin, & Bongar, 2000). The combined participant sample for these 23 investigations totaled nearly 2,000 and was comprised of both in-patients and out-patients. Diagnoses were varied across studies as were treatment modalities and treatment formats. Relatedly, various psychosocial treatments and pharmacological treatments were administered by investigators.

For more specific and detailed information on measures employed, types of treatments, sample characteristics, and outcomes from the numerous studies described briefly in the foregoing sections on coping style, functional impairment, reactance, subjective distress, social support, and problem complexity, the interested reader is directed to Beutler, Clarkin, and Bongar (2000) and Beutler, Malik, Talebi, Fleming, and Moleiro (2004).

## Applications of an Empirically-based Treatment-Selection Model

In recent years, Beutler and Williams co-developed the Systematic Treatment Selection model in a computer-based internet-distributed application that allows for more detailed and easily accessible information on treatment elements such as prognosis, change trajectories, optimal selection of therapist, therapist performance data, optimal selection of treatment principles and strategies, patient demographics, diagnostic information, and the assessment of treatment relevant patient qualities. The first rendition of the STS system in computer application was developed primarily for large health care organizations (e.g., HMOs) and for private practitioners (Harwood & Williams, 2003). Therapists and patients could interface with the STS system via web browser, multiple SQL servers, or by a telephone (interactive voice-response, IVR) intake-update system.

In its second rendition (i.e., as Systematic Treatment, ST), the system is being reconfigured by Beutler and Williams to be entirely patient-based. In this new application, patients will still be able to access ST directly through the internet or telephone. The ST system will offer a similar level of feedback to both patient and clinician; however, assessment will be entirely self-report and the assessment and intervention procedures will merge more than in the previous rendition. Additionally, conventional treatment will be one of the options provided. Further, the STS-CRF has been translated for use in both systems; within a single framework, the six STS patient dimensions can be easily quantified.

The new ST Patient Self-Report version will be available in both English and Spanish. It will allow patients to access their secure treatment information, select therapists, and track their progress in therapy. With patient consent, treating clinicians may also provide input and take advantage of the treatment-relevant information rendered by the ST system. Clinicians can track patient change and gauge whether or not they are improving at a rate that is faster or slower than patients who are similar on diagnostic, demographic, and other treatment-relevant dimensions. Clinicians can evaluate their own effectiveness and make necessary changes based on the information provided by the ST system—patient tracking/awareness of change enhances the likelihood and magnitude of positive treatment outcome (Harwood & Williams, 2003).

Although an updated data-base and revised application is in the works, some clinicians may wish to learn more about the earlier version which has features that are somewhat similar to those included in the upcoming revision. The interested reader is directed to Harwood and Williams (2003) for a detailed description of the STS system—the result of a nine-year evolution based on a large data set consisting of patients suffering from depression, anxiety disorders, substance abuse disorders, psychosis, and personality disorders.

## Summary and Conclusions

Systematic Treatment (ST), Systematic Treatment Selection (STS), and Prescriptive Psychotherapy (PT) all represent variations of the same basic patient-treatment matching model. This model has as its core the identification of generalizable principles that can be applied to predicting and enhancing psychotherapeutic outcomes. The principles that are embodied in the STS system are not considered to be exclusive or exhaustive and the system itself is simply a picture at a moment in time of the constructs and relationships that currently achieve sufficient research support to be translated to practice. Thus, the system is open and fluid and able to incorporate additional principles as these become demonstrably valid. While principles can be added, there are a core number of them that have withstood the several tests of the model. These serve as the "core" of the system to which other principles can be added for specific purposes and with specific populations (e.g., Castonguay & Beutler, 2006; Norcross & Beutler, 2007).

Two decided strengths of the STS system are (1) the reliance on empirical findings to define the working and core principles, and (2) the fact that the principles transcend any given therapeutic school and can be applied within any theoretical model. These strengths are illustrated in the history of the development of the STS core principles. This development has occurred within four stages: 1) comprehensive reviews of literature to identify variables that are predictive of therapeutic prognosis or of the differential effectiveness/efficacy of certain procedures or techniques; (2) refining the resulting list of constructs to a finite set of hypotheses regarding the relationship among a limited list of measureable patient variables and observable qualities of treatment that can be tested both through retrospective research and prospective investigations; (3) construction of operational measures of the constructs representing, respectively, either patient characteristics or corresponding qualities of the treatment itself; and (4) applying these operational measures to the test of the initial hypotheses for the prediction of outcomes across a variety of patient groups and conditions.

The first two stages of this process were reliant on informed reviews of literature and the achievement of consensus among colleagues. Thus, through a gradual process of reiterative literature reviews (e.g., Beutler, 1983; Beutler & Clarkin, 1990), and a specific process of reiterative discussions and consensus seeking (Beutler, Clarkin, & Bongar, 2000), a finite list of variables (both patient and treatment) were identified and a set of 15 hypotheses were extracted from the extant literature and stated in such a way as to support independent empirical tests.

The third task was the development of two rating scales, one based upon identifying the extracted patient qualities that were the objects of the hypotheses about patient prognosis and treatment matching (Fisher Beutler, & Williams, 1999; Corbella, Beutler, Fernandez-Alvarez, Botella, Malik, Lane, & Wagstaff, 2003), and the other upon the qualities of treatment that completed the treatment matching hypotheses (Beutler, Clarkin & Bongar, 2000; Malik, et al, 2003). These scales allowed the implementation of the fourth step of the process; that of prospective tests of these measures to testing the 15 original hypotheses. The largest of these latter studies was that previously reviewed and conducted by Beutler, Clarkin, and Bongar (2000). Using a prospective research design on archival data sets, 13 of the original hypotheses were supported. In subsequent prospective studies (e.g., Beutler, Moleiro, et al, 2003; .Kuenzler & Beutler, 2003; Karno, Beutler, & Harwood, 2002), these initial findings have been confirmed.

The end result of these four developmental steps has been to translate the 13 hypotheses that were originally supported into a set of working principles and to add to these five that are based on conventional practice having to do with the protection and treatment of patients who are deemed to be a danger to themselves or others. The addition of the latter five principles was considered necessary to ensure ethical practice based on consensual opinion although empirical evidence that following these principles enhanced effects was lacking. Thus, the core of the STS system is 18 principles that have been found in both retrospective and prospective studies to be valid (13 principles) or which have passed the test of professional consensus (5 principles).

The 18 core principles are built around the six patient-treatment matching dimensions that have been discussed in the foregoing pages (i.e., coping style, functional impairment, reactance level, subjective distress, social support, and problem complexity and chronicity). The interested reader is directed to Beutler, Clarkin, & Bongar (2000) for a complete discussion of these principles including their application and clinical utility. The ten principles from the Prescriptive Psychotherapy manual are those that are specific to the application of individual psychotherapy and may be described as "overarching"—they enhance the development of the treatment relationship, inform level of care, and guide the application of individual therapeutic procedures (Beutler & Harwood, 2000). The complete set of STS core principles are presented here (Beutler, Clarkin, & Bongar, 2000, pp. 183-184, 204-205). Those that are identified as applied to Risk Reduction are the five principles that were added for professional and ethical considerations and have not met the same standard of empirical support as the others.

## Reasonable and Basic Principles

### Prognosis

- The likelihood of improvement (prognosis) is a positive function of social support level and a negative function of functional impairment.
- Prognosis is attenuated by patient complexity/chronicity, and by an absence of patient distress. Facilitating social support enhances the likelihood of good outcome among patients with complex/chronic problems.

### Level and Intensity of Care

- Psychoactive medication exerts its best effects among those patients with a high functional impairment and high complexity/chronicity.
- Likelihood and magnitude of improvement are increased among patients with complex/ chronic problems by the application of multi-person therapy.
- Benefits correspond to treatment intensity among functionally impaired patients.

### Risk Reduction (Consensual Principles)

- Risk is reduced by careful assessment of risk situations in the course of establishing a diagnosis and history.
- Risk is reduced and patient compliance is increased when the treatment includes family intervention.
- Risk reduction and retention are optimized if the patient is realistically informed about the probable length and effectiveness of the treatment and has a clear understanding of the roles and activities that are expected of him or her during the course of the treatment.
- Risk is reduced if the clinician routinely questions patients about suicidal feelings, intent, and plans.
- Ethical and legal principles suggest that documentation and consultation are advisable.

## OPTIMAL PRINCIPLES*

### Relationship Principles

- Therapeutic change is greatest when the therapist is skillful and provides trust, acceptance, acknowledgement, collaboration, and respect for the patient within an environment that both supports risk and provides maximal safety.
- Therapeutic change is most likely when the therapeutic procedures do not evoke patient resistance.

### Principles of Exposure and Extinction

- Therapeutic change is most likely when the patient is exposed to objects or targets of behavioral and emotional avoidance.
- Therapeutic change is greatest when a patient is stimulated to emotional arousal in a safe environment until problematic responses diminish or extinguish.

### Principle of Treatment Sequencing

- Therapeutic change is most likely if the initial focus of change efforts is to build new skills and alter disruptive symptoms.

### Differential Treatment Principles

Therapeutic change is greatest when the relative balance of interventions either favors the use of skill building and symptom removal procedures among patients who externalize or favors the use of insight and relationship-focused procedures among patients who internalize.

Therapeutic change is greatest when the directiveness of the intervention is either inversely correspondent with the patient's current level of resistance or authoritatively prescribes a continuation of the symptomatic behavior.

The likelihood of therapeutic change is greatest when the patient's level of emotional stress is moderate, neither being excessively high nor excessively low.

The research suggests that adherence to the foregoing principles will improve both the likelihood and magnitude of positive outcomes from treatment (Beutler, Castonguay, & Follette, 2006; Beutler, Clarkin, & Bongar, 2000; Beutler & Harwood, 2000; Beutler et al., 2004; Beutler et al., 2003; Castonguay & Beutler 2006a; Castonguay & Beutler 2006b; Castonguay & Beutler 2006c). As the foregoing statement suggests, each of these principles has received empirical support and constitutes empirically based practices. Continued investigation into relationship factors, specific techniques, common factors and their interactions with patient attributes (ATIs) will continue to improve upon outcomes with respect to likelihood and magnitude.

These principles; have been incorporated into a computerized system that is designed to help a patient select and find an appropriate treatment. Systematic Treatment (ST) is a patient driven computerized application of the STS model. STS is designed primarily for clinicians; however, both clinicians and patients can access the system via computer or voice activated interaction. PT is designed with the clinician or academician in mind—the PT manual is presented in a format that allows the clinician to obtain the information necessary to apply Prescriptive Psychotherapy in their own practice and the PT manual can be utilized as a text in any graduate training program.

* Note: the original order of the Optimal Principles have been rearranged to reflect some commonalities.

## References

Beck, A.T., Steer, R.A., & Brown, G.K. (1996). *Manual for the Beck Depression Inventory-II*. San Antonio, TX: Psychological Corporation.

Beck, A.T., Wright, F.D., Newman, C.F., & Liese, B.S. (1993). *Cognitive therapy of substance abuse*. New York: Guilford Press.

Beutler, L.E., Brookman, L., Harwood, T.M., Alimohamed, S. & Malik, M.M. (2002). Functional impairment and coping style. *Psychotherapy, 38*, 437-442.

Beutler, L.E., & Harwood, T.M. (2000). *Prescriptive Psychotherapy: A practical guide to Systematic Treatment Selection.* New York: Oxford University Press.

Beutler, L.E., Blatt, S.J., Alamohamed, S., Levy, K.N., & Angtuaco, L.A. (2006). Participant factors in treating dysphoric disorders. In L.G. Castonguay & L.E. Beutler (Eds*). Principles of therapeutic change that work* (pp. 13-63). New York: Oxford University Press.

Beutler, L.E., Clarkin, J.F., & Bongar, B. (2000). *Guidelines for the systematic treatment of the depressed patient.* New York: Oxford University Press.

Beutler, L.E., Castonguay, L.G., & Follette, W.C. (2006). Integration of therapeutic factors in dysphoric disorders. In L.G. Castonguay & L. E. Beutler (Eds.*). Principles of Therapeutic Change That Work.* New York: Oxford University Press.

Beutler, L.E., Malik, M., Talebi, H., Fleming, J., & Moleiro, C. (2004). Use of psychological tests/instruments for treatment planning. In M. E. Maruish (Ed.) *The Use of Psychological Testing for Treatment Planning and Outcomes Assessment: Volume 1: General Considerations (3rd ed.).* (pp.111-145). Mahwah, NJ: Lawrence Erlbaum Associates Publishers.

Beutler, L.E., Moleiro, C., Malik, M., Harwood, T.M., Romanelli, R., Gallagher-Thompson, D., & Thompson, L. (2003). A comparison of the Dodo, EST, and ATI factors among co-morbid stimulant dependent, depressed patients. *Clinical Psychology & Psychotherapy, 10*, 69-85.

Butcher, J.N. (1990). *The MMPI-2 in psychological treatment.* New York: Oxford University Press.

Butcher, J.N., Dahlstrom, W.G., Graham, J.R., Tellegen, A.M., & Kaemmer, B. (1989). Minnesota Mulphiphasic Personality Inventory-2 (MMPI-2): *Manual for Administration and scoring.* Minneapolis: University of Minnesota Press.

Castonguay, L.G., & Beutler, L.E. (2006a). Principles of therapeutic change: A Task Force on participants, relationships, and technique factors. *Journal of Clinical Psychology, 62, (6)*, 631-638.

Castonguay, L.G., & Beutler, L.E. (2006b). Therapeutic factors in dysphoric disorders. *Journal of Clinical Psychology, 62 (6)*, 639-647.

Castonguay, L.G., & Beutler, L.E. (2006c). Common and unique principles of therapeutic change: What dowe know and what do we need to know? In L.G. Castonguay & Beutler, L.E. (Eds.), *Principles of therapeutic change that work* (pp. 353-369). New York: Oxford University Press.

Chambless, D.L., & Ollendick, T. H. (2001). Empirically supported psychological interventions:

Controversies and evidence. *Annual Review of Psychology, 52*, 685-716/

Corbella, S., Beutler, L. E., Fernandez-Alvarez, H., Botella, L., Malik, M. L., Lane, G., & Wagstaff, N. (2003). Measuring Coping Style and Resistance among Spanish and Argentine Samples: Development of the Systematic Treatment Selection Self-Report (STS-SR) in Spanish. *Journal of Clinical Psychology, 59, 921-932.*

Daldrup, R.J., Beutler, L.E., Engle, D., & Greenberg, L.S. (1988). *Focused Expressive Psychotherapy: Freeing the overcontrolled patient.* New York: Guilford Press.

Dowd, E.T., Millne, C.R., & Wise, S.L. (1991). The Therapeutic Reactance Scale: A measure of psychological reactance. *Journal of Counseling and Development, 69*, 541-545.

Endicott, J., Cohen, J., Nee, J., Fleiss, J., & Sarantakos, S. (1981). Hamilton Depression Rating Scale. *Archives of General Psychiatry, 38*, 98-103.

Fisher, D., Beutler, L.E., & Williams, O.B. (1999). STS clinician rating form: Patient assessment and treatment planning. *Journal of Clinical Psychology, 55* (7), 825-842..

Gaw, K.F., & Beutler, L.E. (1995). Integrating treatment recommendations. In L.E. Beutler & M. Berren (Eds.), *Integrative assessment of adult personality*. (pp 280-319). New York: Guilford Press

Gonçalves, O.F. (1995). Cognitive narrative psychotherapy: The hermeneutic construction of alternative meanings. In M.J. Mahoney (Ed.), *Cognitive and constructive psychotherapies* (pp. 186-245). New York: Pergamon Press.

Harwood, T.M., Beutler, L.E., Castillo, S. & Karno, M. (2006). Common and Specific Effects of Couples Treatment for Alcoholism: A test of the Generic Model of Psychotherapy. *Psychology and Psychotherapy: Theory Research and Practice, 79*, 365-384.

Harwood, T.M., & Williams, O.B. (2003). Identifying treatment-relevant assessment: Systematic Treatment Selection. In L.E. Beutler & G. Groth-Marnat (Eds.), *Integrative assessment of adult personality, 2nd edition* (pp. 65-81). New York: Guilford Press.

Housley, J., & Beutler, L. E. (2007). *Treating victims of mass trauma and terrorism.* Gottengen: Hogrefe & Huber

Karno, M., Beutler, L. E., & Harwood, T. M. (2002). Interactions Between Psychotherapy Process and Patient Attributes that Predict Alcohol Treatment Effectiveness: A Preliminary Report. *Addictive Behaviors, 27,* 779-797.

Karno, M.P. & Longabaugh, R. (2005). An examination of how therapist directiveness interacts with patient anger and reactance to predict alcohol use. *Journal of Studies on Alcohol, November, 2005, 825-832.*

Kuenzler, A., & Beutler, L. E. (2003). Couple alcohol treatment benefits patients' partners. *Journal of Clinical Psychology, 59,* 791-806.

Machado, P.P.P., Beutler, L.E., & Greenberg, L.S. (1999). Emotion recognition in psychotherapy: Impact of therapist level of experience and emotional awareness. *Journal of Clinical Psychology, 55*, 39-57.

McLellan, A.T., Luborsky, L., Woody, G.E., & O'Brien, C.P. (1980). An improved diagnostic instrument for substance abuse patients: The Addiction Severity Index. *Journal of Nervous and Mental Disease, 168*, 26-33.

Norcross, J.N. (Ed.). (2002). *Psychotherapy relationships that work.* New York: Oxford University Press.

Paul, G.L. (2006). Psychotherapy Outcome can be Studied Scientifically. In S. O. Lillienfield & W.O. Donohue (Eds.). *The Great Ideas of Clinical Science: The 17 Concepts Every Mental Health Researcher and Practitioner should Understand* (pp. 117-145). New York: Brunner-Routledge.

Sarason, I.G., Levine, H.M., Basham, R.B., & Sarason, B.R. (1983). Assessing social support: The Social Support Questionnaire. *Journal of Personality and Social Psychology, 44*, 127-139.

Sobell, L.C. & Sobell, M.B. (1992). Timeline follow-back: A technique for assessing self-reported alcohol consumption. In R.Z. Litten, & J.P. Allen (Eds.), *Measuring alcohol consumption: Psychological and biochemical methods* (pp. 41-72). Treatment Handbook Series, Number 4. Bethesda, MD: National Institute of Alcohol Abuse and Alcoholism.

Spielberger, C.D., Gorsuch, R.L., Lushene, R., Vagg, P.R., & Jacobs, G.A. (1993). *State-Trait Anxiety Inventor*y. Palo Alto, CA: Consulting Psychologists Press.

Weersing, R.V. (2005). Benchmarking the effectiveness of psychotherapy: Program evaluation as acomponent of evidence based practice. *Journal of the American Academy of Adolescent Psychiatry, 44:10, October, 2005*, 1058-1062.

In: Toward a Science of Clinical Psychology
Editor: Luciano L'Abate, pp. 177-196
ISBN: 978-1-60456-062-6


*Chapter X*

# MEASURING AND IMPROVING PSYCHOTHERAPY OUTCOME: LABORATORY METHODS IN ROUTINE CLINICAL PRACTICE

*Michael J. Lambert and Jason L. Whipple*

## ABSTRACT

Since the initial attempts to empirically evaluate client outcome in the 1920s, the quality and quantity of outcome research has steadily increased over the course of many decades. Once the general effectiveness of psychotherapy was established, outcome research began to focus more on comparative studies in which differences in effectiveness between therapies were examined. Such research, which included large meta-analytic reviews, supported the conclusion that psychotherapy is generally effective and that, with few notable exceptions, different therapies are equally effective in treating most problems (Lambert & Ogles, 2004).

## OUTCOME MEASUREMENT

One issue that is consistently at the forefront of outcome research is the measurement of client outcome. For decades, many researchers have argued that the central issue in all social science research is measurement (Nunnaly, 1978). In psychotherapy outcome research, the ability to accurately assess client response to treatment throughout the course of therapy, at termination, and/or at follow-up is directly related to the quality and appropriateness of the measure(s) being used for this purpose. In fact, when client changes are not detected on an outcome measure, either treatment did not work or the instrument was inadequate in detecting changes that occurred (Guyatt, 1988). Therefore, it is imperative that appropriate measures of outcome are used, else treatment gains may go undetected, a mistake that clinicians and researchers can ill afford to make in an age of increased accountability.

Of the thousands of psychological tests that have been published to date, most have been specifically designed to serve one or more of the following purposes: discrimination, prediction, and evaluation (Kirshner & Guyatt, 1985). A discriminative measure is one which is used for the purpose of distinguishing between individuals or groups on the basis of an underlying dimension when no external criterion or gold standard is available. Intelligence tests such as the WAIS and personality tests such as the MMPI are examples of discriminative measures. Discriminative measures are often used as diagnostic instruments because they are specifically designed to discriminate between different individuals (based on their scores on a measure) at a single point in time. A predictive measure is one which is used for the purpose of classifying individuals into categories when a gold standard is available, either concurrently or prospectively, in order to determine whether individuals have been classified correctly. This type of measure is generally used as a screening instrument to identify which specific individuals have or will develop a target condition. When a measure is used to assist in assessing whether or not a client is appropriate for a specific type of treatment (e.g., using a measure to assess a client's ego strength for the purpose of predicting whether he or she will be able to meaningfully participate in brief dynamic therapy), it is being used for predictive purposes. An evaluative measure is one which is used for the purpose of measuring change over time (e.g., pre- and post- treatment, weekly change over the course of treatment) in an individual or group on the dimension(s) of interest. Tests designed to assess treatment benefits or outcomes are examples of evaluative measures. The desired qualities of outcome measures may be quite different from assessments used for discriminative and predictive purposes because they are designed to measure intraindividual change over time via repeated administrations, rather than to discriminate between different individuals at a single point in time (Kirshner & Guyatt, 1985).

Given the importance of outcome measurement, clinicians would benefit from being aware of the qualities associated with sound outcome measures. The development of selection criteria (i.e., characteristics of instruments that will lead to the most accurate measurement of client change) for outcome measures to be implemented in practice has received increased attention in recent years (Trabin, 1995). Because professional practices may come to rely heavily on the demonstration of measured effects of treatments, it is imperative that outcome measures possess characteristics that will lead to the most accurate reflection of client improvement. Synthesizing and building upon the available literature, Lambert, Horowitz, and Strupp (1997) suggested that the following 13 criteria consistently emerge as an appropriate means of selecting methods and measures of outcome for research purposes: relevance to target group; simple, teachable methods; use of measures with objective referents; use of multiple respondents when possible; psychometric strengths and the availability of norms; low measure costs relative to its use; understanding by nonprofessional audiences, easy feedback, and uncomplicated interpretation; useful in clinical services; compatibility with a wide variety of clinical theories and practices; the possibility of multiple administrations; comprehensiveness; ties to a diagnostic classification system (e.g., DSM); and most important sensitivity to change (i.e., the ability of an outcome measure to detect change following an intervention). Attention to the aforementioned criteria will increase the likelihood of selecting a measure that provides the most accurate reflection of client outcome. Accurate assessment of client outcome will, in turn, allow clinicians to demonstrate treatment effectiveness more convincingly and alter treatment strategies in response to client change if needed.

## From Outcome Measurement and Monitoring to Management

A major emerging trend in psychotherapy outcome research is the shift from merely *measuring* or *monitoring* outcome to *managing* outcome (Evans, Mellor-Clark, Barkham, & Mothersole, 2006). For many decades, and even to the present day, psychotherapy outcome research, with the notable exception of the behavior therapies, has relied heavily on study designs that measure client outcome at pre-treatment and post-treatment. While such designs have proven beneficial in establishing the general efficacy and effectiveness of the treatments under investigation, they are limited in that outcome data from these studies (since it is collected following termination from treatment) cannot be used to positively influence the treatment process of the individual clients under investigation. Pre- and post- treatment assessments, then, are essentially a "post-mortem" analysis of outcome, since clients have already terminated treatment and nothing can be done to improve their outcomes, even if they experienced no change or even deteriorated in treatment.

Outcome management extends the practice of measuring and monitoring client progress throughout the course of treatment by then using data collected in real time to positively influence the treatment process and outcome of the clients under investigation. The major advantage of psychotherapy outcome management is that outcome data can be regularly gathered and fed back to clinicians in real time for the purpose of making needed alterations in intervention strategy if clients are either unresponsive to or deteriorating in treatment, which is a primary concern of clinicians. Several psychotherapy outcome management systems have been developed and implemented in clinical service delivery settings worldwide, such as in the United States (Lambert, Hansen, & Finch, 2001; Lueger, et al., 2001), Germany (Kordy, Hannover, & Richard, 2001), and Great Britain (Barkham et al., 2001). While the specific procedures employed in each of these quality management systems vary, a common feature across all of them is the monitoring of client outcome throughout the course of treatment and the use of these data to improve individual client outcomes (Howard, Moras, Brill, Martinovich, & Lutz, 1996).

The value of monitoring and systematic feedback through psychological assessments hinges on the degree to which the information provided goes beyond what a clinician can observe and understand about patient progress without such information. A reasonable conclusion from research in this area is that clinicians have a limited capacity to make accurate predictions, particularly with clients who are failing to improve (e.g., Hannan, et al., 2005). This is not surprising, given the complexity of persons and a treatment context that calls for considerable commitment and determination on the part of the therapist, who actually has very little control over the patient's life circumstances and personal characteristics. Helping with the task of identifying potential treatment failures and feeding back this information to therapists might well be a welcome advance in the practice of psychotherapy.

In many fields researchers and clinicians have provided outcome-related feedback to improve the impact of interventions (most notably, education & medicine; Millenson, 1997; Sapyta, Riemer, & Bickman, 2005). In general, this research supports the conclusion that feedback improves patient outcome. Sapyta (2004) for example, conducted a meta-analysis of

30 randomized clinical trials where health professionals received feedback about client health status in community settings and reported an effect size of .21; a small effect indicating improved outcomes when feedback information was available. This review suggests that the effectiveness of feedback is likely to vary as a function of the degree of discrepancy between expected progress and actual progress; the greater the discrepancy the more likely feedback will be helpful. This finding is consistent with feedback theories and the role of negative feedback in regulatory systems (Bandura, 1997; Lord & Hanges, 1987), feedback about poor progress is expected to have a greater impact than feedback indicating positive progress.

In the remainder of this chapter, one specific psychotherapy quality management system that has been developed, implemented, and empirically evaluated in multiple investigations is described. The methodology employed endeavors to improve psychotherapy outcome by monitoring client progress in relation to expected progress and providing this information to clinicians in order to guide ongoing treatment, particularly for the client who is not having a favorable response to treatment (signal-alarm cases). This methodology is an extension of quality assurance and represents one effort to bridge the gap between efficacy and effectiveness research and clinical practice, while enhancing patient outcome before treatment termination (Lambert, 2001). It is also well suited to models of care in which clinicians attempt to step-up or step-down treatments after assessing patient treatment response (e.g., Otto, Pollack & Maki, 2000).

## The OQ Psychotherapy Quality Management System

Patient outcome can be conceptualized and measured in myriad ways. Strupp and Hadley (1977) proposed a tripartite model for mental health outcomes. They suggested that the three interested parties concerned with therapy outcomes were society, the client, and the mental health professional. Based on this viewpoint, Lambert (1983) suggested the most important aspect of outcome is the subjective experience of the client, including symptoms of anxiety and depression. In addition, the functioning of persons in their social roles (e.g., work) and intimate relationships can be seen as very important for the well being of the person, family, and society in general. In the material that follows we conceptualize outcome mainly with regards to these three areas. But as the reader will see, outcome-focused quality management systems require several compromises to ideal assessment practices.

Quality management systems, as applied in routine practice, demand efficient outcome assessment rather than the more ideal alternative of comprehensive assessment. Outcome measurements that are typically employed in efficacy studies often require hours of assessment from multiple perspectives of change. In contrast, outcome-focused research uses weekly assessments with a single brief measure (Howard, Moras, Brill, Martinovitch, & Lutz, 1996). Thus, assessment in this type of research is much more frequent, with a greater diversity of patients, and large final sample sizes; but less comprehensive, and lacking multiple perspectives of change. To a large degree this methodology is essential to use for two reasons. The first is that unlike clinical trials, where number of treatment sessions a patient is expected to attend is predetermined (usually around 14 sessions), routine practice lengths are indeterminate and largely based on client and therapist preferences. In clinical trials progress can be assessed at preset times during the course of treatment (e.g., at weeks zero, 6, and 12) and especially at termination. In routine care the outcome measure is collected prior to each treatment session, so that the effects of the final session are infrequently collected, but outcome data are available for every session up to that point in time. The second reason is related to repeated measurement. While patients have no problem tolerating a weekly assessment that takes about 5 minutes, they cannot be expected to undergo lengthier, multi-scale, multi-source assessments on a frequent basis.

Given the demand for regular and efficient outcome assessment in psychotherapy outcome management, a suitable but brief measure was selected for implementation in the psychotherapy quality management system under consideration. The Outcome Questionnaire-45 (OQ-45; Lambert et al., 2004) is a 45-item, self-report measure designed for repeated administration throughout the course of treatment and at termination. In accordance with several reviews of the literature (e.g., Lambert, 1983), the OQ was conceptualized and designed to assess four domains of client functioning: symptoms of psychological disturbance, particularly anxiety and depression; interpersonal problems, social role functioning, and quality of life. Consistent with this conceptualization of outcome, the OQ-45 provides a Total Score, based on all 45 items, as well as Symptom Distress, Interpersonal Relations, and Social Role subscale scores. Higher scores on the OQ-45 are indicative of greater levels of psychological disturbance. Research has indicated that the OQ-45 is a psychometrically sound instrument, with excellent internal consistency (Cronbach's alpha = .93), adequate three-week test-retest reliability ($r=.84$), and strong concurrent validity estimates ranging from .55-.88 (all significant at $p<.01$) when the measure was correlated with the MMPI-2, SCL-90R, BDI, Zung Depression Scale, Taylor Manifest Anxiety Scale, State-Trait Anxiety Inventory, Inventory of Interpersonal Problems, and Social Adjustment Scale. Furthermore, the OQ-45 has been shown to be sensitive to changes in multiple client populations over short periods of time while remaining relatively stable in untreated individuals (Vermeersch, Lambert, & Burlingame, 2000; Vermeersch et al., 2004). In short, the OQ-45 is a brief measure of psychological disturbance that is reliable, valid, and sensitive to changes clients make during psychotherapy. It is well suited for assessing initial levels of client distress and tracking client status during and following treatment.

## Defining a Positive and Negative Outcome

A key element in psychotherapy quality management research is defining and operationalizing the concepts of positive and negative outcome for the individual patient. Jacobson and Truax (1991) offered a methodology by which a client's change on an outcome measure can be classified in the following categories: recovered, reliably improved, no change, deteriorated. There are two pieces of information necessary in order to make these client outcome classifications: a Reliable Change Index (RCI) and a normal functioning cutoff score. Clinical and normative data were analyzed by Lambert and colleagues (2004) to establish a Reliable Change Index (RCI) and a cutoff score for the OQ-45. The RCI obtained on the OQ-45 was 14 points, indicating that client changes of 14 or more points on the OQ-45 can be considered reliable (i.e., not due to measurement error). The cutoff score for normal functioning on the OQ-45 was calculated to be 63, indicating that scores of 64 or higher are more likely to come from a dysfunctional population than a functional population, and scores of 63 or lower are more likely to come from a functional population than a dysfunctional population. Using this information, clients can be placed in the following categories based on the change observed in their OQ scores:

- Recovered (i.e., clinically significant change) – Clients whose score decreases by 14 or more points and passes below the cutoff score of 64
- Improved (i.e., reliably changed) – Clients whose score decreases by 14 or more points but does not pass below the cutoff score of 64
- No Change – Clients whose score changes by less than 14 points in either direction
- Deteriorated – Clients whose score increases by 14 or more points

Support for the validity of the OQ-45's reliable change and cutoff score has been reported by Lunnen and Ogles (1998) and Beckstead et al. (2003). Having a method to classify each client's treatment response is an essential component of outcome-focused research, given that the primary purpose of psychotherapy outcome management is to understand and improve the gains each individual is making during the course of treatment. Furthermore, the ability to classify individual client change further bridges the gap between traditional efficacy and effectiveness studies (that focus on changes made by groups of clients) and clinical practice (Kendall, Marrs-Garcia, Nath & Sheldrick, 1999).

## Prediction of Treatment Failure

A core element of outcome management systems is the prediction of treatment failure. In order to improve outcomes of clients who are responding poorly to treatment, such clients must be identified before termination from treatment, and ideally, as early as possible in the course of treatment. Though many studies have investigated the value of several client, therapist, client-therapist interaction, and extratherapeutic variables in predicting outcome, very few of the variables explored are consistently highly predictive of outcome. Research utilizing the OQ-45 has indicated that the best predictors of outcome are initial severity of distress (i.e., pretreatment OQ-45 total score) and change score following separate sessions early in the course of treatment. In fact, Brown & Lambert (1998) found that pretreatment OQ-45 total score and change scores from sessions 1-3 accounted for approximately 40% of the variance in final outcome, and that after taking these variables into account, all other variables combined (e.g., diagnosis, client demographics, therapist demographics, therapist theoretical orientation, etc.) accounted for less than 1% of the variance in final outcome. In other words, in prior studies using the OQ-45, the best way to predict outcome was to know how distressed clients were prior to treatment and whether or not the changes they made early in the treatment process were positive or negative.

Given research on the variables most predictive of outcome, an empirically-derived signal-alarm system (which plots a statistically-generated expected recovery curve for differing levels of pre-treatment distress on the OQ-45 and uses this as a basis for identifying clients who are not making expected treatment gains and are at risk of having a poor outcome) was developed to alert clinicians to potential treatment failures. The accuracy of this signal-alarm system has been evaluated in a number of empirical investigations (Ellsworth, Lambert, & Johnson, 2006; Lambert, Whipple, Bishop, et al., 2002; Lutz, et al 2006; Spielmans, Masters, & Lambert, 2006), and though an extensive discussion of the results of these studies is beyond the scope of this chapter, it is important to note that the signal-alarm system is highly sensitive in that it is able to accurately predict a poor outcome in 88% of cases that actually end with a negative outcome, and it is also far superior to clinical judgment in its ability to identify clients who are at risk of having a negative treatment outcome (Hannan, et al., 2005).

Unlike some medical decisions where the cost of over identification of signal cases may result in intrusive and even health threatening interventions, the signal-alarm in psychotherapy merely alerts the therapist to the need for reconsidering the value of ongoing treatment, rather than mandating specific changes. Thus, we see the signal-alarm as supporting clinical decision-making, rather than supplanting it. Since the signal-alarm alerts therapists to the possible need for action, rather than triggering a negative chain of events such as termination or referral, the current level of misidentification would seem to be tolerable.

## The Provision of Feedback and Clinical Support Tools

The signal-alarm system has been used as an intervention for preventing deterioration and enhancing positive outcomes in clients, in that it alerts clinicians to potential treatment failures and allows them to modify their treatment approach in an attempt to improve the outcomes of clients who are having a poor response to treatment and are predicted to have a poor outcome. Once a client takes the OQ-45, commences treatment, and completes a session of treatment, the signal-alarm system can be used to generate feedback regarding the client's progress. The feedback to therapists consists of several components, among which are a progress graph that includes all the client's OQ-45 total scores from pretreatment to the current session and a color-coded message (white, green, yellow, red) that indicates the status of client progress. The specific language of the feedback messages varies not only as a function of client progress, but also as a function of the session at which the feedback is provided (i.e., a red message at session 2 is not as urgent as a red message at session 20). An illustrative summary of each feedback message follows:

White Message— "The client is functioning in the normal range. Consider termination."

Green Message— "The rate of change the client is making is in the adequate range. No change in the treatment plan is recommended."

Yellow Message— "The rate of change the client is making is less than adequate. Recommendations: consider altering the treatment plan by intensifying treatment, shifting intervention strategies, and monitoring progress especially carefully. This client may end up with no significant benefit from therapy."

Red Message— "The client is not making the expected level of progress. Chances are he/she may drop out of treatment prematurely or have a negative treatment outcome. Steps should be taken to carefully review this case and decide upon a new course of action such as referral for medication or intensification of treatment. The treatment plan should be reconsidered. Consideration should also be given to presenting this client at case conference. The client's readiness for change may need to be re-assessed."

Over the last 25 years, methodologies have been used in medical research and practice to manage clinical interventions in areas such as drug dosage, diagnosis, and preventive care. These interventions are often used in a stepwise approach that assists physicians in clinical decision making and provides recommendations to improve the quality of patient health care (Hunt, Haynes, Hanna, & Smith, 1998). Similarly, a set of Clinical Support Tools (CST) was developed and integrated into the existing psychotherapy quality management system in an attempt to augment the feedback provided to therapists and further improve outcomes of nonresponding and deteriorating patients (Whipple et al., 2003). As such, the CSTs are intended to be utilized by therapists when one of their clients is predicted to have a poor outcome (i.e., when a therapist receives a red or yellow warning message, indicating that client is not responding or deteriorating in treatment).

The CSTs are composed of a problem-solving decision tree designed to systematically direct therapists' attention to certain factors that have been shown to be consistently related to client outcome in the empirical literature, such as the therapeutic alliance, social support, readiness to change, diagnostic formulation, and need for psychiatric referral. Specific measures aimed at assisting therapists to assess the quality of the therapeutic alliance, client readiness for change, and client perceptions of social support are also included. These measures have included the Revised Helping Alliance Questionnaire (HAq-II; Luborsky et al., 1996), Multidimensional Scale of Perceived Social Support (MSPSS; Zimet, Dahlem, Zimet, & Farley, 1988), and Stages of Change Scale (SCS; McConnaughy, Prochaska, & Velicer, 1983). Furthermore, the CST Manual provides specific intervention strategies that could be used by therapists if problems were detected in the aforementioned domains. Figure 10.1 depicts the CST problem-solving decision tree provided to therapists in cases in which their clients were predicted to have a poor outcome.

When the signal-alarm rules identified a client as Not-On-Track (red or yellow warning) therapists had the option of using the clinical support tools (CST), which included the CST measures, a decision tree that ordered variables hierarchically, a list of possible interventions, and a tracking form. If a therapist asked the client to take the included measures, they were scored by a research assistant and returned to the therapist with a brief message about the results prior to the client's next therapy session. For example, if a NOT client was given the clinical support measures and scored below average on the helping alliance measure, the therapist then examined the list of suggestions for strengthening the relationship (e.g., discuss the clients ratings of the relationship, explore relationship ruptures). If the client's

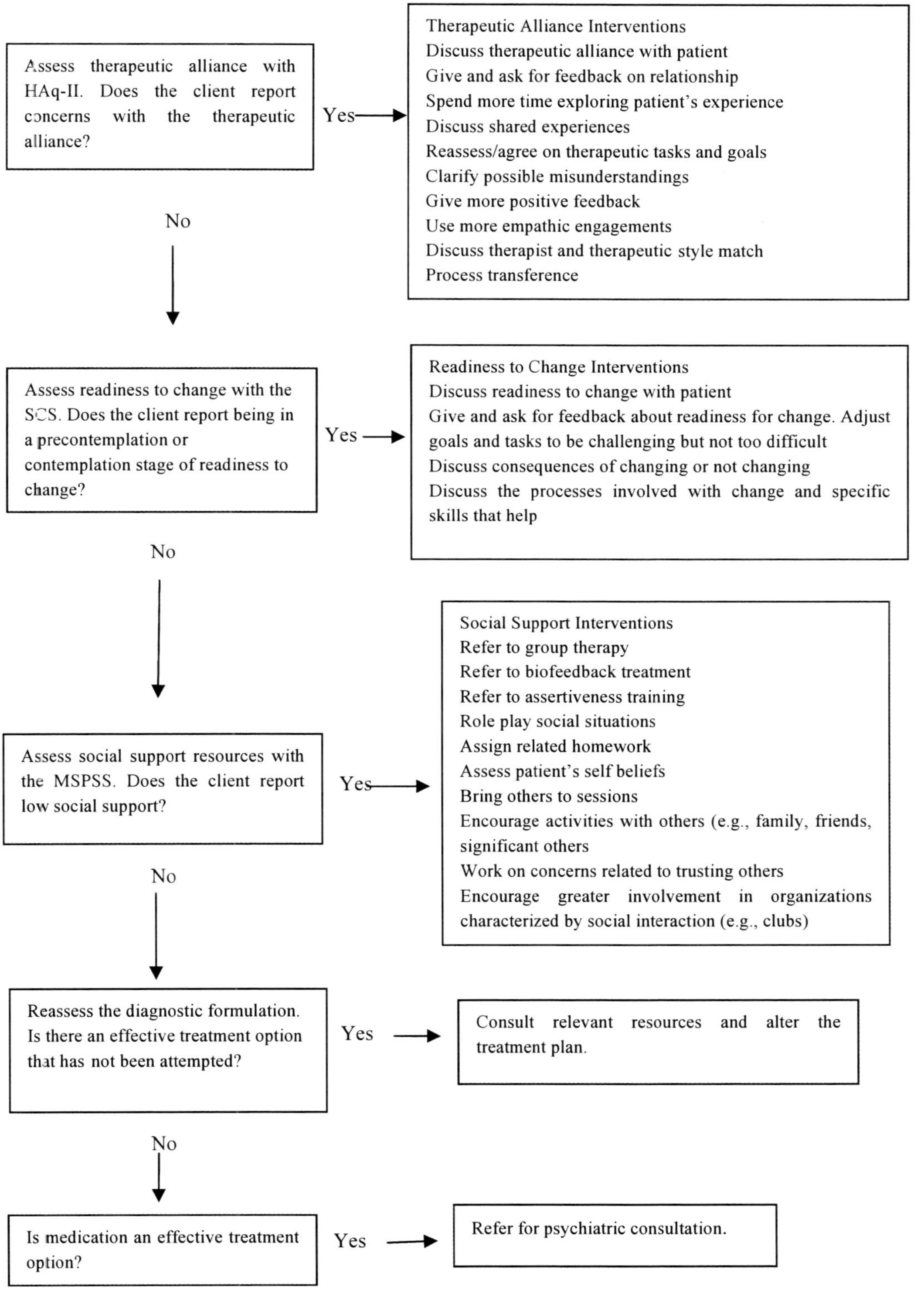


Figure 10.1. Clinical Support Tool (CST) problem-solving decision tree

alliance rating was not below average the therapist would proceed to evaluation of the client stage of motivation and so forth. It should be noted that the procedures used in the Whipple, et al. (2003) study resulted in a client group that was Not-On-Track, whose therapists received feedback, and then used their clinical judgment to decide if they wanted to use the clinical tools with a particular case. Clients who made up this group were selected by their therapist. To further influence therapists' decisions and actions as recipients of feedback, a tracking form was given to therapists as soon as a client was identified as NOT. This survey form was seen as part of the experimental manipulation, as it listed actions that might be taken by therapists and, therefore, could affect the way therapists treated clients who were not showing adequate progress.

In addition to providing feedback regarding client progress and CSTs to therapists, feedback can also be provided directly to clients. Client feedback messages (i.e., white, green, yellow/red) that correspond to the aforementioned therapist feedback messages have been developed in an effort to directly inform clients of their progress in treatment and enhance client/therapist collaboration in treatment (Harmon, et al., 2007; Hawkins et al., 2004). A summary of a *client* feedback message (that can be provided between sessions 2-4) follows:

> Yellow/Red Message- Please note that the following information is based on your responses to the questionnaire that you have completed prior to each therapy session. It appears that you have not experienced a reduced level of distress. Because you may not be experiencing the expected rate of progress, it is possible that you have even considered terminating treatment, believing that therapy may not be helpful for you. Although you have yet to experience much relief from therapy, it is still early in treatment and there is the potential for future improvement. However, we **urge** you to openly discuss any concerns that you may be having about therapy with your therapist because there are strategies that can be used to help you receive the most out of your therapy. It may also require your willingness to complete additional questionnaires that may shed light about why you are not experiencing the expected rate of progress.

Unlike the written messages and graphs provided to therapists, which were similar across studies (e.g., Lambert, Whipple et al., 2001; Lambert, Whipple, Vermeersch et al., 2002), the written messages used to communicate patients' progress to patients were created specifically for the two direct patient feedback studies. Consistent with the findings of prior research (Flowers, 1979; Kivlighan, 1985; Kluger & DeNisi, 1996), the messages designed for patients were a blend of positive and negative language. Effort was made to avoid message content potentially perceived as threatening or discouraging to patients' self-esteem. Patients were informed of their self-reported level of distress according to the OQ-45, progress since beginning therapy, and likelihood of benefiting from treatment given the present course of progress. Additionally, patients identified as potential treatment failures were encouraged to discuss personal concerns about their progress, alternative courses of action, and goals of therapy with their therapists to further facilitate the collaborative alliance.

The administration of the OQ-45 (whether via paper-pencil or computerized), scoring, application of the signal–alarm system, and generation of feedback reports (for therapists and/or clients) can all be integratively and almost instantaneously processed through software called OQ-Analyst (administration of the measure & generation of the feedback report takes approximately 5-7 minutes). Figure 10.2 depicts a screen shot of a therapist feedback report generated by the OQ-Analyst software. This feedback report illustrates the progress of a client from intake to Session 9. At session 9, the client's degree of deterioration (i.e., an increase of 21 points, from a 58 at pre-treatment to a 79 at session 9) prompted a RED feedback message to be given to the therapist. The feedback report also allows the therapist to view all prior OQ-45 scores and associated feedback messages (e.g., this therapist first received a RED feedback message at session 3, then again at sessions 5 and 9). At every session the therapist is able to look below the graph and read the message that is provided. Feedback messages vary depending on the size of the deviation from expected treatment response (the dark sloping line) and amount of therapy. Client scores are also displayed in the graph in relation to the horizontal line at a score of 63, which as previously mentioned, represents the cutoff score between client and nonclient populations on the OQ-45. The feedback report also provides information about the client's answer to five critical items, as well as other information (e.g., whether or not the client's change at the current session meets clinical significance criteria for recovery, improvement, no change, or deterioration) that may potentially be helpful to a therapist working with such a client.

## Impact of Feedback on Client Outcome

Five controlled studies have been published that examine the effects of providing client progress feedback to therapists and clients using the methodology described above (Harmon, et al., 2007; Hawkins, Lambert, Vermeersch, Slade, & Tuttle, 2004; Lambert, Smart, Hawkins, Nielsen, Slade, & Lutz, 2007; Lambert, Whipple, Smart, et al., 2001; Lambert, Whipple, Vermeersch, et al., 2002; Whipple et al., 2003). Each of the studies required about one year of daily data collection and evaluated the effects of providing feedback about a client's improvement through the use of progress graphs and warnings about clients who were not demonstrating expected treatment responses (signal-alarm cases). The primary question in each of these studies was: Does formal feedback to therapists (and in two studies, clients) on client progress improve psychotherapy outcomes? The hypothesis in each of these studies was: Clients identified as signal-alarm cases (those predicted to have a poor final treatment response) whose therapist received feedback will show better outcomes than similar clients whose therapists did not receive feedback.

The five studies shared many things in common: 1) Each included consecutive cases seen in routine care regardless of client diagnosis or co-morbid conditions (rather than being disorder specific); 2) Random assignment of client to experimental (feedback) and treatment as usual conditions (no feedback) was made in all but one of the studies; 3) Psychotherapists provided a variety of theoretically guided treatments with more clinicians adhering to cognitive behavioral and eclectic orientations followed by psychodynamic and experiential orientations; 4) A variety of clinicians were involved—post-graduate psychotherapists represented about 50%, with graduate students representing the remainder of the therapists; 5) Therapists saw both experimental (feedback) and treatment as usual (no feedback) cases, thus limiting the likelihood that outcome differences between conditions could be due to therapist effects; 6) The outcome measure as well as the methodology rules/standards for identifying signal-alarm clients (failing cases) remained constant; 7) The length of therapy (dosage) was determined by client and therapist rather than by research design or arbitrary insurance limits; and 8) Client characteristics such as gender, age, and ethnicity were generally similar across four of the studies and came from the same university counseling center, while the fifth sample (Hawkins et al., 2004) was older, more disturbed, and treated in a hospital-based outpatient clinic.

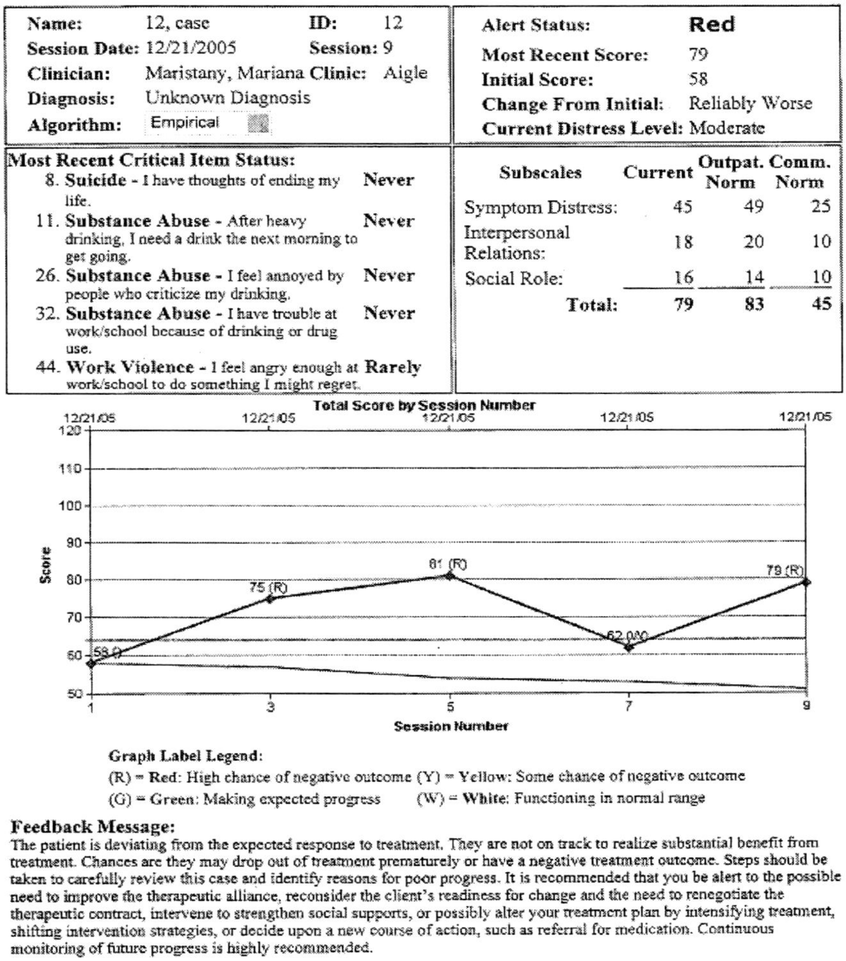
OQA: OQ Clinician Feedback Report

**Name:** 12, case **ID:** 12
**Session Date:** 12/21/2005 **Session:** 9
**Clinician:** Maristany, Mariana **Clinic:** Aigle
**Diagnosis:** Unknown Diagnosis
**Algorithm:** Empirical

**Alert Status:** Red
**Most Recent Score:** 79
**Initial Score:** 58
**Change From Initial:** Reliably Worse
**Current Distress Level:** Moderate

**Most Recent Critical Item Status:**

|  |  |
|---|---|
| 8. **Suicide** - I have thoughts of ending my life. | **Never** |
| 11. **Substance Abuse** - After heavy drinking, I need a drink the next morning to get going. | **Never** |
| 26. **Substance Abuse** - I feel annoyed by people who criticize my drinking. | **Never** |
| 32. **Substance Abuse** - I have trouble at work/school because of drinking or drug use. | **Never** |
| 44. **Work Violence** - I feel angry enough at work/school to do something I might regret. | **Rarely** |

| Subscales | Current | Outpat. Norm | Comm. Norm |
|---|---|---|---|
| Symptom Distress: | 45 | 49 | 25 |
| Interpersonal Relations: | 18 | 20 | 10 |
| Social Role: | 16 | 14 | 10 |
| **Total:** | **79** | **83** | **45** |



**Graph Label Legend:**
(R) = **Red:** High chance of negative outcome (Y) = **Yellow:** Some chance of negative outcome
(G) = **Green:** Making expected progress (W) = **White:** Functioning in normal range

**Feedback Message:**
The patient is deviating from the expected response to treatment. They are not on track to realize substantial benefit from treatment. Chances are they may drop out of treatment prematurely or have a negative treatment outcome. Steps should be taken to carefully review this case and identify reasons for poor progress. It is recommended that you be alert to the possible need to improve the therapeutic alliance, reconsider the client's readiness for change and the need to renegotiate the therapeutic contract, intervene to strengthen social supports, or possibly alter your treatment plan by intensifying treatment, shifting intervention strategies, or decide upon a new course of action, such as referral for medication. Continuous monitoring of future progress is highly recommended.

Figure 10.2. OQ-Analyst screen shot illustrating feedback report of client progress provided to therapist

Another notable difference in the studies was that two of the studies (Harmon et al., 2007; Whipple et al., 2003) extended the design of the first two studies by including a second experimental condition. This was intended to strengthen the feedback intervention by encouraging therapists to use the aforementioned Clinical Support Tools (i.e., problem-solving decision tree, additional measures and cutoffs, and suggestions for alternative clinical interventions) with signal-alarm cases. The Harmon et al. (2007) and Hawkins et al. (2004) studies also included two experimental conditions aimed at comparing treatment as usual with feedback to therapists, and feedback to therapists and clients. Design features of the five studies are detailed in Table 10.1.

**Table 10.1 Summary of Design Characteristics of Controlled Outcome Studies Aimed at Reducing Deterioration and Enhancing Positive Outcome**

| Study | Clients/ Therapists N | TAU | Therapist Feedback | Therapist/ Client Feedback | Clinical Support Tools |
|---|---|---|---|---|---|
| Lambert, Whipple, et al. (2001) | 609/31 | X | X | | |
| Lambert, Whipple, et al. (2002) | 1020/49 | X | X | | |
| Whipple et al. (2003) | 981/48 | X | X | | X |
| Hawkins et al. (2004) | 201/5 | X | X | X | |
| Harmon et al. (2007) | 1374/47 | | X | X | X |

Results from the combined studies are presented graphically in Figure 10.3. As can be seen, the clients identified as Not-on-Track (signal-alarm clients) had a different outcome course depending on assignment to the no feedback or feedback treatment conditions. Up to the point that these signal-alarm cases were first signaled (or in the case of the no feedback treatment as usual condition could have been signaled) the graph illustrates an average worsening of around 10 points (about one-half a standard deviation on the OQ-45). From the point of the signal-alarm, all the experimental (feedback) groups (NOT-Fb, NOT-Fb+CST, and NOT-Th & PT) improved while the no feedback control (treatment as usual; TAU) cases improved to an average score near 80 but were, as a group, slightly worse off than when they entered treatment. Also displayed is the outcome for On-Track (OT) cases where therapists did (OT- FB) and did not get feedback (OT-TAU). As can be seen these clients made steady progress and left treatment, as a group, well within the ranks of normal functioning. It appeared to make little difference in outcome for feedback (Green or White messages) to have been given.

In the individual studies themselves, the effect sizes (standardized mean differences) for the difference between various feedback conditions for the NOT clients and TAU controls ranged from .34 to .92. Such effect sizes are surprisingly large when one considers an average effect for comparative studies (active treatments) typically falls between .00 and .20 (Lambert & Ogles, 2004) and is widely considered important enough to lead to a recommendation of a "best practice".

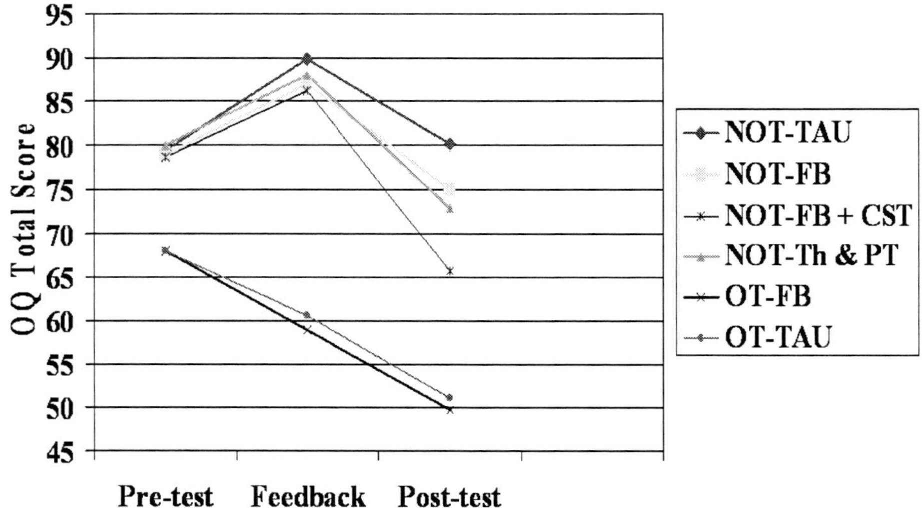


Figure 10.3. Change from pre- to post-testing of Not-On-Track (signal-alarm) and On-Track patients.

Note: Not-NFb = Signal-alarm cases whose therapist got no signal or message; NOT-Fb = Signal-alarm cases whose therapist got a red or yellow signal, indicating they were at risk for treatment failure; OT-NFb = Patients who were making satisfactory progress and whose therapist never received any information about their progress; OT-Fb = Patients whose therapist got a green or white signal and message and who were predicted to have a positive outcome; NOT-Fb+CST = Signal-alarm cases whose therapist got feedback and used the Clinical Support Tools; T/Pat Fb = All patients who entered treatment and were assigned to receive feedback and whose therapist also received feedback; Pre OQ = average patient scores on the OQ-45 at intake; Warn OQ = average patient score on the OQ-45 at the point at which a patient qualified for a yellow or red message (the time of warning varied across patients); Post OQ = Average patient OQ-45 score at the session they terminated treatment (number of sessions until termination occurred varied).

Across the five studies some inconsistent results have been found. Usually the provision of NOT feedback increases the number of sessions that clients attend by about 2-3 sessions and decreases sessions for OT cases by 2/3 a session, but this was not found in the Hawkins et al. (2004) study where feedback to both NOT and OT were equal. In about half the studies, feedback to OT cases improved outcomes despite reducing treatment length. Direct feedback to clients in the form of a written message improved outcomes dramatically in the Hawkins et al. (2004) study, but had no impact in the Harmon et al. (2007) replication.

Table 10.2 presents a classification of signal-alarm clients based on their final treatment status at termination. As shown, 20% of the signal-alarm cases seen by therapists who received no feedback (TAU) showed a negative treatment outcome at termination. In contrast, when therapists received feedback that identified their client as not-on-track, only 15%, 12%, and 8% depending on treatment condition deteriorated. The rates for signal-alarm cases (NOT) showing clinically significant or reliable change were also markedly different, with the highest rates of improvement in the T-Fb+CST condition (45%), compared to 22% in the TAU condition. These data suggest the improved outcomes for clients in the experimental conditions are not only statistically significant but are of considerable clinical meaning for the individual client.

**Table 10.2 Percent of Not-On-Track (Signal-Alarm) Cases Meeting Criteria for Clinically Significant Change at Termination Summed Across Five Studies**

| | TAU[a] | T-Fb[b] | T-Fb+CST[c] | T/C-Fb[d] |
|---|---|---|---|---|
| Outcome Classification | n (%) | n (%) | n (%) | n (%) |
| Deteriorated[e] | 64 (20%) | 90 (15%) | 12(8%) | 19(12%) |
| No Change | 184 (58%) | 316 (53%) | 73(47%) | 71(46%) |
| Reliable/or Clinically Significant Change[f] | 70 (22%) | 196 (33%) | 169(45%) | 57(37%) |

[a]TAU = patients who were not on track and whose therapist was not given feedback
[b] T-Fb = patients who were not on track and whose therapist received feedback
[c] T-Fb+CST = patients who were not on track and whose therapist received feedback and used clinical support tools
[d] T/C-Fb = therapist feedback plus written direct feedback to clients
[e] Worsened by at least 14 points on the OQ from pre-treatment to post-treatment
[f] Improved by at least 14 points on the OQ or improved and passed the cut-off between dysfunctional and functional populations

Feedback was also hypothesized to affect dose of psychotherapy as well as outcome. In this context it was anticipated that those patients who were OT (i.e., received green or white messages without ever receiving a yellow or red warning) would receive less therapy than the control patients who were OT and whose therapists received no feedback. In contrast, patients who were NOT were expected to stay in therapy longer if feedback was given than patients whose therapists did not receive feedback. Signal-alarm cases whose therapist received feedback stayed in therapy longer (attended more sessions of therapy) than the signal-alarm patients where no feedback was given. On average they attended about one and one-half additional sessions. This increase in attendance occurred after the warning was given (or could have been given). In contrast, the OT patients of therapists who received no feedback participated in more sessions than the OT feedback group. Although only slightly greater, this session difference reached statistical significance. The pattern is consistent with cost-effective psychotherapy since the decrease in attendance for the large number of OT-Fb cases offsets the additional costs of increasing dosage for the NOT-Fb feedback cases.

## SUMMARY AND CONCLUSIONS

The program of research described in this chapter has taken over a decade to complete. It began with the simple aim of applying research to practice with the goal of enhancing client outcomes. Outcome was defined conceptually as including symptoms of psychopathology, interpersonal difficulties, social role functioning, and well-being. The elements of these constructs were operationally defined through a 45-item self-report scale that could be administered on a session-by-session basis throughout the course of psychotherapy. The scale was constructed and validated with particular attention to including items that remained constant over time if a person went untreated, but demonstrated positive change with increasing doses of psychotherapy.

Following the progress of thousands of clients over the course of treatment allowed for the study of longitudinal trends of change over time. These longitudinal data led to the generation of expected recovery curves and the determination of the amount of deviation from expected recovery that is predictive of a poor outcome. From this information, an empirically-derived signal-alarm system for providing ongoing feedback to therapists (with particular emphasis placed on providing feedback about potential treatment failure) was developed and its predictive accuracy was tested and supported. This signal-alarm system ultimately led to the creation of software that made providing this information to therapists and clients nearly instantaneous.

Perhaps most importantly, the signal-alarm system has been successfully implemented in five clinical trials that clearly demonstrate that feedback provided to therapists about impending treatment failure improves the outcome for clients at risk for having no response to treatment or a poor outcome. The practical difficulties of adding monitoring and managing activities to busy practices can be an important barrier to implementation. Fortunately, recent developments in software programs make the possibility of instantaneous feedback to clinicians easy to implement. If the client takes the OQ-45 immediately prior to the scheduled psychotherapy session, feedback through the OQ-Analyst is available to the therapist prior to beginning that session. Despite limitations and challenges, it is hoped that the research results convince practitioners that systematically monitoring their clients with the methods described in this chapter is in the best interest of clients.

## REFERENCES

Bandura, A. (1997). Social cognitive theory of self regulation. *Organizational Behavior and Human Decision Processes, 50*, 248-287.

Barkham, M., Margison, F., Leach, C., Lucock, M., Mellor-Clark, J., Evans, C., Benson, L., Connell, J., Audin, K., & McGrath, G. (2001). Service profiling and outcomes benchmarking using the CORE_OM: Toward practice-based evidence in the psychological therapies. *Journal of Consulting and Clinical Psychology, 69,* 184-196.

Beckstead, D. J., Hatch, A. L., Lambert, M. J., Eggett, D. L., Goates, M. K., & Vermeersch, D. A. (2003).Clinical significance of the Outcome Questionnaire (OQ-45.2). *The Behavior Analyst Today, 4,* 79-90.

Brown, G. S., & Lambert, M. J. (1998, June). Tracking patient progress: Decision making for cases who are not benefiting from psychotherapy. Paper presented at the annual meeting of the Society for Psychotherapy Research, Snowbird, UT.

Ellsworth, J. R., Lambert, M. J., & Johnson, J. (2006). A Comparison of the Outcome Questionnaire-45 and Outcome Questionnaire-30 in classification and prediction of treatment outcome. *Clinical Psychology and Psychotherapy, 13 380-391..*

Evans, R., Mellor-Clark, J., Barkham, M., &. Mothersole,G. ( 2006). Developing the resources and management support for routine evaluation in counselling and psychological therapy service provision: Reflections on a decade of core development. *European Journal of Psychotherapy & Counselling ,8,* 141-161.

Finch, A. E., Lambert, M. J., & Schaalje, B. G. ( 2001). Psychotherapy quality control: The statistical generation of expected recovery curves for integration into an early warning system. *Clinical Psychology and Psychotherapy, 8,* 231-242.

Flowers, J. V. (1979). The differential outcome effects of simple advice, alternatives and instructions in group psychotherapy. *International Journal of Group Psychotherapy, 29* (3), 305-316.

Guyatt, G. (1988). Measuring health status in chronic airflow limitation. *European Respiratory Journal, 1,* 560-564.

Haas, E., Hill R., Lambert, M. J.,& Morrell, B.(2002). Do early responders to psychotherapy maintain treatment gains? *Journal of Clinical Psychology, 58,* 1157-1172.

Hannan, C., Lambert, M. J., Harmon, C., Nielsen, S. L., Smart, D. W., Shimokawa, K., & Sutton, S. W. (2005). A lab test and algorithms for identifying clients at risk for treatment failure. *Journal of Clinical Psychology: In Session, 61,* 155-63.

Hansen, N. B., Lambert, M. J., & Forman, E. V. (2002). The psychotherapy dose-response effect and its implications for treatment delivery services. *Clinical Psychology: Science and Practice, 9,* 329-343.

Harmon, S. C., Lambert, M. J., Smart, D. W., Hawkins, E. J., Nielsen, S. L., Slade, K., & Lutz, W. (2007). Enhancing outcome for potential treatment failures: Therapist/client feedback and clinical support tools. Psychotherapy Research, 17, 379-392.

Hatfield, D. R., & Ogles, B. M. (2004). The current climate of outcome measures use in clinical practice. *Professional Psychology:Research & Practice, 35, 485-491.,*

Hawkins, E. J., Lambert, M. J., Vermeersch, D. A., Slade, K., & Tuttle, K. (2004). The effects of providing patient progress information to therapists and patients. *Psychotherapy Research, 14,* 308-327.

Howard, K. I., Kopta, S. M., Krause, M. S., Orlinsky, D. E. (1986). The dose-effect relationship in psychotherapy. *American Psychologist, 41,* 159-164.

Howard, K. I., Moras, K., Brill, P. L., Martinovich, Z., & Lutz, W. (1996). Efficacy, effectiveness, and client progress. *American Psychologist, 51,* 1059–1064.

Hunt, D. L., Haynes, B., Hanna, S. E., & Smith, K. (1998). Effects of computer-based clinical decision support systems on physician performance and patient outcomes. *Journal of the American Medical Association, 280,* 1339-1346.

Jacobson, N. S., & Truax, P. (1991). Clinical significance: A statistical approach to defining meaningful change in psychotherapy research. *Journal of Consulting and Clinical Psychology, 59,* 12–19.

Kadera, S.W., Lambert, M.J., Andrews, A.A. (1996). A session-by-session analysis of the psychotherapy dose-effect relationship. *Journal of Psychotherapy Practice and Research, 5,* 132-151.

Kendall, P. C., Marrs-Garcia, A., Nath, S. R., & Sheldrick, R. C. (1999). Normative comparisons for the evaluation of clinical significance. *Journal of Consulting and Clinical Psychology, 67*, 285-299.

Kirshner, B., & Guyatt, G. (1985). A methodological framework for assessing health indices. *Journal of Chronic Diseases, 38*, 27-36.

Kivlighan, D. M. (1985). Feedback in group psychotherapy: Review and implications. *Small Group Behavior, 16*(3), 373-385.

Kluger, A. N., & DeNisi, A. (1996). The effects of feedback interventions on performance: A historical review, a meta-analysis, and a preliminary feedback intervention theory. *Psychological Bulletin, 119*, 254-284.

Kordy, H., Hannöver, W., & Richard, M. (2001). Computer-assisted feedback-driven quality management for psychotherapy: The Stuttgart-Heidelberg model. *Journal of Consulting and Clinical Psychology, 69,* 173-183.

Lambert, M.J. (1983). Introduction to assessment of psychotherapy outcome: Historical perspective and current issues. In M.J. Lambert, E.R. Christensen, & S.S. DeJulio (Eds), *The assessment of psychotherapy outcome*. New York, NY: Wiley.

Lambert, M. J., Burlingame, G. M., Umphress, V. J., Hansen, N. B., Vermeersch, D., Clouse, G., & Yanchar, S. (1996). The reliability and validity of the Outcome Questionnaire. *Clinical Psychology and Psychotherapy, 3,* 106–116.

Lambert, M. J., Hansen, N. B., & Finch, A. E. (2001). Client-focused research: Using client outcome data to enhance treatment effects. *Journal of Consulting and Clinical Psychology, 69,* 159-172.

Lambert, M. J., Horowitz, L. M., & Strupp, H. H. (1997). Conclusions and recommendations. In H. H. Strupp, L. M. Horowitz, & M. J. Lambert (Eds.), *Measuring patient changes in mood, anxiety, and personality disorders: Toward a core battery* (pp. 491-502). Washington, DC: American Psychological Association.

Lambert, M. J., Morton, J.J., Hatfield, D., Harmon, C., Hamilton, S., Reid, R. C., Shimokowa, K., Christopherson, C., and Burlingame, G. M. (2004). *Administration and Scoring Manual for the Outcome Questionnaire -45.* SLC, UT: OQ Measures.

Lambert, M. J., & Ogles, B. M. (2004). The efficacy and effectiveness of psychotherapy. In M. J. Lambert (Ed.), *Bergin and Garfield's handbook of psychotherapy and behavior change* ($5^{th}$ ed., pp. 139-193). New York: Wiley.

Lambert, M. J., Whipple, J. L., Bishop, M. J., Vermeersch, D. A., Gray, G. V., & Finch, A. E. (2002). Comparison of empirically derived and rationally derived methods for identifying clients at risk for treatment failure. *Clinical Psychology and Psychotherapy, 9,* 149-164.

Lambert, M. J., Whipple, J. L., Harmon, C., Shimokawa, K., Slade, K., Christofferson, C. (2004). *Clinical Support Tools Manual*, Department of Psychology, Brigham Young University, Provo UT.

Lambert, M. J., Whipple, J. L., Hawkins, E. J., Vermeersch, D. A., Nielsen, S. L., & Smart, D.W. ( 2003). Is it time for clinicians to routinely track patient outcome?: A meta-analysis. *Clinical Psychology: Science & Practice, 10,* 288-301.

Lambert, M. J., Whipple, J. L., Smart, D. W., Vermeersch, D. A., Nielsen, S. L., & Hawkins, E. J. (2001). The effects of providing therapists with feedback on client progress during psychotherapy: Are outcomes enhanced? *Psychotherapy Research*, 11, 49-68.

Lambert, M. J., Whipple, J. L., Vermeersch, D. A., Smart, D. W., Hawkins, E. J., Nielsen, S. L., & Goates, M. K. (2002). Enhancing psychotherapy outcomes via providing feedback on client progress: A replication. *Clinical Psychology and Psychotherapy, 9,* 91-103.

Luborsky, L., Barber, J., Siqueland, L., Johnson, S., Najavits, L., Franks, A., & Daley, D. (1996). The revised helping alliance questionnaire (HAq-II). *Journal of Psychotherapy Practice and Research, 5,* 260-271.

Lueger, R. J., Howard, K. I., Martinovich Z., Lutz, W., Anderson, E.E., & Grissom, G. (2001). Assessing treatment progress of individual clients using expected treatment response models. *Journal of Consulting and Clinical Psychology, 69,* 150-158.

Lunnen, K. M., & Ogles, B. M. (1998). A multiperspective, multivariable evaluation of reliable change. *Journal of Consulting and Clinical Psychology, 66*, 400-410.

Lutz, W., Lambert, M. J., Harmon, S. C., Stulz, N., Tschitsaz, A.,& Schürch, E. (2006). The probability of treatment success, failure and duration – what can be learned from empirical data to support decision making in clinical practice? *Clinical Psychology & Psychotherapy, 13*, 223-232.

McConnaughy, E. A., Prochaska, J. O., & Velicer, W. F. (1983). Stages of change in psychotherapy: Measurement and sample profiles. *Psychotherapy: Theory, Research & Practice, 20*(3), 368-375.

Millenson, M. L. (1997). *Demanding medical excellence*. Chicago:University of Chicago Press.

Nunnaly, J. C. (1978). *Psychometric Theory*. New York: Mcgraw-Hill.

Otto, M. W. Pollack, M. H., & Maki, K. M. (2000). Empirically supported treatments for panic disorder: Costs, benefits, and stepped care. *Journal of Consulting and Clinical Psychology, 68,* 556-563.

Sapyta, J., Riemer, M, & Bickman, L. (2005). Feedback to clinicians: Theory, research, and practice. *Journal of Clinical Psychology, 62*(2), 145-153.

Spielmans, G. I., Masters, K. S., & Lambert, M. J. (2006). A comparison of rational versus empirical methods in prediction of negative psychotherapy outcome. *Clinical Psychology & Psychotherapy, 13,* 202-214.

Trabin, T. (1995). Making quality and accountability happen in behavioral healthcare. *Behavioral Healthcare Tomorrow, 4(3)*, 5-6.

Umphress, V. J., Lambert, M. J., Smart, D. W., Barlow, S. H., & Clouse, G. (1997). Concurrent and construct validity of the Outcome Questionnaire. *Journal of Psychoeducational Assessment, 15,* 40-55.

Vermeersch, D. A., Lambert, M. J., & Burlingame, G. M. (2000). Outcome Questionnaire: Item sensitivity to change. *Journal of Personality Assessment, 74*, 242-261.

Vermeersch, D. A., Whipple, J. L., Lambert, M. J., Hawkins, E. J., Burchfield, C. M., & Okiishi, J. C. (2004). Outcome Questionnaire: Is it sensitive to changes in counseling center clients? *Journal of Counseling Psychology, 51,* 38-49.

Whipple, J. L., Lambert, M. J., Vermeersch, D. A., Smart, D. W., Nielsen, S. L., & Hawkins, E. J. (2003). Improving the effects of psychotherapy: The use of early identification of treatment failure and problem solving strategies in routine practice. *Journal of Counseling Psychology, 58,* 59-68.

Zimet, G. D., Dahlem, N. W., Zimet, S. G., & Farley, G. K. (1988). The multidimensional scale of perceived social support. *Journal of Personality Assessment, 52*, 30-41.

In: Toward a Science of Clinical Psychology
Editor: Luciano L'Abate, pp. 197-209
ISBN: 978-1-60456-062-6


*Chapter XI*

# Evaluating and Treating the Psychological Consequences of Chronic Pain

*T.M. McClanahan*

## Abstract

Patients who suffer from chronic pain are often forced to face the stigma of the perception that the vast majority of patients who report that they suffer from chronic pain are malingering in order to substantiate an outside claim with Worker's Compensation or in a civil action. In fact, it has been estimated that approximately 42% of patients who report a minor head injury and file litigation are malingering and that approximately 33% of patients who complain of pain and who file a claim or litigation are in fact malingering (Mittenberg et al., 2002). Others have predicted that the prevalence of malingering in patients who present for personal injury claims ranges from 20 to 59% (Guriel and Frenouw, 2003). Another common belief is that the patient who suffers from chronic pain doesn't want to get better.

In order to better understand chronic pain one must differentiate it from acute pain. Chronic pain is often described as a pain state that is persistent due to the fact that the source of the pain can not be removed or otherwise effectively treated within a medical model. Thus, the patient may experience a constellation of symptoms that have no clearly established etiology which of late has been labeled chronic pain syndrome (Searight, 1998). This vagueness often leads health care providers to question the authenticity of the patient's complaints and generates feelings of frustration for both the provider as well as the patient. Acute pain, on the other hand, most often has a definite etiology and identifiable source. It also resolves within a few weeks of onset or following the completion of an intervention designed to ameliorate the symptoms.

One of the earliest epidemiological studies that examined the phenomenon of chronic pain was conducted by Bonica (1990). This study estimated that more than one third of the American population suffers from chronic pain. Given the prevalence of chronic pain, it is only logical that the economic consequences of chronic pain are astronomical. In fact, Bonica (1990) estimated that chronic pain lead to a loss of 400 million work days to the American workforce in 1986, the year that was examined. The burden to the American economy due to health care cost, lost productivity, litigation, and compensation totaled $79 billion for that year.

More recent data estimate that reduced productivity while at work accounts for a greater percentage (76.6%) of lost productive time and accounts for an estimated $61.2 billion per year (Stewart et al., 2003). Researchers have even estimated that chronic pain syndrome may account for up to 80% of patient visits to physicians (Searight, 1998).

## INTERVENTION

There are various rationales for intervening with a patient and various measures of successful treatment. The patient may want to eliminate their pain and increase the quality of their life. Conversely, if they are involved in litigation they may need to remain in a place of pain in order to not jeopardize their case. The latter scenario is one which the medical field is most interested in and which creates much of the negative stigma that patients must also deal with in their treatment. This conflict of interest is often an exclusionary criterion that is covered elsewhere in this chapter. The healthcare provider, or Healthcare Maintenance Organization (HMO) may want to reduce the number of visits to the Primary Care Physician (PCP), or to reduce the number of mentions to the Emergency Department, or to reduce the number of medications that the patient is prescribed. The patient's employer may want to reduce absenteeism and to increase productivity.

Treatment for chronic pain often includes pharmacological agents, surgical procedures, neuroaugmentative (e.g., epidural injections, nerve blocking agents), physical therapy (e.g., TENS, ultrasound, traction, body mechanics, stretching exercises, strengthening exercises), adjunct therapies (e.g., acupressure, acupuncture), and Cognitive Behavioral Therapy.

The two leading psychological explanations, thus treatment, of chronic pain are the gate control theory (Melzack and Wall, 1965) and the behavioral model (Fordyce, 1976). The gate control model was the first model that posited that chronic pain was not simply a function of tissue damage. Rather, it is influenced by central nervous system phenomena that included motivation, attention, and emotional states. According to this model, the spinal column includes neural mechanisms in the dorsal horns and act as a "gate" that can either increase or decrease the flow of nerve impulses from peripheral fibers to the spinal cord cells which transmit these signals to the brain. Emotions affect the reticulolimbic area as well as the frontal cortex and can either inhibit or amplify the perception of pain.

One of the first to apply a behavioral perspective to chronic pain was Fordyce (1976). According to Fordyce's initial postulation, chronic pain generally follows the principles of operant learning and is maintained by the consequences of pain behavior in the patient. For instance, back pain may be reinforced by receiving attention from another family member. Fordyce also posited that secondary gain from litigation, worker's compensation cases, or veteran's benefits would increase the peripheral source of pain. There is some evidence that supports the position that patients engaged in litigation or other financial gain report a higher subjective pain experience and greater functional impairment (Rohling, Binder, & Langhinrichsen-Rohling, 1995).

More recent behavioral application in the treatment of chronic pain is Cognitive Behavioral Therapy (CBT). CBT has been used to treat various age groups (e.g., children, adults, couples, geriatric populations, inpatient populations, and outpatient populations) as well as various disorders (e.g., depression, anxiety, thought disorders, personality disorders, suicidal behaviors, trauma survivors, etc.).

The treatment protocol used to treat patients suffering from chronic pain in this examination is as L'Abate earlier in this volume describes as being "systematic, replicable, and progressive". The treatment was systematic in that it was structured and delivered to each treatment cohort in similar manner with the same participant being given exact duplicates. It is replicable in that the format can be delivered by any clinician who meets the state's statutes, which in the state of this population is doctoral level. The State has determined that this level of training is required in order to formulate a diagnosis and to develop a treatment plan for patients in a hospital setting. The treatment is progressive in that each stage of treatment from evaluation to treatment to discharge is based upon empirical evidence.

## Group Intervention

The group treatment was structured in that each cohort met once per week for nine weeks, and each group session lasting for 2 ½ hours. Each group had a maximum of 10 participants and each group member was given identical materials (e.g., syllabus, participant workbook, handouts, relaxation tape, homework, etc).

Session 1 provided an orientation to the 9-week treatment and a general overview of chronic pain which included understanding chronic pain (thoughts, behaviors, emotions), the impact of chronic pain, a stress management exercise that examined stressors in participant's lives and how the sympathetic and parasympathetic nervous systems respond to stress, and the logistics of the 9-week group treatment (e.g., format of the session, expectations, and completion of assessment questionnaires). The first homework assignment was completion of a pleasant activity (Lewinsohn, Munoz, Youngren, and Zeiss, 1978) and followed the general format of identifying and participating in one pleasant activity in the upcoming week for each participant

Session 2 consisted of educating the participant regarding the neurophysiology of chronic pain and presenting the two leading theories: gate control and behavioral theory. The physician then presented information on medications that are used in the treatment of chronic pain. This session addressed the use of Nonsteroidal Anti-Inflamatory Drugs (NSAIDs, aspirin, ibuprofen, Indocin, Relafen), Acetaminophen, narcotics and opiates (Vicodin, Percocet, morphine, fentanyl, etc.), muscle relaxants (Robaxin, Flexeril, Soma), benzodiazepines/sedatives (Valium, lorazepam, oxazepam, alprazolam), antidepressants (amitriptyline, nortriptyline, trazodone), anti-seizure medications (Neurontin, Depakote, Tegretol). This session also included a discussion of the stigmas associated with certain medications. It also included the presentation and discussion of use, habituation, dependence, and addiction.

Session 3 covered sleep hygiene and how the participant could develop a self-management approach to improving their sleep patterns. This session covered areas such as caffeine and its effects on sleep, negative sleep thoughts and how to challenge these negative patterns, sleep medications, and ten recommendations for improving sleep (e.g., regular schedule, regular exercise, using the bed for sleeping, investing in a good bed, not taking worries to bed, sleep and meals, quality versus quantity of sleep, pre-sleep routine, reducing sleep expectations, and reducing daytime naps).

Session 4 introduced the participant to the concept of what is referred to as the 3Ps of chronic pain (Prioritizing, Planning, and Pacing). Each of these concepts is interrelated. For instance, prioritizing each activity that the participant may need to attend to enables them to plan on how each activity can be completed and pacing is assisting the participant in identifying ways to break each activity into components in order that flare-ups and break through pain can be either reduced or eliminated.

Session 5, 6, & 7 expanded upon the concept of Cognitive Behavioral Therapy for the participant. The first of these three sessions began by educating the participants on the effect that thoughts have on a person's emotions, and how each of these dictates a person's behaviors. The participants were then taken through an experiential exercise where they were asked to diagram their particular pain using different colors, figures, etc but no words to describe their pain to others. As each person explained their depiction of their pain, a "pain vocabulary" was developed. This would enable each participant to better describe their pain to family, friends, health care providers, and others in a more descriptive and quantifiable fashion versus the ambiguous manner that many persons who suffer from chronic pain often do. The next two sessions were devoted to educating the participants on how they can manage their belief systems through an examination of their negative thought processes. For instance, a person might have the thought "I am going to have this pain forever", which in turns makes the person depressed, which in turns causes the patient to withdraw from their family, friends, and life obligations. The participant was first asked to monitor and track their thoughts daily for a week, and the subsequent session helps the participant to categorize their thoughts (i.e., generalizations, personalizations, catastrophizing, mental filtering, etc.). The participant was then taught how to challenge the negative thought with their own particular clinical data. This often comes in the participant being able to rely upon the fact that they do not know if the pain will be present forever. They also have, in the vast majority of cases, never used any of the techniques covered in the 9-week treatment group previously. They may also rely upon the new information where they learn that pain-free pathways can be developed which might enable them to not experience their chronic pain. The categorization and challenging of negative thought processes draws from Ellis (1986), Beck (1979), Burns (1999).

Session 8 covered communication styles and how communication patterns are often negatively affected when someone experiences chronic pain. This session educated the participant on the difference between passive, assertive, and aggressive communication styles. It also helps the individual identify situations that may cause them to act passively until they reach a certain level of frustration and then to act aggressively. This understanding on the part of the participant often enables them to change their behavioral patterns in order to be able to better meet their individual needs. They are also taught how to use "I" statements in a more effective manner also in an attempt to have their needs met.

Session 9 is the final session and was devoted to a review of progress that each participant accomplished during the 9-week treatment. The participant also participated in a collaborative approach to treatment planning. Three post-treatment options are available: (1) if the participant successfully completed the requirements and feels comfortable in their newly learned skills and are eligible to attend the "Alumni Group" which meets once per week (this group uses the same skills and handouts that are originally presented during the 9-week treatment and the participant can attend the Alumni Group for up to two years post completion of the 9-week group intervention), (2) if the participant attended each group, but for a variety of reasons did not master the material in a manner sufficient to incorporate them into their daily lifestyles in a level that reduces the level of pain, they can choose to repeat the 9-week group intervention, (3) and the final treatment option is where the participant, either due to psychological or to physical reasons, requires a higher level of care which generates a referral to the next level of care. Once the decision has been reached for which aftercare treatment is most appropriate, time is spent on relapse prevention, and finally upon having the participant complete the post-treatment outcome questionnaire.

## Method

Conducting formalized and standardized evaluations is becoming more commonplace in the various practices of clinical psychology. Researchers and academics alike have been advocating the use of standardized testing across domains for many years, however, data continually indicate that clinicians who use standardized assessments remain in the minority (Patterson and McClanahan, 1999).

The medical community is adopting multidisciplinary evaluation which incorporates the principle of standardized evaluations as the universal standard of care for determining disposition of complex medical issues (Simon & Folen, 2001). These evaluations typically consist of a physician, a psychologist, and one other discipline which in this study is a physical therapist. Within a multidisciplinary team evaluation the professional psychologist is relied upon to unravel the patient who is ambivalent about treatment or the patient who is experiencing "delayed recovery". The medical community has long known that psychological factors can aide as well as hinder recovery from an illness or injury, but have been reluctant to join with psychologists in order to facilitate the healing process. This reluctance is giving way to integrated assessment and treatment.

Professional psychologists are relying upon multimodal psychological evaluation while trying to unravel the complexities of medical patients. For instance, the use of the clinical interview is widely used to glean information from a patient (McClanahan & Antonuccio, 2002). Standardized instruments such as depression scales and anxiety scales yield symptoms and severity of symptoms. This information is vital to the practitioner who targets interventions toward ameliorating these specific symptoms. Standardized instruments such as objective measures of personality can yield a patient's openness to treatment, thus treatment outcome and tailoring treatment to the specific personality traits of that participant (Simon & Folen, 2001).

## Participants

The sample used in this study consisted of 76 individuals who participated in and completed an outpatient chronic pain management program. Informed consent was obtained from each participant prior to being admitted into the Chronic Pain Management Program.

## Measures

The multimodal psychological evaluation used in this study incorporated the standardized and structured clinical interview, the D-Ark (Depression Scale University of Arkansas), and the Pain Outcomes Questionnaire (POQ, Clark, Gironda, & Young, 2003).

## Structured Clinical Interview

The structured clinical interview was developed by Regional Program Offices who required that each patient be evaluated with this format. The structured clinical interview was administered by the principal investigator to each participant and was scheduled for fifty minutes. The structured clinical interview included the evaluation of each of the following areas: identifying information (demographical data), pain location and subjective score (1 to 10), current medications, problem areas associated with pain (vegetative signs – difficulty falling or staying asleep, non restorative sleep, low energy, increase or decease in appetite, anorexia, bulimia, decreased libido)(stressors – problems with relationships, social environment, education, occupational, housing, economic, health, legal, acculturation) (psychiatric history – self and family for depression, anxiety, bipolar, schizophrenia, substance abuse, suicide attempts or successes), functional status (no changes, normal routine, occupational functioning, academic functioning, social functioning), health habits (tobacco use, alcohol use, caffeine use, physical activity, OTC drugs or herbs), treatment adherence issues (Pain Stage of Change), level of distress, mental status evaluation (appearance, behavior, demeanor, speech, mood, affect, thought process, thought content, orientation, attention, concentration, memory, impulse control, insight, judgment), risk assessment (suicide, homicide, other risk issues), impression (full five Axis diagnosis), disposition (invite to participate in this treatment program, refer to higher level of care, refer to psychiatry, refer to chemical dependency services, follow up visit with case manager/physical therapist/psychologist/MD, trial of acupuncture, no further treatment, patient contemplating treatment, patient declines treatment).

## Depression-Arkansas Scale

The Depression Arkansas Scale (D-Ark, Netoutcomes, 1997) was the only scale authorized to be used to assess depressive symptoms in medical patients for the medical center. The developers of the D-Ark report that the D-Ark's reliability with regard to depressive symptom severity range from .85 to .92, suicidality reliability coefficients ranged from .56 to .70, and classification of remission of Major Depressive Disorder at follow-up had a .51 reliability coefficient. The D-Ark had a reliability coefficient of .41 as compared to the Hamilton Depression Scale. The D-Ark is reported to have a reliability coefficient of .56 to the DIS Interview when the number of depression symptoms was compared.

## Pain Outcomes Questionnaire

The primary instrument used to collect data outcome was the Pain Outcomes Questionnaire (POQ, Clark, Gironda, & Young, 2003). The POQ was developed over a five year time frame under the Veteran's Health Administrative's National Pain Initiative in order to evaluate the effectiveness of treatment for veterans experiencing chronic non-cancer pain. The normative sample included two samples. Sample 1 consisted of 248 inpatients, and Sample 2 consisted of both inpatient (n=367) and outpatient (n=342). In order to evaluate validity of the instrument, items were compared to the Minnesota Multiphasic Personality Inventory-II (MMPI-II), the Sleep Problems Questionnaire (Jenkins, Stanton, Niemcryk, & Rose, 1988), the Tampa Scale of Kineisiophobia (Crombez, Vlaeyen, Heuts, Lysesns, 1999), Sickness Impact Profile (Williams, 1988), the Pain Visual Analog Scale, and the Physical Capabilities Evaluation (Woods, 1989).

The POQ consists of six domains (Pain, Mobility, Activities of Daily Living (ADLs), Vitality, Negative Affect, and Fear. A score is derived for each patient for each domain as well as a Total Score. The POQ is reported to have a $7^{th}$ to $8^{th}$ grade readability index, which indicates that it is acceptable for clinical usage.

The authors report stability coefficients (reliability) range from a low of .63 on the Pain subscale to a high of .89 on the ADL subscale. Alpha coefficients ranged from a low of .59 on the Fear subscale to a high of .90 on the ADLs subscale. Regarding validity, the authors report a generalizability coefficient ranging from a low of .78 on the Pain subscale to a high of .93 on the ADL subscale.

## Procedure

Participants were referred to this chronic pain management program by their primary care physicians (PCP). Each participant was required to have experienced chronic pain for over three months prior to the referral by the PCP. Once a referral was received by this program, each participant was contacted by a case manager who scheduled them to attend a free one-hour overview of the chronic pain management program. If the participant attended this seminar, they were given a pain questionnaire that asked questions regarding demographic information, location of pain, length of pain, previous as well as current medications being taken, a diagraph of the participant's pain, questions relating to stage of change, etc.). If the pain questionnaire was completed and returned, then the patient was scheduled for the multidisciplinary team evaluation (physician, psychologist, and physical therapist). During the multidisciplinary team evaluation, each potential participant was evaluated by the physician, psychologist, and physical therapist. Each treatment provider formulated a diagnosis and treatment plan within their discipline. Once each potential participant was individually evaluated, the treatment providers conferred to determine if the potential participant would be invited to participate in the program. If the potential participant agreed to participate, then that individual would be placed on a waiting list for the next available group.

**Table 1: Demographic characteristics.**

| | Variables | n=76 | % |
|---|---|---|---|
| Gender | Male | 18 | 23.68% |
| | Female | 58 | 79.32% |
| Age | M (SD) | 54.0 | 12.02 |
| Ethnicity | Caucasian | 67 | 88.16% |
| | Hispanic | 5 | 6.58% |
| | African-American | 2 | 2.63% |
| | Pacific Rim | 2 | 2.63% |
| Education | M (SD) | 13.47 | 2.82 |
| | Doctorate | 2 | 2.63 |
| | Masters Degree | 3 | 3.95 |
| | Bachelors Degree | 17 | 22.37% |
| | High School (equiv) | 52 | 68.42% |
| | < High School | 2 | 2.63% |
| Length of pain experience | M (SD) | 8.35 | 10.36 |

## Exclusionary Criteria

Potential participants could be excluded due to either the physical or the psychological evaluation. If during the physical examination, the patient had not received a complete medical work-up that included diagnostic imaging (e.g., MRI, x-Ray, CT scan), a failed trial of physical therapy, a failed trial of pain medication, or pending surgery then the patient would be excluded from participating in the chronic pain management program. Similarly, if the patient was actively suicidal, psychotic, manic, severely depressed, or severely anxious then the patient would be referred to the department of psychiatry and would be excluded from participation.

## Inclusionary Criteria

Potential participants who had received a complete medical work-up and medical interventions would meet the physical requirements to be invited to participate in the program. Likewise, if a patient was free of significant psychopathology they would be invited to participate in the program.

# Results

## Demographic Data

The demographic characteristics of the participants are presented in Table 1. The sample consisted of 58 females (79.32%) and 18 males (23.68%) with a mean age for treatment completers of 54.0 years (SD 12.02). The ethnic breakdown tracked with local County census data and was comprised of 67 Caucasian (88.16%), 5 Hispanic/Latino (6.58%), 2 African-American (2.63%, and 2 Pacific Rim (2.63%). The mean educational level was 13.47 years, with 28.95% holding a college degree. The mean length of time that patients suffered from pain was 8.35 years (SD 10.36). The mean length of time that participants were on the waitlist was 35.74 days (SD=23.20).

**Table 2: Primary location of pain as reported by patient.**

| Variables | n=76 | % |
|---|---|---|
| Low back | 29 | 38.16 |
| Neck | 15 | 19.75 |
| Fibromyalgia | 10 | 13.16 |
| Leg | 4 | 5.26 |
| Knee | 3 | 3.95 |
| Hand | 3 | 3.95 |
| Hip | 2 | 2.63 |
| Foot | 2 | 2.63 |
| Pelvic | 2 | 2.63 |
| Myofascial | 2 | 2.63 |
| Scoliosis | 1 | 1.32 |
| Shoulder | 1 | 1.32 |
| Post Polio | 1 | 1.32 |
| Cancer | 1 | 1.32 |

## Source of pain & psychiatric co-morbidity

Table 2 indicates that the most common primary location of pain was: low back (38.16%), neck or cervical pain (19.75%), and fibromyalgia (13.16%). Table 3 indicates that 65.79% of the patients who completed the outpatient chronic pain management program had a comorbid psychiatric diagnosis. Depression was the most common psychiatric diagnosis (38.16%), with personality disorders (9.21%) being the second most common psychiatric diagnosis. Table 4 indicates that of the 76 treatment completers, 93.43% were either in the Precomtemplative Stage of Change (17.11%) or in the Contemplative Stage of Change (76.32%).

**Table 3: Psychiatric diagnosis.**

| Variables | n=76 | % |
|---|---|---|
| Depression | 29 | 38.16 |
| Personality Disorder | 7 | 9.21 |
| Anxiety | 3 | 3.93 |
| Alcohol Abuse/Addiction (current) | 2 | 2.63 |
| Polysubstance addiction (in rem.) | 2 | 2.63 |
| Malingering | 2 | 2.63 |
| Bipolar Disorder | 1 | 1.32 |
| Thought Disorder | 1 | 1.32 |
| Impulse Control Disorder | 1 | 1.32 |
| TOTAL | 50 | 65.79 |

**Table 4. Pain Stages of Change for Treatment Completers.**

| Variables | n=76 | % |
|---|---|---|
| Precontemplative | 13 | 17.11 |
| Contemplative | 58 | 76.32 |
| Preparation | 1 | 1.32 |
| Action | 4 | 5.26 |
| Maintenance | 0 | 0.00 |

**Table 5. Treatment outcomes for All Treatment Completers (n=76) as measured by The Pain Outcomes Questionnaire.**

| Variables | Waitlist Control + Pre-treatment | | | | | Post-treatment | Post-pre |
|---|---|---|---|---|---|---|---|
| | M | SD | M | SD | M | SD | % change |
| Pain | 5.43 | 2.11 | 5.57 | 1.93 | 4.40 | 1.67 | -26.50 |
| Mobility | 15.33 | 9.88 | 16.26 | 10.13 | 13.49 | 10.60 | -20.60 |
| ADLs | 4.63 | 6.55 | 5.14 | 6.95 | 3.76 | 5.93 | -36.53 |
| Vitality | 17.67 | 5.39 | 16.15 | 5.52 | 16.40 | 6.05 | 1.52 |
| Neg. Affect | 21.11 | 11.03 | 22.35 | 13.47 | 17.57 | 10.01 | -27.19 |
| Fear | 10.57 | 10.57 | 4.39 | 10.32 | 4.19 | 8.60 | -20.03 |
| Total score | 74.74 | 25.24 | 75.79 | 29.62 | 64.22 | 27.89 | -24.75 |

## Outcome Data

Table 5 represents the outcome data for all treatment completers and indicates that for the participants who completed the program pain scores improved on average by 26.50%. The participants reports that their mobility improved by 20.60%, their ADLs improved by 36.53%, their vitality improved by 1.52%, their negative affect improved by 27.19%, their fear improved by 20.03%, and their total score improved by 24.75%. These improvements represent a significant clinical improvement in the quality of life for these patients.

**Table 6. Treatment compliance for all Treatment Completers.**

| Variables | n=76 | % |
|---|---|---|
| Not compliant | 0 | 0 |
| Not very compliant | 21 | 27.63 |
| Somewhat compliant | 17 | 22.37 |
| Very compliant | 24 | 31.58 |
| Fully compliant | 14 | 18.42 |

## Treatment Compliance

Table 6 represents treatment compliance for the treatment completers. This data indicates that of the treatment completers (n=76), 27.63% of the participants (n=21) met the criteria for being "not very compliant" with treatment, 22.37% (n=17) were "somewhat compliant" with treatment, 31.58% (n=24) were "very compliant" with treatment, and 18.42% (n=14) were "fully compliant" with treatment. No participant met the criteria for being "not compliant" with treatment. "Not compliant" was measured as missing more than two of the group psychotherapy sessions, complying with none of the homework assignments, and participating in none of the in-session assignments. "Not very compliant" was measured as missing two group psychotherapy sessions, complying with 25% of the homework assignments, and participating in 25% of the in-session assignments. "Somewhat compliant" was measured by missing two group psychotherapy sessions, complying with 50% of the homework assignments, and participating in 50% of the in-session assignments. "Very compliant" was measured by missing one group psychotherapy session, complying with 75% of the homework assignments, and participating in 75% of the in-session assignments. "Fully compliant" was measured by missing none of the group psychotherapy sessions, complying with 90% of the homework assignments, and participating in 90% of the in-session assignments.

**Table 7: Treatment outcomes for Fully Compliant Treatment Completers (n=14) as measured by The Pain Outcomes Questionnaire.**

| Variables | Waitlist Control + Pre-treatment | | | | Post-treatment | | Post-pre |
|---|---|---|---|---|---|---|---|
| | M | SD | M | SD | M | SD | % change |
| Pain | 4.86 | 2.07 | 5.07 | 2.20 | 2.93 | 1.07 | -73.17 |
| Mobility | 14.36 | 8.81 | 15.36 | 8.90 | 9.21 | 7.33 | -66.67 |
| ADLs | 3.43 | 4.26 | 5.14 | 6.88 | 1.57 | 3.46 | -227.27 |
| Vitality | 16.50 | 5.02 | 16.14 | 5.33 | 12.79 | 5.74 | 26.26 |
| Neg. Affect | 20.50 | 12.40 | 25.14 | 22.64 | 10.86 | 7.64 | -131.58 |
| Fear | 10.49 | 4.68 | 10.79 | 4.54 | 6.43 | 4.45 | -67.78 |
| Total score | 70.43 | 26.81 | 77.64 | 34.97 | 43.79 | 19.01 | -77.32 |

### Outcomes for "Fully Compliant" treatment completers

Table 7 depicts treatment outcome for the treatment completers (n=76) for participants who were "fully compliant" with the treatment regimen. This data is perhaps the most informative of the outcome data. Of the participants who were "fully compliant" ($90^{th}$ percentile)(n=14), an average improvement of 73.17% was reported in the area of pain, a 66.67% improvement in mobility, a 227.27% improvement in ADLs, a 26.26% improvement in vitality, a 131.58% improvement in negative affect, a 67.78% improvement in fear, and a total improvement of 77.32%. These changes proved to be life altering for these patients.

As predicted, the participants who were "not very compliant" yielded a flat outcome overall, yet even this group yielded improvement in their pain scores (-6.32%) as well as their fear score (-19.62%). For the participants who were "somewhat compliant" ($50^{th}$ percentile)(n=17), improvements were made in each of the measured domains with the exception of no change in the fear subscale. Outcomes indicated that for the "very compliant" treatment completers (n=24) improvements in the each of the subscales was clinically significant. For instance this sub-population reported a 41.05% improvement in pain score, a 39.34% improvement in mobility, an 80.88% improvement in ADLs, a 3.59% improvement in vitality, a 39.15% improvement in negative affect, a 16.33% improvement in fear, and a total average improvement of 26.58%.

## Findings and Conclusions

The two major assumptions in the general population and many argue amongst treatment providers is that: (1) the majority of patients who report that they experience chronic pain are malingering, and (2) that patients who report that they suffer from chronic pain either don't know how to get better or don't want to take an active role in improving. The data from this study indicates that the first premise is inaccurate. Only 2.63% of the treatment completers were diagnosed with malingering. The second assumption, however, was borne out by virtue of the fact that the vast majority of the patients who entered the program were ambivalent about treatment at least at the beginning (Table 4).

### Future Directions

The results of this study indicate that regardless of the pre-treatment stage of change, the most crucial aspect of treatment is treatment compliance. The treatment completers who were not treatment compliant reported virtually no change in treatment outcome as measured pre- versus post-treatment. Likewise, for those treatment completers who followed the treatment recommendations made to them, the changes were dramatic. Anecdotally this comes as no surprise to the treatment provider, however, this study empirically establishes this fact for the ambivalent patient.

## REFERENCES

Bonica, J.J. (1990), *The management of pain ($2^{nd}$ ed.),* Philadelphia: Lea & Febiger.

Beck, A. T. (1979). *Cognitive therapy and the emotional disorders.* New York: Meridian.

Burns, D. D. (1999). The feeling good handbook. New York: Penguin.

Clark, M.E., Gironda, R.J., & Young, R.W. (2003). Development and validation of the Pain Outcomes Questionnaire-VA. *Journal of Rehabilitation Research and Development 40*(5), 381-395.

Crombez, G., Vlaeyen, J.W., Heuts, P.H., Lysens, R. (1999). Pain-related fear is more disabling than pain itself: Evidence of the role of pain-related fear in chronic back pain disability. Pain, 35(3), 329-339.

Ellis, A. (1986). *Handbook of rational-emotive therapy.* New York: Springer.

Fordyce, W. E. (1976). *Behavioral methods for chronic pain and illness.* St. Louis: Mosby.

Guriel, J. and Fremouw, W. (2003). Assessing malingered posttraumatic stress disorder: a critical review. *Clinical Psychology Review, 23,* 881.

Jenkins, C.D., Stanton, B.A., Niemcryk, S.J., & Rose, R.M. (1988). A scale for the estimation of sleep problems in clinical research. *Journal of Clinical Epidemiology 41*, 313-321. Lewinsohn, P. M., Munoz, R. F., Youngren, M. A., & Zeiss, A. M. (1978). *Control Your Depression.* New York: Fireside. McClanahan, T. M. & Antonuccio, D. O. (2002). Cognitive-Behavioral treatment of panic attacks. *Clinical Case Studies, 1*(3), 211-223.

Melzack, R. and Wall, P. D. (1965). Pain mechanisms: a new theory. *Science, 150,* 971-979.

Mittenberg, W., Patton C., Canyock, E. M., and Condit, D. C. (2002). Base rates of malingering and symptom exaggeration. *Journal of Clinical Experimental Neuropsychology, 24*(8), 1094-1102

Patterson, T. and McClanahan, T. M. (1999). *The Couple and Family Clinical Documentation Sourcebook.* New York: Wiley.

Rohling, M. L., Binder, L. M. & Langhinrichsen-Rohling, J. (1995). A meta-analytic review of the association between financial compensation and the experience and treatment of chronic pain. *Health Psychology, 14,* 537-547. Searight, H. R. (1998). *Behavioral Medicine: A Primary Care Approach* (pp. 162-173). Philadelphia: Brunner-Mazel.

Simon, E. P. & Folen, R. A. (2001). The role of the psychologist on the multidisciplinary pain management team. *Professional Psychology: Research and Practice, 32*(2), 125-134.

Stewart, W.F., Ricci, J. A., Chee, E., Morganstein, D., & Lipton, R. (2003). Lost productive time and cost due to common pain conditions in the US workforce, *Journal of the American Medical Association* (290, 2371).

Williams, R.C. (1988). Toward a set of reliable and valid measures for chronic pain assessment and outcome research. *Pain, 35*(3), 239-251.

Woods, D.A. (1989). Rehabilitation aquatics for low back injury: Functional gains or pain reduction? *Journal of Clinical Kinesiology, 43,* 96-102.

In: Toward a Science of Clinical Psychology
Editor: Luciano L'Abate, pp. 211-228
ISBN: 978-1-60456-062-6


*Chapter XII*

# MANUALIZED TREATMENTS FOR PEOPLE WITH PERSONALITY DIFFICULTIES

***Mary McMurran***

## ABSTRACT

The treatments described in this chapter are designed for people with personality difficulties, and much of the research reported here is with offender populations. The term 'personality difficulties' is not one found in any diagnostic system, but it does permit the inclusion in treatment of those whose problems are related to their personality but who are not officially diagnosed as personality disordered. Personality disorder is defined in the American Psychiatric Association's (1994) Diagnostic and Statistical Manual of Mental Disorders as 'an enduring pattern of inner experience and behavior that deviates markedly from the expectations of the individual's culture, is pervasive and inflexible, has an onset in adolescence or early adulthood, is stable over time, and leads to distress or impairment' (p. 629). The personality disorders and their key characteristics are listed in Table 1. In psychiatric diagnostic systems, if these features are present to a certain degree, then a personality disorder diagnosis may be made. However, this diagnostic cut-off point is somewhat arbitrary and often excludes people who have difficulties. Instead of diagnostic cut-offs, personality difficulties can be looked at as existing on a continuum, where the problems are experienced by the person concerned, or others in his or her social world, to a greater or lesser degree. So, personality difficulties would be said to exist where a person has 'a history of emotional problems and problematic behaviour that leads to distress, difficulties in relating to other people, and poor social functioning'.

Having a personality disorder or personality difficulties does not equate with being an offender. Most people with personality difficulties do not offend, however many offenders do have personality difficulties. The reason that offenders are focused upon in this chapter is quite simply that the author is reporting her own work as a forensic clinical psychologist. It is, however, true to say that treatments for offenders with personality disorders have until recently attracted the greater share of attention, at least in the United Kingdom. Indeed, the main expenditure has been on personality disordered offenders detained in secure facilities under mental health legislation. This situation is now changing, since the publication of a health service guidance document entitled, Personality Disorder: No Longer a Diagnosis of Exclusion (National Institute of Mental Health for England, 2003).

Whatever the client group and whatever the therapy, evidence-based practice is the only ethical approach to offering psychological therapies. The gold standard outcome evaluation is the randomized controlled trial, and it has been suggested that psychotherapies should show better outcomes than either a no treatment or a placebo condition in at least two independent, controlled studies before being considered effective (Beutler, 2000; Chambless & Hollon, 1998). Clearly, for independent trials to be possible, the therapy in question needs to be replicable, which is a considerable challenge where complex interventions are concerned.

## TREATMENT MANUALS

Treatment manuals are essentially technical guidelines describing how to conduct a given treatment by operationalizing the therapy and clarifying the procedures involved (Chambless & Ollendick, 2001; Wilson, 1996). Despite the advantages, the standardization of therapy in treatment manuals has attracted criticism, with some commentators arguing that the use of manuals limits the art of therapy and reduces the ability to be responsive to clients' individual needs (Garfield, 1998). There are a number of responses to this criticism, and one is that it rather depends on how a treatment manual is configured (Hickling & Blanchard, 1997). Some manuals are highly detailed, offering specific instructions for each procedure within each session, whereas others provide only a general outline of treatment. Indeed, many practitioners admit to being unclear about what a treatment manual actually is (Addis & Krasnow, 2000). It seems likely that the utility of manuals and the effectiveness of manualized treatments will vary depending upon the therapist, the type of manual, the target problem, the treatment programme, and the type of client (McMurran & Duggan, 2005). Among psychologists, Addis and Krasnow (2000) found that manuals were favored most by cognitive-behavioral therapists, perhaps because cognitive-behavioral interventions are particularly amenable to a manualized approach.

The purpose of this chapter is to describe two interventions which have been developed using different styles of treatment manual. Evaluations of these therapies and experience with the different approaches will be given. The first intervention is *Stop & Think!*, a social problem solving therapy which has been used in mental health settings. Although the format of sessions is structured, the content of each session varies according to the participants' current problems. Hence, in *Stop & Think!* there is considerable latitude to be responsive to the individual's unique problems. The second intervention is COVAID, which is an acronym for Control of Violence for Angry Impulsive Drinkers. This has largely been used in criminal justice settings. The COVAID manual is highly structured, with introductions, exercises, discussions, and assignments all specified. This is typical of the detailed manuals that are in use in correctional services worldwide, where treatments are often implemented by personnel who are less experienced in delivering therapies, for example prison officers.

**Table 12.1 Personality disorders**

| Personality disorder | Key characteristics |
|---|---|
| *Cluster A* | |
| Paranoid | Distrust, suspiciousness |
| Schizoid | Socially and emotionally detached |
| Schizotypal | Unusual perceptions, odd beliefs, socially anxio |
| *Cluster B* | |
| Antisocial | Disregards rights of others |
| Borderline | Unstable mood, relationships, and self-image |
| Histrionic | Excessively emotional, attention-seeking |
| Narcissistic | Grandiose, lacks empathy, needs admiration |
| *Cluster C* | |
| Avoidant | Socially inhibited, feels inadequate, oversensitive |
| Dependent | Clinging, submissive |
| Obsessive-compulsive | Perfectionist, inflexible |

## Stop & Think!

*Stop & Think!* is a form of social problem solving therapy based upon the work of psychologists Thomas D'Zurilla, Arthur M. Nezu, and Christine Maguth Nezu (D'Zurilla & Nezu, 2007) which is used with people with personality difficulties to help them improve their social functioning. *Stop & Think!* aims to deal with people's current concerns rather than tackle problems in the abstract, since people's current concerns are 'hot' topics and working towards a solution has real meaning in the here and now. If by using *Stop & Think!* a client solves or ameliorates a current problem, then not only has a real problem been solved, but the effectiveness of the procedure has also been demonstrated. This should encourage that person to try *Stop & Think!* with other problems. *Stop & Think!* is, therefore, designed not only to help people tackle problems that they are currently experiencing, but also to help them learn, practise, and generalise the skills required for problem solving. In time, the client will be able to use these skills independently, without the need for professional help.

## Personality, Social Problem Solving, and Problems

Good problem solving skills consist of the ability to recognise problems when they arise, define the problem clearly, set goals for change, produce a diversity of possible solutions, anticipate outcomes, devise effective action plans that have stepwise stages, and carry out those action plans to solve problems effectively. Poor problem solving skills are associated with a range of psychological and behavioural problems, including substance abuse (Herrick & Elliott, 2001) and hostility and aggression (Keltikangas-Järvinen & Pakaslahti, 1999;

Matthys, Cuperus, & van Engeland, 1999), which are common amongst people with personality problems.

Poor social problem solving is also directly associated with personality disorders. We used the Social Problem Solving Inventory – Revised (SPSI-R; D'Zurilla, Nezu, & Maydeu-Olivares, 2002) to compare the problem solving abilities of personality disordered offenders, prisoners, and mature students, and found that personality disordered offenders were the most negative, impulsive, and avoidant, and least rational in their approach to problems (McMurran, Blair, & Egan, 2002; McMurran, Egan, & Duggan, 2005; McMurran, Egan, Blair, & Richardson, 2001). Herrick and Elliott (2001) found poor problem solving in personality disordered substance abusers, especially in Cluster A, the so-called 'eccentric' personality disorders (i.e., paranoid, schizoid, and schizotypal) and Cluster C, the 'anxious' personality disorders (avoidant, dependent and obsessive-compulsive).

Evidence exists to suggest that poor social problem solving mediates the relationship between personality traits and psychological and behavioural problems. A mediator is a variable that explains how or why one thing has an effect on another. In this case, certain personality traits are more likely to lead to psychological or behavioural problems in people who have poor social problem solving abilities. In our research, we have found social problem solving to mediate between trait impulsivity and aggression in both men and women (McMurran et al., 2002; Ramadan & McMurran, 2005). That is, impulsive people are more likely to be aggressive if they have poor social problem solving skills. In men, social problem solving also mediated between trait impulsivity and heavy drinking (McMurran et al., 2002). Other research that we have conducted shows that an impulsive/careless problem solving style is associated with borderline and histrionic personality traits, which are typified by emotional instability, and a negative approach to problems is associated with avoidant and dependent personality traits (McMurran, Duggan, Christopher, & Huband, 2007).

Based upon this research, we are developing a testable model of personality difficulties in which the concept of social problem solving is central to adaptive functioning (McMurran et al., 2005). This is outlined in Figure 12.1. Here, innate disopositions are the developmental start-point for behavioural patterns. Certain dispositions limit and bias information processing, interfering with the acquisition of good social problem solving skills and consequently leading to dysfunctional ways of operating in everyday life. Interpersonal dysfunction causes distress, experienced affectively in a number of ways including anxiety, depression, and anger. Stress further impairs problem solving abilities and may also lead to problematic stress-relieving behaviours, such as substance use, which still further impair social problem solving abilities and also potentially create additional interpersonal problems. Persistent dysfunction leads to a negative approach to life's problems and the development of maladaptive self-schemas that have a further deleterious effect on information processing and social problem solving.

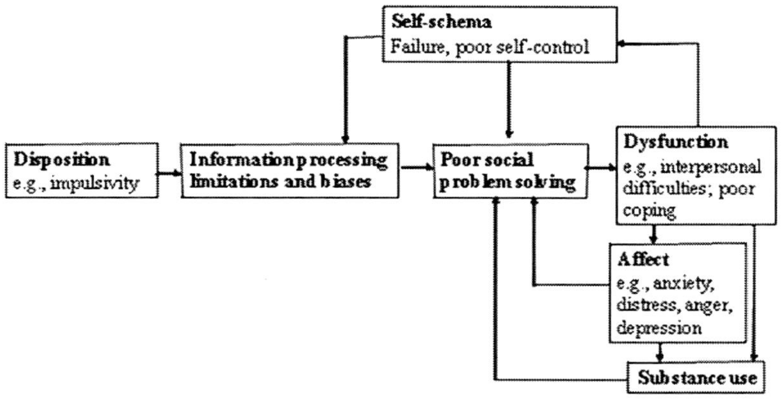


Figure 12.1. A social problem solving model of personality difficulties

Overall, then, this proposed model indicates the importance of targeting social problem solving skills as an important means of tackling the cycle of other emerging difficulties that an individual might experience. This further affirms the relevance of focusing on the person's current concerns and problems as a practical method of dealing with life's difficulties. Also, breaking the cycle of dysfunction and distress can begin to change other aspects of this system, for example reducing feelings of failure, enhancing self-efficacy, and reducing the need to rely on dysfunctional means of coping, such as substance use.

## The Therapy

The skills of social problem solving may be described in seven separate steps. *1. Problem Orientation* is the recognition of 'bad feelings' and using these as a cue to begin the problem solving process. This requires a positive problem orientation, that is the understanding that problems are a normal part of life and that problems can be solved. *2. Problem definition* is the ability to define a problem clearly and accurately. *3. Goal setting* is identification of the desired outcome. *4. Generation of alternatives* is the creative generation of multiple possible ways of achieving the goal. *5. Decision-making* is where the likely consequences of each potential solution is examined. *6. Action* is where one or more of the viable options are selected into an action plan. *7. Evaluation* is a review of the success or otherwise of the action plan. In *Stop & Think!* these steps are translated into six key questions that guide the problem solving process in clinical practice. Bad feelings? What's my problem? What do I want? What are my options? What is my plan? How am I doing? In practice, the six key questions are used every time, without variation. The aim is to teach people a strategy for solving problems. By using the procedure repeatedly, it is more likely to stick in a person's mind, and thus it becomes more likely that that person will use the strategy when problems arise.

## Does Stop & Think! Work?

Problem solving therapy has been used successfully in the treatment a range of problems, including depression (Biggam & Power, 2002; Townsend et al., 2001), aggressiveness in children (Frey et al., 2000), self-harm (Salkovskis, Atha, & Storer, 1990), and offending (Friendship, Blud, Erikson, Travers, & Thornton, 2003). Based on the evidence and the empirically-derived model described earlier, it is reasonable to suppose that problem solving therapy might benefit people with personality difficulties.

The main measure we used to examine the effectiveness of *Stop & Think!* was the Social Problem-Solving Inventory -Revised (SPSI-R; D'Zurilla et al., 2002). This is a 52-item, self-report questionnaire which provides a total score as well as scores on five scales. The scales of the SPSI-R are as follows:

- *Positive Problem Orientation* (PPO; 5 items). This is a 'cognitive set' (i.e., a person's perspective) where there is a constructive approach to problems, with problems seen as a challenge rather than a threat. There is optimism about the solvability of problems and a belief in one's own personal ability to solve problems. There is an understanding that problems take time and effort to solve.
- *Negative problem orientation* (NPO; 10 items). This is a cognitive-emotional set where problems are viewed as a threat to well-being. Problems are viewed as unsolvable and there is a low expectation of one's own ability to solve problems. When confronted with problems, people become frustrated and upset.
- *Rational Problem Solving* (RPS; 20 items). This is a systematic approach to solving problems that includes problem definition, goal setting, generation of alternatives, thinking of the consequences, and forming an action plan.
- *Impulsivity/Carelessness Style* (ICS; 10 items). This is where attempts to solve problems are impulsive, hurried, and careless. Insufficient information is gathered in defining the problem, achievable goals are not set, only a few options are generated, the consequences of each option are incompletely thought through, and the effectiveness of the action plan is not monitored.
- *Avoidance Style* (AS; 7 items). This is where problem-solving is deferred. There is a hope that the problem will solve itself or that other people will solve it.
- *Social Problem Solving* (SPS). This is a total score derived by averaging each scale and reversing the scores of the negative scales (NPO, ICS, and AS).

*Stop & Think!* groups were first piloted with nine male patients (six mentally ill and three personality disordered) in a UK regional secure unit for mentally disordered offenders. Using the SPSI-R, we found that only six weekly sessions of 1½ hours' duration produced statistically significant improvements in patients' overall problem solving scores, and significant reductions in impulsivity and negative problem orientation (McMurran, Egan, Richardson, & Ahmadi, 1999). The effectiveness of *Stop & Think!* was then examined further with personality disordered offenders in the secure unit. After three months in treatment, personality disordered offenders ($N$=14) showed positive change on all scales of the SPSI-R except PPO (McMurran, Fyffe, McCarthy, Duggan, & Latham, 2001).

More recently, the effectiveness of a combination of *Stop & Think!* along with a psychoeducation component which taught participants about their personality problems was examined in a randomised controlled trial (Huband, McMurran, Evans, & Duggan, 2007). Participants were 176 community-dwelling men and women with personality disorders in several sites across the East Midlands of England, who were randomly allocated to either treatment or a wait-list control. The treated group received, on average, 9 groups sessions and a further 3 individual sessions, and they showed significantly greater improvement on SPSI-R scales, on a Social Functioning Questionnaire (SFQ; Tyrer et al., 2005), which measures functioning in the domains of home, work, leisure, and relationships, and on anger expression, as measured by the State-Trait Anger Expression Inventory (STAXI-2; Spielberger, 1999).

In summary, *Stop & Think!* is an intervention that seems to work well with people with personality disorders, although most of the evaluation to date has been self-reported improvements. The common sense nature of the intervention appeals to both practitioners and clients alike. Our research into social problem solving with this client group has developed along more theoretical lines, culminating to date in a testable model that will guide future research and practice.

## Control of Violence for Angry Impulsive Drinkers

Alcohol misuse and personality disorders are commonly co-occurring problems. In a recent analysis of a sample the US general population (*N*=43,093), 15% had at least one personality disorder, and of these 16% had current alcohol use problems (Grant et al., 2006). Analysis of data from a sample of the UK general population (*N*=626) estimated a prevalence of personality disorder of 4%, with the odds of alcohol dependence being substantially increased over those with no disorder for those in Clusters A (odds ratio 1.61) and B (odds ratio 4.21) (Coid, Yang, Tyrer, Roberts, & Ullrich, 2006). In substance misusing populations, the co-occurrence of personality disorders may be as high as 61%, as identified in a review of 50 studies (Verheul, van den Brink, & Hartgers, 1995). Among those with an alcohol use disorder, the prevalence of personality disorder has been identified as 29% in the US general population study (Grant et al. 2006) and as many as 53% in a UK study of alcohol-dependent patients (Bowden-Jones et al., 2004). It seems, then, that alcohol use disorders are common among people with personality disorders, and that the association is strongest with Cluster B personality disorders, namely the externalising disorders.

There is a strong association between alcohol and violence, with estimates that around half of violent crimes involve alcohol. Epidemiological studies show that increased alcohol consumption is associated with increased homicide and violence, and this is strongest in those countries where binge drinking is the typical pattern (Room & Rossow, 2001; Rossow, 2001). Correlational studies show that offenders are heavy drinkers, and violent offenders are the heaviest drinkers of all (McMurran, 2005; Singleton, Farrell & Meltzer, 1999). Longitudinal studies indicate that heavy drinkers are more likely to be violent than light drinkers (Farrington, 1995; Fergusson, Lynskey, & Horwood, 1996). Laboratory studies show that alcohol has the effect of eliciting aggression most markedly in men, and in those who have an aggressive disposition (Giancola, 2006). Dispositional aggressiveness is a personality difficulty associated with several personality disorders.

Alcohol-related violence is, therefore, a common and serious problem amongst offenders that deserves some attention from criminal justice and forensic mental health professionals. Offender treatment programmes generally address either drinking or violence, rather than alcohol-related violence together. However, in their review of intoxicated aggression, Graham and colleagues (1998) concluded that there is a need for interventions that "not only employ standard treatment techniques (e.g., anger management), but also use knowledge of the effects of alcohol and the process of aggression in treating violent individuals" (p. 670). The development and preliminary evaluation of a treatment programme for alcohol-related violence is described here. COVAID, the acronym for Control Of Violence for Angry Impulsive Drinkers, is a comprehensively manualized, structured, cognitive-behavioural treatment programme, in line with what is known to be effective in offender treatments (see review by McGuire, 2001). Based upon a developmental risk factor model of alcohol-related violence (McMurran, 1996), aggression and violence are the principal treatment targets, and these are addressed by tackling the mediators of anger, impulsivity, and drinking.

There is evidence that early impulsivity and hyperactivity are associated with adult alcohol problems and violence (Af Klinteberg, Andersson, Magnusson, & Stattin, 1993). Impulsivity may also militate against the acquisition of behavioural self-control (McMurran et al., 2002). Furthermore, under-control in childhood may lead to hostile attributional biases through frequent chastisment by authority figures and lack of popularity with pro-social peers. Hostile attributional biases correlate with anger and aggression in children and adolescents (Dodge, Price, Bachorowski, & Newman, 1990). Heavy drinking by people who are impulsive, undercontrolled, and hostile may exacerbate the likelihood of aggression and violence.

In COVAID, these risk factors are dealt with using six principal components:

- *The 'personal scientist' approach* (Mahoney & Thoresen, 1974). Clients are taught a cognitive-behavioral model as a means of understanding the need to tackle a range of issues to reduce the risk of aggression and violence. 'Personal scientists' are then encouraged to SEE, that is 'Study' triggers to their behaviour, 'Experiment' with change, and 'Evaluate' outcomes. COVAID aims to help clients identify and enhance their existing methods of control, as well as to provide new control strategies.
- *Information gathering and feedback.* Clients monitor their anger, aggression, and violence to identify triggers to aggression. Drinking is monitored simultaneously, assisting with the exploration of the relationship between drinking and aggression, as well as assessing quantities consumed. A number of psychological tests are administered, with feedback on each being provided. Within a motivational framework, assessment of the problem behaviour and feedback of results has been shown effective in reducing drinking (Miller & Sovereign, 1989).
- S*tress and anger management.* This is based upon the principle that the more stressed and angry a person is, the more likely is a provocation to trigger aggression and violence. Stress reduction, anger control, and hostile thinking styles are addressed in this component. Meta-analyses of the effectiveness of treatments for anger problems

show medium to large effect sizes for cognitive-behavioral treatments, with relaxation, social skills training, cognitive-relaxation, and cognitive treatment all showing positive and sustained effects (Beck & Fernandez, 1998; Edmondson & Conger, 1996).

- *Thinking and problem-solving skills training.* The aim here is to counter impulsivity using the *Stop & Think!* problem solving approach described earlier. Additionally, the expectancy that alcohol causes violence is attenuated using Socratic challenge, whereby the therapist aims to elicit evidence, or lack of it, for a client's belief through questioning the client about his or her observations and experiences (Beck, Wright, Newman, & Liese, 1993).
- *Modifying drinking.* Reducing alcohol consumption is tackled by behavioral self-control training, an approach that can be successful for drinkers who choose either to abstain from alcohol or to moderate their consumption (Miller, Leckman, Delaney, & Tinkcom, 1992). Additionally, efforts are made to change drinking patterns in order to avoid trouble. Relapse prevention is included to help people maintain change over time by recognising and coping with situations that present a high risk of relapse to problem drinking (Marlatt, 1996; Marlatt & Gordon, 1985). Relapse prevention is effective in reducing the intensity of relapses, particularly for those who show deficits in coping skills (Carroll, 1996).
- *Lifestyle maintenance.* The aim is to build up a lifestyle that is supportive of moderate drinking and prosocial behaviour to assist with maintenance of gains. Walters (1998) suggests attention to involvements (i.e., routines, activities, and relationships), commitments (i.e., goals, values, and priorities), and identity (i.e., self-image). Resocialisation into pro-social networks is a strong predictor of positive outcome in both substance users and criminals (Meyers & Smith, 1995; Walters, 1998).

These six components are interwoven throughout COVAID, the session outline for which is presented in Table 12.2.

## Is COVAID Effective?

The version of COVAID on which some preliminary evaluation data have been collected is an individual intervention for people resident in the community (i.e., have unrestricted access to alcohol). A group treatment version, applicable in both institutions and the community is under development.

In one study of men on Probation Orders (McMurran & Cusens, 2003), 17 referrals were received in the year between August 2001 and July 2002. Six of these completed COVAID: one was not accepted for COVAID because of low literacy; one was still in treatment at the time of the evaluation; three did not attend for the first interview because they were detained in prison or hospital; three did not attend for the first interview without giving any reason; and three dropped out during COVAID because it was not meeting their needs. Participants were between 21 and 31 years old, all but one were single, four were unemployed, and all had criminal histories of alcohol-related violence. One participant had already decided to abstain from drinking. The other five participants reported drinking on average 123 units[2] (SD=39) of alcohol in the week prior to starting COVAID.

The measures used before and after COVAID were: the *State-Trait Anger Expression Inventory - 2* (STAXI-2; Spielberger, 1999); the *Conflict Resolution, Impulsivity and Aggression Questionnaire* (CRIAQ; Honess, Maguire, & Vanstone, 2001); the *Barratt Impulsiveness Scale - 11* (BIS-11; Barratt, 1994); the *Social Problem-Solving Inventory - Revised* (SPSI-R; D'Zurilla et al., 2002); the *Alcohol Abstinence Self-Efficacy Scale* (AASE; DiClemente, Carbonari, Montgomery, & Hughes, 1994), and the *Alcohol-Related Aggression Questionnaire* (ARAQ; McMurran, Egan, Cusens, van den Bree, Austin, & Charlesworth, 2006). Additionally, self-report measures of quantity and frequency of alcohol consumption, incidents of anger, intoxicated aggression, and violence were taken throughout. Information about offending was gathered from Probation officers.

With such small numbers of participants, there were no statistical analyses of the data. However, as an indicator of where COVAID had an effect, improvement was most uniform on alcohol-related aggression beliefs, as measured by the ARAQ, and overall social problem solving. Although more variable, improvement was also apparent on the STAXI-2 anger control (in and out) scales, and impulsivity as measured by the CRIAQ. Of the five drinkers, three decreased their drinking and one's drinking repeatedly rose and fell. One participant's reported alcohol consumption increased considerably, perhaps because he felt more able to make an accurate report, and he expressed concern about his inability to control his drinking; he was referred for specialist help.

No participants were convicted of any violent offending during COVAID. Data on offending were collected from the Probation Service on the six men who had completed COVAID and the ten who had been referred for COVAID but did not complete the programme, although these do not form a comparable control group. Follow-up from the time of referral to COVAID, which averaged 18.50 weeks (SD=12.59, range 3–35), indicated that one of the six COVAID participants was convicted of a violent offence (17%), whereas three of the ten non-participants of COVAID were convicted (30%). For aggressive and violent offending, the relative risk is 1.62 (95% confidence interval 0.20 – 12.78), meaning that without COVAID treatment the chances are 1.62 times higher that an offender will be reconvicted compared with those who participate in COVAID, although with such a small number of participants the confidence interval is extremely wide.

This preliminary study suggested that COVAID has promise as an intervention for offenders whose violence is alcohol-related. In developing our research, we introduced a more rigorous single case approach, a useful method in the developmental stage of a programme in that it provides information about who improved, who remained unchanged, and who deteriorated as a result of treatment (Jacobson, Roberts, Berns & McGlinchey, 1999). The methods used were to examine clinical significance and reliability of change on psychometric tests. In the second study (McCulloch & McMurran, under review), there were ten participants, recruited from social services, probation services, and a community alcohol and drug service, each of which had a trained COVAID facilitator. All participants were

[2] 1 unit = 8 grams of alcohol

male, between 21 and 32 years of age, and most were employed ($N$=7). The median alcohol consumption for the week prior to intervention was 50 units, ranging from 22 to 147 units.

**Table 12.2. COVAID session**

| Session | Content |
|---|---|
| Pre-programme introduction | Information about COVAID<br>Screening interview<br>Participant consent |
| Assessment and introduction | Participant assessment<br>Motivation enhancement<br>Introduction to 'Personal Scientist' |
| Explaining drunken aggression | Introduction to anger-aggression system<br>How drink affects the system |
| Crime harm reduction | Consider harm reduction methods for triggers, thought and anger<br>Physical relaxation techniques |
| Managing stress and arousal | Increase awareness of the need to manage stress<br>Consider different methods of stress management<br>Psychological and physical relaxation techniques |
| Altering triggers | Identify common triggers for aggression<br>Consider methods for tackling triggers |
| Weakening beliefs aboutthe effects of alcohol | Identify alcohol-outcome expectancies<br>Challenge expectancies<br>Beliefs about abstainers |
| High risk situations | Identify future high risk situations<br>Methods for dealing with risk<br>Maintaining positive change |
| Problem Solving (1) | Identifying problems<br>Stop & Think! method of problem solving<br>Problem solving practice |
| Problem Solving (2) | Apply Stop & Think! to negative moods<br>Consider the effect of good moods<br>Develop an action plan for the future |
| Synthesis and evaluation | Review progress<br>Action plan for the future |

The measures used were the *Alcohol-Related Aggression Questionnaire* (ARAQ; McMurran et al., 2006), and the *Controlled Drinking Self- Efficacy Scale* (CDSES; Sitharthan et al., 2003). The latter was introduced as an optional alternative to the *Alcohol Abstinence Self-Efficacy Scale* (AASE; DiClemente, Carbonari, Montgomery, & Hughes, 1994) because most of the COVAID clientele were not aiming for abstinence. A pragmatic decision was made to omit tests which were available only at a cost from test publishers (STAXI-2, CRIAQ, and SPSI-R), and the BIS which did not detect change in the earlier study. As before, participants were asked to report their weekly alcohol consumption, anger incidents, and alcohol-related aggression and violence, and programme facilitators were asked for information about criminal convictions after COVAID had been completed.

With regard to psychometric evaluations, Jacobson and Truax (1991) suggest that the best definition of clinical significance of change is that post-intervention scores are closer to the mean of the functional population than the dysfunctional population. This is the definition adopted for the ARAQ, a scale for which both functional and dysfunctional norms are available (McMurran et al., 2006). This requires the calculation of the score that the participant's post-treatment score must cross for change to be considered clinically significant using the equation: (SD functional population x M dysfunctional population) + (SD dysfunctional population x M functional population)/ SD functional population + SD dysfunctional population. A less rigorous definition of clinical significance was used for CDSES scores, for which functional norms are not a logical proposition. This is simply that post-treatment scores should fall into the functional range.

Additionally, since change on psychometric tests may result from unreliability of the tests themselves, Jacobson and Truax (1991) recommend that reliability of change should also be calculated. Reliable change (RC) refers to whether change over time is greater than the change that would be expected due to the unreliability of the measure. RC was calculated on the ARAQ only using the formula: (Post intervention score – Pre-intervention score)/Standard difference. The standard difference is calculated as follows: $\sqrt{2}$(Standard error of measurement)$^2$. The standard error of measurement is: SD of normal population/$\sqrt{}$ 1-test-retest reliability. RC is a z score, with a score greater than 1.96 indicating reliable change (Collie, Maruff, McStephen, & Darby, 2003). This means that the likelihood of change having occurred due to measurement error is less than five percent. If the change is reliable but the score still remains in the non-functioning range, then the client is deemed to have improved; if the change is both reliable and clinically significant, then the client is considered to have recovered (Jacobson et al., 1999).

Nine of the participants showed a reduction in ARAQ scores, with five of these demonstrating both clinically significant and reliable change (i.e., recovered), a sixth showed clinically significant change that did not meet the reliability criterion, and three showed reductions that were in the right direction but neither clinically significant nor reliable. One participant's ARAQ score increased, but this was neither clinically significant nor reliable. Nine participants changed in the desired direction on both CDSE subscales: (1) Overall confidence and (2) Confidence in controlling the frequency and amount consumed. One participant demonstrated clinically significant change on both scales; three showed clinically significant change on the Confidence in controlling frequency and amount subscale; and two showed clinically significant change on the Overall confidence subscale.

Mean weekly self-reported alcohol consumption was calculated for the first five weeks in treatment and compared with that for the second five weeks in treatment. Six of the ten participants showed a reduction in alcohol consumption. Self-reports of aggression and violence were low throughout COVAID. In the week prior to COVAID, five participants reported having been aggressive or violent, and in the week prior to the final session only two participants reported aggression or violence. Follow up conviction data were available for eight of the participants at a mean of 29.13 weeks (SD = 24.93) after completing COVAID. None of these participants had been reconvicted for a violent offence since completing COVAID.

The results of these single case evaluations provide some further support for COVAID in reducing proneness to alcohol-related violence, as measured by the ARAQ, improvements in perceived ability to control their alcohol consumption, as measured by the CDSES, a reduction in drinking, and few incidents of aggression and violence.

## Comparisons Between the Interventions

One realisation during the course of this work was that, although manuals are widely used, there is very little information about what practitioners find useful in a treatment manual. To rectify this, at least partially, we conducted a Delphi survey of trainers of correctional practitioners, asking them what they thought made a good treatment manual (McCulloch & McMurran, 2007). The main preferences are presented in Table 12.3. Detail in the manual was what trainers of practitioners wanted. Although trainers are typically experienced practitioners who have moved into training, active correctional services practitioners may have different opinions, and so too may mental health service practitioners.

Whatever the style of the manual, staff training and supervision were of paramount importance. Structure and detail in a manual make training easier to design and deliver, since it is clear what the therapeutic aims and activities are. Where less detailed manuals are used, there is a challenge in conveying the 'spirit' of the intervention in training without detailing every therapeutic strategy. Adherence to the treatment protocol as it is manualized is easier to check in highly structured programmes, simply by observing a session to see if it is being delivered in accordance with the recipe. However, the quality of the delivery may be missed by this actuarial approach, and supervision is essential to ensure that practitioners understand the therapeutic aims and the methods of achieving those aims.

Highly structured treatment programmes are more commonly used in criminal justice settings and less structured approaches are more typical of mental health settings. Recipients of structured treatments in correctional services say they benefit from these, as long as the programmes tackle whatever concern they have at the time (McMurran & McCulloch, 2007). Where there is dissatisfaction, it is not at the programme itself but rather because it is mistimed in relation to the offenders current concerns. These observations support the view that the effectiveness of manualized treatments will vary depending upon the therapist, the type of manual, the target problem, the treatment programme, and the type of client (McMurran & Duggan, 2005). It is probable that no one treatment is superior, but that a variety of treatments, manualized in different ways, will be useful for a range of problems at particular stages in a person's contact with services. Opportunities to be innovative, both as a therapist and a researcher, abound. Most importantly, the varied needs of a wide range of clients may be best met through developing a range of treatments and delivery formats.

**Table 12.3. Preferences in cognitive-behavioral treatment manuals**

1. There is a clear statement of theory
2. Theory and practice are linked
3. There are clearly stated aims and objectives
4. Advice is given on how to prepare for each session
5. Specific learning points are listed throughout
6. Realistic timing suggestions should be given for exercises.
7. Troubleshooting suggestions should be included.
8. Examples should be culturally diverse.
9. The sessions are not too prescriptive
10. Creativity is permitted within boundaries of integrity
11. There is information on style of delivery
12. Assessment materials are integral
13. Materials are available on CD
14. Plain English is used
15. The layout is clear, e.g., large font; different types of activity distinguished by icons

# REFERENCES


Addis, M. E., & Krasnow, A. D. (2000). A national survey of practising psychologists' attitudes toward psychotherapy treatment manuals. *Journal of Consulting and Clinical Psychology, 68,* 331-339.

Af Klinteberg, B. A., Andersson, T., Magnusson, D., & Stattin, H. (1993). Hyperactive behavior in childhood as related to subsequent alcohol problems and violent offending: A longitudinal study of male subjects. *Personality and Individual Differences, 15,* 381-388.

American Psychiatric Association (1994) *Diagnostic and Statistical Manual of Mental Disorders.* 4th Ed. Washington: American Psychiatric Association.

Barratt, E. S. (1994). Impulsiveness and aggression. In J. Monahan and H.J. Steadman (eds). *Violence and mental disorder: Developments in risk assessment.* Chicago: University of Chicago Press.

Beck, A. T., Wright, F. D., Newman, C. F., & Liese, B. S. (1993). *Cognitive therapy of substance abuse.* New York: Guilford Press.

Beck, R., & Fernandez, E. (1998). Cognitive-behavioral therapy in the treatment of anger: A meta analysis. *Cognitive Therapy and Research, 22*, 63-74.

Beutler, L. E. (2000). David and Goliath. When empirical and clinical standards of practice meet. *American Psychologist, 55,* 997-1007.

Biggam, F. H., & Power, K. G. (2002). A controlled, problem-solving, group-based intervention with vulnerable incarcerated young offenders. *International Journal of Offender Therapy and Comparative Criminology, 46*, 678-698.

Bowden-Jones, O., Iqbal, M. Z., Tyrer, P., Seivewright, N., Cooper, S., Judd, A., & Weaver, T. (2004). Prevalence of personality disorder in alcohol and drug services and associated comorbidity. *Addiction, 99,* 1306-1314.

Carroll, K. M. (1996). Relapse prevention as a psychosocial treatment: A review of controlled clinical trials. *Experimental and Clinical Psychopharmacology, 4,* 46-54.

Chambless, D. L., & Hollon, S. D. (1998). Defining empirically supported therapies. *Journal of Consulting and Clinical Psychology, 66,* 7-18.

Chambless, D. L., & Ollendick, T. H. (2001). Empirically supported psychological interventions: controversies and evidence. *Annual Review of Psychology, 52,* 585-716.

Coid, J., Yang, M., Tyrer, P., Roberts, A., & Ullrich, S. (2006). Prevalence and correlates of personality disorder in Great Britain. *British Journal of Psychiatry, 188,* 423-431.

Collie, A., Maruff, P., McStephen, M., & Darby, D. (2003). Are reliable change (RC) calculations appropriate for determining the extent of cognitive change in concussed athletes? *British Journal of Sports Medicine, 37,* 370-376.

DiClemente, C. C., Carbonari, J. P., Montgomery, R. P. G., & Hughes, S. O. (1994). The alcohol abstinence self-efficacy scale. *Journal of Studies on Alcohol, 55*, 141-148.

Dodge, K. A., Price, J. M., Bachorowski, J., & Newman, J. P. (1990). Hostile attributional bias in severely aggressive adolescents. *Journal of Abnormal Psychology, 99,* 385-392.

D'Zurilla, T. J., & Nezu, A. M. (2007). *Problem solving therapy: A positive approach to clinical intervention.* 3rd edition. New York: Springer Publishing Company.

D'Zurilla, T. J., Nezu, A. M., & Maydeu-Olivares, A. (2002). *Social Problem Solving Inventory – Revised (SPSI-R): Technical manual.* North Tonawanda, NY: Multi-Health Systems, Inc.

Edmondson, C. B., & Conger, J. C. (1996). A review of treatment efficacy for anger problems:

Conceptual, assessment, and methodological issues. *Clinical Psychology Review, 16*, 251-275.

Farrington, D. P. (2005). Childhood origins of antisocial behaviour. *Clinical Psychology and Psychotherapy, 12,* 177-190.

Fergusson, D. M., Lynskey, M. T., & Horwood, L. J. (1996). Alcohol misuse and juvenile offending in adolescence. *Addiction, 91,* 483-494.

Frey, K. S., Hirschstein, M. K., & Guzzo, B. A. (2000). Second step: Preventing aggression by promoting social competence. *Journal of Emotional and Behavioral Disorders, 8*, 102-112.

Friendship, C., Blud, L., Erikson, M., Travers, R., & Thornton, D. (2003). Cognitive-behavioural treatment for imprisoned offenders: An evaluation of H M Prison Service's cognitive skills programmes. *Legal and Criminological Psychology, 8,* 103-114.

Garfield, S. L. (1998). Some comments on empirically supported treatments. *Journal of Consulting and Clinical Psychology, 66,* 121-125.

Giancola, P. R. (2006). Influence of subjective intoxication, breath alcohol concentration, and expectancies on the alcohol-aggression relationship. *Alcoholism: Clinical and Experimental Research, 30,* 844-850.

Graham, K., Leonard, K. E., Room, R., Wild, T. C., Pihl, R. O., Bois, C., & Single, E. (1998). Current directions in research on understanding and preventing intoxicated aggression. *Addiction, 93*, 659-676.

Grant, B. F., Stinson, F. S., Dawson, D. A., Chou, S. P., Ruan, W. J., & Pickering, R. P. (2006). Co-occurrence of 12-month alcohol and drug use disorders and personality disorders in the United States. *Archives of General Psychiatry, 61,* 361-368.

Herrick, S. M., & Elliott, T. R. (2001). Social problem-solving abilities and personality disorder characteristics among dual diagnosed persons in substance abuse treatment. *Journal of Clinical Psychology, 57*, 75-92.

Honess, T., Maguire, M., and Vanstone, M. (2001). CRIAQ: A new Conflict Resolution, Impulsivity and Aggression Questionnaire. Swansea: M&A Research.

Huband, N., McMurran, M., Evans, C., & Duggan, C. (2007). Social problem solving plus psychoeducation for adults with personality disorder: A pragmatic randomised controlled trial. *British Journal of Psychiatry, in press.*

Hickling, E. J., & Blanchard, E. B. (1997). The private practice psychologist and manual-based treatments: Post-traumatic stress disorder secondary to motor vehicle accidents. *Behaviour Research Therapy, 35,* 191-203.

Jacobson, N. S., Roberts, L. J., Berns, S. B., & McGlinchey, J. B. (1999). Methods for defining and determining the clinical significance of treatment effects: Description, application, and alternatives. *Journal of Consulting and Clinical Psychology, 67,* 300-307.

Jacobson, N. S., & Truax, P. (1991). Clinical significance: A statistical approach to defining meaningful change in psychotherapy research. *Journal of Consulting and Clinical Psychology, 59*, 12-19.

Keltikangas-Järvinen, L., & Pakaslahti, L. (1999). Development of social problem solving strategies and changes in aggressive behaviour: A 7-year follow-up from childhood to late adolescence. *Aggressive Behavior, 25,* 269-279.

Mahoney, M. J., & Thoresen, C. E. (1974). *Self-control: Power to the person.* Monterey, CA: Brookes Cole.

Marlatt, G. A. (1996). Taxonomy of high-risk situations for alcohol relapse: Evolution of a cognitive-behavioral model. *Addiction, 91* (Supplement), S37-S49.

Marlatt, G. A. & Gordon, J. R. (Eds). (1985). *Relapse prevention.* New York: Guilford.

Matthys, W., Cuperus, J. M., & van Engeland, H. (1999). Deficient social problem-solving in boys with ODD/CD, with ADHD, and with both disorders. *Journal of the American Academy of Child and Adolescent Psychiatry, 51,* 215-224.

McGuire, J. (2001). What works in correctional intervention? Evidence and practical implications. In G. A. Bernfield, D. P. Farrington, & A. W. Leschied (eds). *Offender rehabilitation in practice.* (pp.25-43). Chichester, UK: Wiley.

McCulloch, A., & McMurran, M. (2007). The features of a good treatment manual: A Delphi survey of experts. *Psychology, Crime, and Law,13,* 265-274.

McCulloch, A., & McMurran, M. (under review). Evaluation of a treatment programme for alcohol-related aggression.

McMurran, M. (1996). Substance use and delinquency. In C.R. Hollin & K. Howells (Eds). *Clinical Approaches to Working with Young Offenders.* Chichester, UK: Wiley.

McMurran, M. (2005). Drinking, violence, and prisoners' health. *International Journal of Prisoner Health, 1,* 25-29.

McMurran, M., Blair, M., & Egan, V. (2002). An investigation of the correlations between aggression, impulsiveness, social problem solving, and alcohol use. *Aggressive Behavior, 28,* 439-445.

McMurran, M., & Cusens, B. (2003). Controlling alcohol-related violence: A treatment programme. *Criminal Behaviour and Mental Heath, 13,* 59-76.

McMurran, M. & Duggan, C. (2005). The manualization of a treatment programme for personality disorder. *Criminal Behaviour and Mental Health, 15,* 17-27.

McMurran, M., Duggan, C., Christopher, G., & Huband, N. (2007). The relationships between personality disorders and social problem solving in adults. *Personality and Individual Differences, 42,* 145-155.

McMurran, M., Egan, V., Blair, M., & Richardson, C. (2001). The relationship between social problem-solving and personality in mentally disordered offenders. *Personality and Individual Differences, 30*, 517-524.

McMurran, M., Egan, V., Cusens, B., van den Bree, M., Austin, E., & Charlesworth, P. (2006). The Alcohol-Related Aggression Questionnaire. *Addiction Research and Theory, 14,* 323-343.

McMurran, M., Egan, V., & Duggan, C. (2005). Stop & Think! Social problem-solving therapy with personality disordered offenders. In M. McMurran & J. McGuire (Eds). *Social problem solving and offending: Evidence, evaluation, and evolution.* Chichester, UK: Wiley.

McMurran, M., Egan, V., Richardson, C., & Ahmadi, S. (1999). Social problem-solving in mentally disordered offenders: A brief report. *Criminal Behaviour and Mental Health, 9,* 315-322.

McMurran, M., Fyffe, S., McCarthy, L., Duggan, M., & Latham, A. (2001). 'Stop & think!': Social problem-solving therapy with personality disordered offenders. *Criminal Behaviour and Mental Health, 11,* 273-285.

McMurran, M., & McCulloch, A. (2007). Why don't offenders complete treatment? Prisoners' reasons for non-completion of a cognitive skills programme. *Psychology, Crime and Law.13,* 345-354.

Meyers, R. J., & Smith, J. E. (1995). *Clinical guide to alcohol treatment: The community reinforcement approach.* New York: Guilford Press.

Miller, W. R., Leckman, A. L., Delaney, H. D., & Tinkcom, M. (1992). Long-term follow-up of behavioral self-control training. *Journal of Studies on Alcohol, 53,* 249-261.

Miller, W. R., & Sovereign, R. G. (1989). The Check-Up: A model for early intervention in addictive behaviours. In T. Loberg, W.R. Miller, P.E. Nathan, & G.A. Marlatt (Eds). *Addictive Behaviors: Prevention and Early Intervention.* Amsterdam: Swets & Zeitlinger.

National Institute of Mental Health for England (2003). *Personality disorder: No longer a diagnosis of exclusion.* London: Department of Health.

Ramadan, R., & McMurran, M. (2005). Alcohol and aggression: Gender differences in their relationships with impulsiveness, sensation-seeking, and social problem-solving. *Journal of Substance Use, 4,* 215-224.

Room, R., & Rossow, I. (2001). The share of violence attributable to drinking. *Journal of Substance Use, 4,* 218-228.

Rossow, I. (2001). Alcohol and homicide: A cross-cultural comparison of the relationship in 14 European countries. *Addiction, 96 (Suppl. 1),* S77-S92.

Salkovskis, P. M., Atha, C., & Storer, D. (1990). Cognitive-behavioural problem solving in the treatment of patients who repeatedly attempt suicide. a controlled trial. *British Journal of Psychiatry, 157*, 871-876.

Singleton, N., Farrell, M., & Meltzer, H. (1999). *Substance misuse among prisoners in England and Wales.* London: Office for National Statistics.

Sitharthan, T., Job, R. F. S., Kavanagh, D. J., Sitharthan, G., & Hough, M. (2003). Development of a controlled drinking self- efficacy scale and appraising its relation to alcohol dependence. *Journal of Clinical Psychology, 59,* 351-362.

Spielberger, C.D. (1999) *STAXI-2: State-Trait Anger Expression Inventory-2.* Odessa, FL: Psychological Assessment Resources, Inc.

Townsend, E., Hawton, K., Altman, D. G., Arensman, E., Gunnell, D., Hazell, P., House, A., & van Heeringen, K. (2001). The efficacy of problem-solving treatments after deliberate self-harm: Meta-analysis of randomized controlled trails with respect to depression, hopelessness, and improvement in problems. *Psychological Medicine, 31*, 979-988.

Tyrer, P., Nur, U., Crawford, M., Karlsen, S., McLean, C., Rao, B., & Johnson, T. (2005). The social functioning questionnaire: A rapid and robust measure of perceived functioning. *International Journal of Social Psychiatry, 51,* 265-275.

Verheul, R., van den Brink, W., & Hartgers, C. (1995). Prevalence of personality disorders among alcoholics and drug addicts: An overview. *European Addiction Research, 1*, 166-177.

Walters, G. D. (1998). *Changing Lives of Crime and Drugs.* Chichester: Wiley.

Wilson, T. G. (1996). Manual-based treatments: The clinical application of research findings. *Behaviour Research and Therapy, 34,* 295-314.

In: Toward a Science of Clinical Psychology
Editor: Luciano L'Abate, pp. 229-260
ISBN: 978-1-60456-062-6


*Chapter XIII*

# INTEGRATIVE EVIDENCE-BASED CLINICAL PSYCHOLOGY: A FIELD-TESTED PROTOCOL

***Roland A. Carlstedt***

## ABSTRACT

This chapter introduces a field-tested evidence-based psychological assessment, psychotherapy/mental training and intervention efficacy protocol (Carlstedt Protocol) and the *Universal Clinical Trial* (UCT) project. It was designed to integrate into the clinical practice an accessible and user-friendly research component that can be routinely engaged in by most practitioners. One of the goals of the protocol is to encourage clinicians to better delineate and quantify assessments and interventions in terms of their neuropsychophysiological underpinnings in the context of more ecologically valid settings and situations and in relationship to objective outcome measures, longitudinally. The ultimate goal of this evidence-based protocol is to integrate practitioners into a massive universal "clinical trial" (UCT) in which standardized measurement, monitoring, efficacy testing and databasing procedures are used to better document the diagnostic and intervention process.

## INTEGRATIVE EVIDENCE-BASED CLINICAL PSYCHOLOGY: A FIELD-TESTED PROTOCOL

This chapter introduces a field-tested evidence-based psychological assessment, psychotherapy/mental training and intervention efficacy protocol (Carlstedt Protocol, CP; 2007) and the *Universal Clinical Trial* (UCT) project. It can be implemented on varying levels by most practitioners irrespective of their clinical orientation, training, or preferred intervention modality. It was designed to integrate into the clinical practice an accessible and user-friendly research component that can be routinely engaged in. One of the goals of the protocol is to encourage practitioners to better delineate and quantify assessments and interventions in terms of their neuropsychophysiological underpinnings, in the context of more ecologically valid settings and situations and in relationship to objective outcome measures, longitudinally.

The CP is especially applicable to the diagnosis and treatment of psychophysiological disorders such as anxiety, phobias, ADD/HD, depression and neurocognitive dysfunction/ learning disabilities but can also be used to better illuminate the patient evaluation and treatment process relative to most diagnoses.

The ultimate goal of this evidence-based protocol is to integrate practitioners of many orientations, however divergent, into a massive universal "clinical trial" (UCT) in which standardized measurement, monitoring, efficacy testing and databasing procedures are used to better document mind-body processes that are involved in or mediate mental disorders and determine how they may change as a function of interventions to treat them.

Within the intervention efficacy component of the protocol neuropsychophysiological measures can used both as independent/predictor and dependent/criterion variables. Depending upon the design or methodology associated with the research question certain mind-body measures may predict outcome at baseline (intake-testing/assessment) or reflect and provide evidence that an intervention has resulted in mind-body changes when compared to baseline. For example, a psychoanalyst, prior to commencing with a series of sessions would take his or her patient through a standardized neurocognitive testing and an autonomic nervous system stress test battery to establish baseline measures of, for example, frontal lobe functioning and heart rate variability and then determine to what extent resulting measures may be associated with a particular diagnosis and importantly, assess changes in these measures over time, during the course of and after an intervention (in this case psychodynamic therapy).

When using such an assessment strategy certain mind-body measures are likely to emerge as predictors (mediators) of later treatment outcome (dependent/criterion variables) that reflect intervention induced change (compared to baseline/intake). While such an approach may seem too empirical or reductionistic for those practitioners who are more comfortable with their own clinical intuition than with objective tests, and some clinicians may be reluctant to employ procedures that they may not have been trained in (e.g., psychophysiology; ambulatory monitoring) the methods and techniques that this protocol advances can easily be engaged in by most therapists on some level with basic training. Sophisticated instruments for monitoring patient responding in and out of the office have become user friendly and affordable and patient reports can be generated quickly and reliably with data being centrally stored for analytic, comparative, interpretation and research purposes.

Data-driven and quantitatively based clinical assessment and intervention protocols need not be incompatible with philosophical or practical concerns that some practitioners may have. If anything clinicians should welcome the opportunity to utilize and participate in a protocol that may better support anecdotal contentions that they may have about their intervention orientation and importantly provide their patients with evidence that a therapy works that transcends mere self-report. In fact, patients should demand and dictate such and one could argue that not providing a patient with objective evaluative and outcome evidence is unethical and negligent. Augmenting interventions that are frequently not readily transparent as to their methods and outcome should be encouraged, since at minimum, the acquisition of pre and post information on patient mind-body measures can lead to unprecedented insight into a particular therapeutic process.

Another goal of the protocol is to foster interdisciplinary understanding, information sharing and integrative approaches to patient assessment, treatment and outcome studies. Such is made necessary by the fact that mental health practice has become increasingly specialized with the majority of practitioners working in relative isolation and in the context of unidimensional assessment and intervention paradigms that may no longer meet the gold standard for patient care or client services (Drake, Goldman, Leff, Lehman, Dixon, Mueser & Torrey, 2001). Practitioners tend to practice the way they were trained and often go through an entire career married to an assessment and intervention approach that is either antiquated, obsolete, or needs to be augmented with the best emerging evidence-based practices.

While many practitioners may welcome being able to augment or upgrade their practice approaches most are mired in the clinical realities associated with having to survive as a practitioner. Time is scarce, with little available to keep up with advances across numerous sub-domains of psychology, psychiatry and behavioral medicine. In the end we all suffer from this state of affairs, with patients frequently not receiving the highest standard of care available today. Consequently, a road-map is needed, a blue-print for a truly integrative evidence-based clinical psychology that is designed to disseminate vast amounts of critical emerging research in an efficient and understandable manner, as well as expose practitioners to sophisticated methods and procedures that need to be integrated into *all* clinical practices, regardless of orientation or specialty. The psychoanalyst needs to be aware that sophisticated brain imaging techniques are revealing things that appear reconcilable with Freudian theory that have been previously discounted (Slipp, 2000). The psychiatrist needs to know about practices being used by psychologists who are demonstrating, for example, that heart rate variability biofeedback may be a viable alternative for treating anxiety in patients who cannot safely tolerate anti- anxiety medications or that neurofeedback may be the modality of choice for treating ADD in select patients (Nolan, Kamath, Floras, Stanley, Pang, Picton, & Young, 2005; Holtman & Stadler, 2006). Conversely, many psychologists and psychotherapists are not familiar with the neuorochemistry of psychotropic medications, leading to an oftentimes radical bias against certain drugs that have been shown to be highly efficacious (Verdoux & Begaud, 2004). Cardiologists need to be made aware of alternative evidence-based psychological interventions that may help ameliorate refractory functional arrhythmias that frustrate patients (Lehrer, Vaschillo, Vaschillo, Lu, Eckberg, Edelberg, Shih, Lin, Kuusela, Tahvanainen & Hamer, 2003). Virtually all practitioners need to consider issues of ecological validity and the temporal dynamics of an intervention or longitudinal impact of a treatment before marrying themselves to a psychotherapy method (Fahrenberg & Myrtek, 1996). Sophisticated assessment and monitoring methods are capable of revealing things that previously were unobservable including qEEG and in-the-field ambulatory wireless monitoring of psychophysiological processes (Jovanov, Raskovic, Price, Chapman, Moore, Krishnamurthy, 2001). These are a few of many procedures that are leading to revealing research, information and methods that are critical to optimal patient care that are not being used across clinical specialties and especially, at the level of private practice.

## PATIENT ASSESSMENT AND INTERVENTION USING THE CARLSTEDT PROTOCOL: CASE STUDIES

To better demonstrate how the CP is applied two case studies are presented throughout the remainder of this chapter (one in abbreviated form). Readers are encouraged to contemplate how they could apply the procedures that they will be exposed to, within their practices.

### Case I

A thirteen year-old male was referred to the author by his mother in the context of youth baseball team's sport psychology program (hereafter referred to as "our patient," "patient," "patient-athlete" or "athlete.") He had been diagnosed with ADD/HD and was taking a psycho-stimulant. Since his diagnosis emanated from his family's primary care physician I was very cautious in accepting such a diagnosis uncritically[3]. When seeing a patient who has been diagnosed with ADD or when suspecting such, extensive further assessment is indicated. It should be noted that regardless of previous diagnoses or reasons for seeing a client or patient, the CP approach requires that routine investigative assessment, monitoring and efficacy testing should take place at intake and pre, during and post intervention. As such, while the presented case study involves a disorder that dictates and even mandates extensive further testing to confirm its existence, information and data that transcend mere clinical judgment and intuition should be obtained on *all* patients regardless of the diagnosis or clinical orientation.

## ASSESSMENT OF PATIENT'S PRIMARY HIGHER ORDER CLINICAL PREDICTOR FACTORS

The first step of the CP involves administering the Tellegen Absorption Scale (TAS) or Stanford Scale of Hypnotic Susceptibility-A (SSHS-A), Eysenck Personality Inventory (EPI) or NEO Five-Factor Inventory (NEO) neuroticism scales and Marlowe Crowne (MC) scale to measure a patient's level of absorption/hypnotic susceptibility (A/HS), neuroticism (N) and repressive coping respectively (RC; Tellegen & Atkinson, 1974; Hilgard, 1965; Eysenck & Eysenck, 1968; Costa & McRae, 1992; Crowne & Marlowe, 1960). Sport specific analogues of the above measures, Subliminal Attention (SA-hypnotic susceptibility), Subliminal Reactivity (SR-neuroticism) and Subliminal Coping (SC-repressive coping) can also be concurrently administered to patients who are also athletes using the Carlstedt Subliminal Attention-Reactivity-Coping Scale-A (CSARCS-A; Carlstedt, 2008.). This validated sport-specific scale purports to measure attention, physiological reactivity and cognitive processing

---

[3] Physicians routinely arrive at a diagnosis of ADD on the basis of cursory symptom check lists that are provided by pharmaceutical companies.

during competition and has high convergent validity with their parallel clinical constructs (Carlstedt, 2008).

The above personality and behavioral measures are emerging as potent clinical and performance mediators and predictors of style of information processing/perception of threat, physiological reactivity, cognitive processing of affect, placebo, nocebo, pain threshold tendencies, as well as intervention amenability and compliance and a broad spectrum of other performance measures (e.g., critical moment performance in sports; Wickramaskera, 1988; Fortino, 2002; Carlstedt, 2001; Carlstedt, 2004; Carlstedt, 2008). Their predictive potency can be attributed to their intimate role in the mediation of key neuropsychophysiological processes that underlie numerous mind-body processes and disorders, including attention/focus (perception of threat), physiological reactivity and neurocognitive processing (Wickramasekera, 1988, 2003; Carlstedt, 2004). These measures were isolated and extracted from the *High Risk Model of Threat Perception* (HRMTP; Wickramasekera, 1988) a theoretical and applied model that attempts to assess and predict the risks specific mind-body interactions pose for the development of psychological and physical symptoms and illness. This model has isolated a set of primary higher order (PHO) behavioral and personality risk factors (predictor variables) that have been shown to, depending upon their level and constellation, interactively and differentially affect stress responding and drive physical symptoms. The constellation of PHO factors that has been shown to be the most potent predictor of psychophysiological disorders is 1) either high or low hypnotic susceptibility and/or absorption (high HS and low HA or high A); 2) high neuroticism/negative affect (high N/NA) and 3) high or low repressive coping (RC). The model's hypothesized dynamics in both clinical and performance contexts have been conceptualized and are further elucidated in the *Theory of Critical Moments and Clinical Mind-Body Reactivity Profile* (Athlete's Profile in athletes; Carlstedt, 2004) models as illustrated on the next page.

It should be noted that the above PHO factors have emerged as key clinical measures on the basis of extensive research that has linked them to mind-body processes that underlie or mediate psychophysiological disorders namely, attention to external and internal stimuli and the perception of threat, physiological reactivity and cognitive processing and subliminal coping (Wickramasekera, 1988, 2003; Carlstedt, 2004, 2007, 2008).

The following charts depict the hypothesized neuropsychophysiological dynamics of the HRMTP isolated PHO measures at baseline (first chart) when a patient encounters routine life situations or innocuous stimuli/situations, compared to encountering real or perceived stressors/stimuli as a function of the most reactive (detrimental) versus protective constellations of hypnotic susceptibility-neuroticism-repressive coping (charts two and three). It is beyond the scope of this chapter to elucidate these dynamics to a greater extent. Essentially, differential constellations of these measures are thought to be mediators of mind-body processes that can protect or make individuals more vulnerable to psychophysiological pathogenesis (see Wickramasekera, 1988 for a complete review of the HRMTP).

## I. Hypothesized Relative Brain Hemispheric Activation as a Function of a Context-Specific Tasks Carried Out Under Stress-Free Conditions

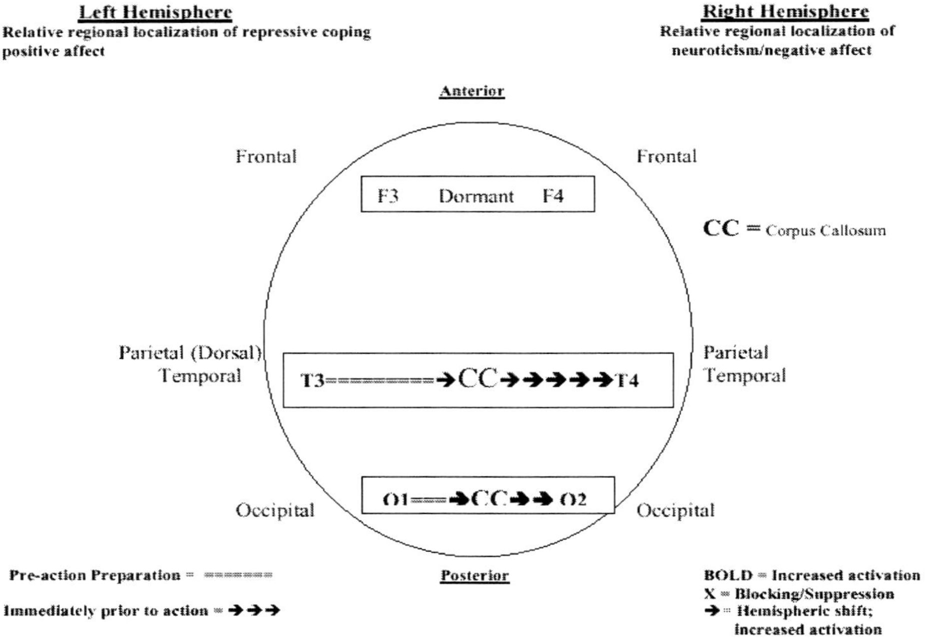


**Neurophysiological dynamics during routine moments: Stress Free**

1. **In the absence of critical moments constellations of or individual PHO factors (hypnotic ability/absorption, neuroticism and repressive coping) will remain dormant ot contribute positively to technical performance.**
2. **Pre-action mental preparation will be marked by greater relative activation of the left-hemisphere especially in the region spanning T3 to O1.**
3. **Immediately prior to action a relative left to right hemisphere shift will occur marked by decreasing activation in the general T3 and O1 regions. Increased activation will occur in the general T4 and especially O2 regions.**
4. **A brief period of internal focus gives way seamlessly to right brain hemisphere external stimulus oriented focus.**

**Heart Rate Deceleration Pattern During Routine Moments of Competition**

**I_I_I__I__I___I____I_____I______I_______I________I_________I_I_I**

1. **Heart rate deceleration will always occur during the pre-action preparatory phase during routine moments marked by successively longer cardiac cycles leading up to action when heart rate acceleration occurs. HRD is a psychophysiological concomitant of the above cortical dynamics. This neurocardiologic dynamic can be facilitated or disrupted as a function of constellation of PHO factors, especially during critical moments (see Chart III).**

Figure 1.

## II. Hypothesized Effects of High Neuroticism, High Hypnotic Ability/Absorption and Low Repressive Coping During Critical Moments (task-related) on Cortical Functioning

**Left Hemisphere**

**Hypoactivation in Left-frontal region**
**Repressive coping remains dormant**

**Right Hemisphere**

**Hyperactivation in Right-frontal region**
**Neuroticism generated negative intrusive cognitions**

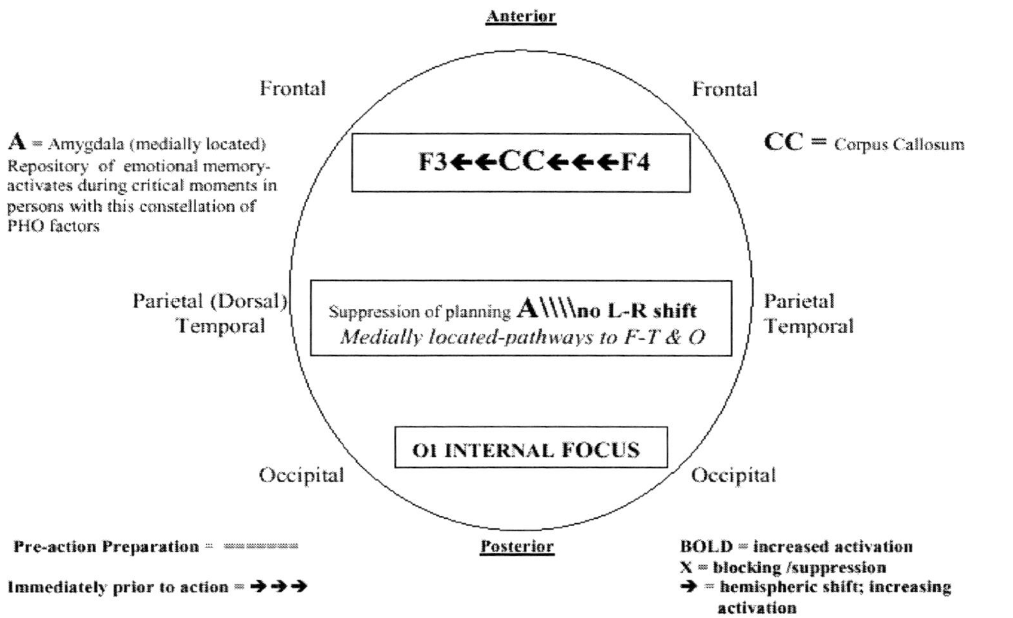


**Neurophysiological dynamics of HN, HHA/A and LRC during critical moments**

1. **Amygdala mediated emotional response activates F4 general region.**
2. **Resulting negative intrusive thoughts infiltrate F3 general region.**
3. **Leads to suppression of pre-planning stage prior to action (left-hypoactivation).**
4. **Increases rumination on negative cognitions.**
5. **Bi-laterally localized hypnotic ability/absorption affects occipital region O1-O2 leading to a disruption of external focus on stimulus (e.g., ball) immediately prior to action as reflected in reduced rCBF, MRI and/or EEG activity in this region when more of such activity should be occurring.**
6. **Results in loss of focus, cognitive and motor control and performance**

**Concurrent Heart Rate Deceleration Pattern Associated HN/HHA/A-LRC-CMs**

**___I___I___I___I___I__I__I_I_I_I_I_I**
**(depiction of heart rate acceleration-shorter cardiac cycle)**

**1. Heart rate deceleration will be lacking due to less baroreceptor control over cortical blood flow to the above brain regions contributing to excessive neuropsychophysiological activation.**

Figure 2.

**Cortical Dynamics of the Ideal Clinical Mind-Body Reactivity Profile: Critical Moments (High or Low Subliminal Attention-Low Subliminal Reactivity-High Subliminal Coping)**

**Left Hemisphere**
Left-hemisphere based repressive coping functionally inhibits the inter-hemispheric transfer of negative intrusive thoughts from the right to the left hemisphere

**Right Hemisphere**
Hypoactivation of right-hemisphere, suppression of negative intrusive thoughts

**Increased activation in the F3-C3 regions**

**Decreased activation in the F4-C4 regions**

Anterior

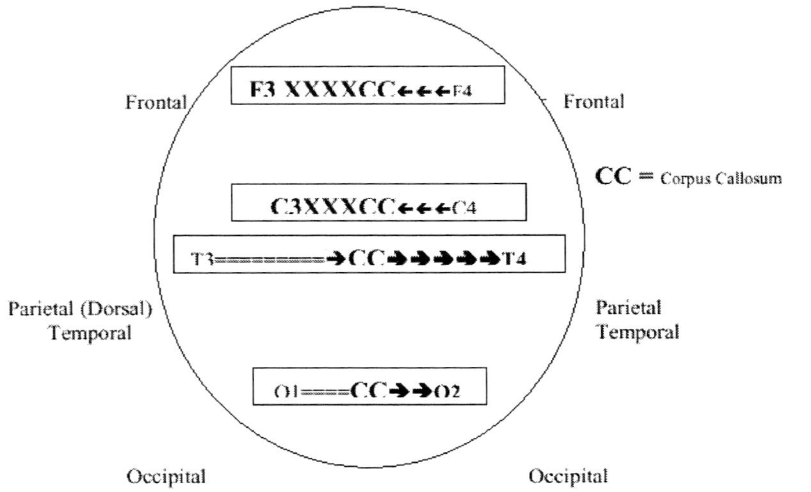


Posterior

**Pre-action Preparation = =======**

**Immediately prior to action = →→→**

**BOLD = increased activation**
**X = Blocking/Suppression**
**→ = Hemispheric shift; increased activation**

**Neurophysiological dynamics of the Ideal CMBR Profile During Crit.-Moments**

1. **Subliminal coping functions to suppress negative intrusive thoughts. Blocks transfer of negative intrusive thoughts from F4 to F3 and C4 to C3.**
2. **This facilitates the pre-action relative left to right hemispheric shift and increased focus on external stimulus (e.g., ball), leading to greater relative activation in the O2 region.**

**Heart Rate Deceleration Pattern During Routine Moments of Competition**

**_I_I_I__I__I___I____I_____I______I_______I________I_________I_I_I**

1. **Heart rate deceleration will occur during the pre-action preparatory phase during critical moments in athletes possessing the above constellation of PHO factors.**

Figure 3.

The CP mandates assessing all patients on these measures as a first step in the intake process. This does not to preclude the inclusion of other psychological measures and tests, so long as there is an empirical basis for doing so and that such can be further supported and justified on the basis of pilot data. However, by the very nature of having been designated *Primary Higher Order* factors in mediating most if not all psychophysiological disorders, it is expected that all other psychological measures will play an ancillary, subordinate or secondary role in the etiology, progression and treatment of psychophysiologically based disorders. Consequently, it may be superfluous, for example, to use a self-report test of anxiety to infer a patient's stress response tendencies, when in effect, a patient's constellation of hypnotic susceptibility-neuroticism-repressive coping is what ultimately drives an individual's level of anxiety. Nevertheless, since nothing is unequivocal in clinical psychology, practitioners are free to incorporate their preferred instruments (to augment the prescribed PHO test measures) within the context of this protocol so long as they follow prescribed methodological procedures for determining their impact on a particular disorder (including ambulatory monitoring and assessment in ecological situations and settings and the incorporation of objective outcome measures longitudinally). Practitioners who are formally affiliated with the UCT are required to assess patients on the above HRMTP-PHO measures.

## CASE STUDY I: PATIENT FINDINGS/PHO MEASURES

1. Patient Constellation of PHO Factors based on the CSARCS-A:

| Measure | Client Score | Range |
|---|---|---|
| ***Subliminal Attention*** | 18 | Medium |
| ***Subliminal Reactivity*** | 2 | Low |
| ***Subliminal Coping*** | 17 | Medium |

Clinical Analogue Rating: Hypnotic Susceptibility (SSHS-A) **Medium**; Neuroticism (NEO; see below) **Low**; Repressive Coping (Marlowe-Crown) **Medium**

***Client:*** *CARL-SQFRE-00054*
***Client ID:*** *CARL-SQFRE-00054*

***Test Date:*** *24 Jun 2006*
***Page*** *3 of 16*

### NEO-FFI Data Table

| Scale | | Raw Score | *T* Score | Range |
|---|---|---|---|---|
| (N) | Neuroticism | 17 | 40 | Low |
| (E) | Extraversion | 26 | 42 | Low |
| (O) | Openness | 22 | 40 | Low |
| (A) | Agreeableness | 32 | 53 | Average |
| (C) | Conscientiousness | 32 | 52 | Average |

Figure 4. Primary Higher Order (PHO) measure scores/profile for patient-client

**Comments:** The PHO constellation Medium-Low-Medium does not raise any red flags nor do any single measures stand out as having negative Mind-Body health implications. The patient's low level of neuroticism (if the diagnosis of ADD is supported) may serve as a protective trait in attenuating heightened physiological reactivity that can result from ADD symptoms and known associated psycho-social problems (Dykman & Ackerman, 1993). However, since the patient profile is more neutral in nature further diagnostics are necessary for exploratory and confirmatory purposes (see 2).

## 2. Psychophysiological Stress Testing

This testing procedure is used in an attempt to concurrently validate stress responses that would be predicted on the basis of a patient's profile of PHO and CSARCS-A measures. In an evidence-based approach assessment is oftentimes multi-tiered in order to check for false positive/false negative findings in initial screenings or for the purpose of further assessment, especially when individuals are found to have more ambiguous *Patient's Profiles*. Recent research has found that excessive physiological reactivity during serial 7s[4] stress testing, as being reflected in *Very Low Frequency* and greater *Low:High Frequency* heart rate variability (HRV) ratios is associated with greater autonomic nervous system (ANS) responsivity to real world stressors and critical moments during competition (Carlstedt, 2004, 2008). More reactive stress test responses are also strongly correlated with the most performance disruptive *Patient's and Athlete's Profile* constellation (High Hypnotic Susceptibility/Subliminal Attention-High Neuroticism/Subliminal Reactivity-Low Repressive Coping/Subliminal Coping; Wickramasekera, 1998; Carlstedt, 2008).

Since this patient-athlete's constellation of PHO factors was not predictive of undue susceptibility to psychophysiological disorders per se or with having developed protective response tendencies, his stress test can be considered an additional layer or level up in the diagnostic evidence chain in that it revealed psychophysiological response tendencies that could not have been predicted or inferred on the basis of his PHO profile alone.

### *Patient Stress Test Results (HRV)*

| Condition/HRV Measure | | | | | | |
|---|---|---|---|---|---|---|
| | HR | SDNN | VLF | LF | HF | LF/HF |
| Baseline | 91 | 142 | 1901 | 939 | 842 | 1.1 |
| Stress Test | 77 | 255 | 2359 | 6327 | 4265 | 1.5 |

**Comments:** The patient's baseline heart rate (HR) was actually higher compared to the stress test condition, a paradoxical response that occurs in less than 10% of all test takers (Carlstedt, 2004, 2008). Similarly, the patient's heart rate variability index (SDNN) did not conform to expectations and while it was high in the baseline condition, it was hyper-inflated

[4] The Serial 7s stress test involves counting backwards from 1000 or other number out loud. This task usually elicits increased cognitively mediated sympathetic nervous system reactivity as evident when monitoring HRV during this assessment of autonomic responses to induced stressors.

in the stress test condition. Arithmetic and counting exercises almost always result in increased heart rate due to cognitive engagement and stress. To assess physiological reactivity to stressors one calculates the difference in change of each HRV measure derived from the stress test compared to baseline response measures. The greater the change, especially increases in HR, VLF and LF:HF ratio reflects greater sympathetic nervous system reactivity (flight response) to cognitive stress. This patient's paradoxical responses must be further explored and may lead to the determination that he does not have ADD. It is also conceivable that HRV in individuals with ADD may result in paradoxical stress test responses and/or that forced conditions (backward counting) that require cognitive engagement lead to better self-regulation and attenuation of lack of focus.

These findings highlight the benefits of engaging in conceptually sound and justified testing that would not routinely be carried out by most practitioners. In this case it was revealed that a supposed ADD patient actually was less reactive to cognitive stress than "normals," which may call into question the diagnosis of ADD. These findings also suggest

that ADD patients may have a unique ANS physiological reactivity signature that should be investigated further (Dykman & Ackerman, 1993). It should be noted that the Serial 7s stress test can easily be administered in less than ten minutes using a user-friendly HRV software package (BioCom Technologies, 2007).

## 3. Neurocognitive Testing: Assessing Subliminal Brain Responses

This test battery is also a routine component of the CP intake process and patient database development. Standard neuropsychological tests ranging from the measurement of *sustained attention* to *motor tapping* and from *choice reaction time* to *go-no-go* tests of inhibition and impulsivity are used to determine clinical and performance relevant neurocognitive processing (Brain Resource Company, 2007). This battery is not merely administered for descriptive or normative purposes, but for analyzing brain functioning at the intra-and inter-individual level in the context of clinical and/or performance outcome and other measures that are documented in the CP assessment process. For example, various neurocognitive measures that reflect cortical processing in certain brain areas, including the frontal lobes and anterior cingulate have been found to be associated with specific constellations of CSARCS-A, PHO and heart rate variability measures in the direction that would be expected on the basis of their hypothesized and documented dynamics (e.g., high executive-strategic planning scores based on the executive maze test and High or Low SA/HS-Low SR/N-High SC/RC and greater low frequency HRV; Carlstedt, 2008). This battery is also an inexpensive alternative to assessment procedure 4. (see below) and can be used to determine pre and post intervention changes in neurocognitive performance (test-retest).

The following chart provides an overview of the tests included in the Brain Resource Company laboratory and internet-based test batteries and the brain regions that are engaged when a specific test is being taken.

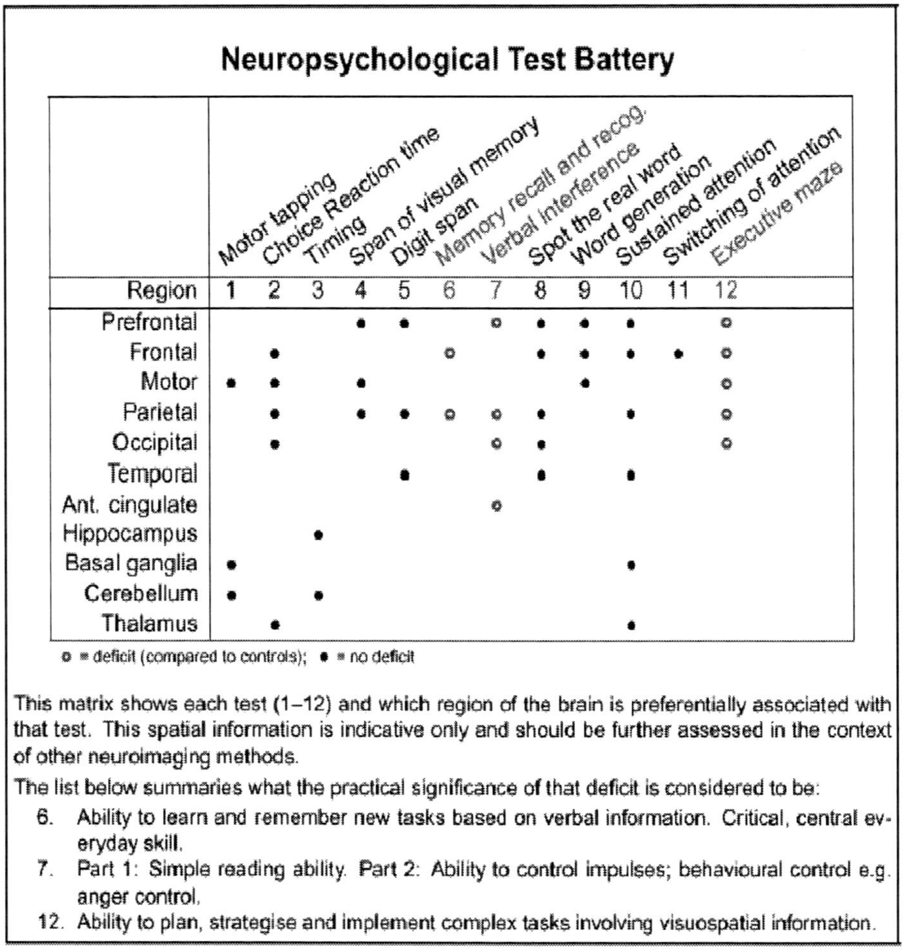

Neuropsychological Test Battery

| Region | 1 Motor tapping | 2 Choice Reaction time | 3 Timing | 4 Span of visual memory | 5 Digit span | 6 Memory recall and recog. | 7 Verbal interference | 8 Spot the real word | 9 Word generation | 10 Sustained attention | 11 Switching of attention | 12 Executive maze |
|---|---|---|---|---|---|---|---|---|---|---|---|---|
| Prefrontal | | | | • | • | | o | • | • | • | | o |
| Frontal | | • | | | | o | | • | • | • | • | o |
| Motor | • | • | | • | | | | | • | | | o |
| Parietal | | • | | • | • | o | o | • | | • | | o |
| Occipital | | • | | | | | o | • | | | | o |
| Temporal | | | | | • | | | • | | • | | |
| Ant. cingulate | | | | | | | o | | | | | |
| Hippocampus | | | • | | | | | | | | | |
| Basal ganglia | • | | | | | | | | | • | | |
| Cerebellum | • | | • | | | | | | | | | |
| Thalamus | | • | | | | | | | | • | | |



Figure 5 Brain areas and structures that are implicated in the listed neurocognitive tests

## Patient Test Results (Neurocognition)

The following charts depict the patient's scores on the BRC neurocognition test, in summary form (1st chart) and comparison form (Z scores relative to normative database).

## Brain Resource Summary Report

**Cognition, CSARCS-A, EI, Personality.**

**Client:** CARL-SQFRE-00054 (birth date 09 Apr 1993; age 13 years; male)

| Test | Level | Function Measured | Functional Significance |
|---|---|---|---|
| ***Cognition*** | | | |
| Memory | Deficit | Working memory recall and recognition | Ability to attend to, learn, remember, store, retrieve and manipulate new information. It includes long and short term memory |
| Attention, Behavioral | Average | Sustained attention<br>Focussed attention<br>Impulsivity<br>Cognitive flexibility | Ability to selectively concentrate during cognitive tasks, detect and respond to change in the environment, sustain attention over time and control impulses |
| Sensory-Motor/Spatial | Average | Hand/eye coordination<br>Accuracy of selecting an appropriate response | Ability to perform motor skills and respond to information in a timely fashion. It includes reaction time |
| Language | Borderline | Word comprehension<br>Verbal fluency<br>Verbal memory | Ability to recognize words, access words and remember what has been heard |
| Executive Function | Borderline | Planning<br>Abstraction<br>Error correction | Ability to plan, strategize and execute complex tasks. It includes planning, abstract thinking, rule acquisition, inhibiting inappropriate actions and ignoring irrelevant sensory information |
| Social Cognition | Average | Emotion recognition | Ability to recognize interpersonal emotions through facial expression |
| ***CSARCS-A*** | | | |
| | Medium<br>Low<br>Medium | Subliminal Attention<br>Subliminal Reactivity<br>Subliminal Coping | Ability to attain peak performance during critical moments |

Deficit ≤-2 standard deviation — Average >-1 and <1 standard deviation

Borderline >-2 and ≤-1 standard deviation — Superior ≥1 standard deviation

**Important Information and Disclaimer**

Feference: PA 0257 8495 Test Date: 24 Jun 2006 Report Date: 27 Jun 2006

This report provides indications of brain function and cognition as compared to a normative database. Its only purpose is to provide evidence based data to assist the decision making process of a competent relevant professional. It must not be used as a basis for action without consideration by a competent relevant professional.

This report is not intended to diagnose or treat any health condition and it must never be used on its own to make any diagnostic or treatment decisions.

This report does not establish any physician-patient relationship or supplant any in-person medical consultation or examination. Appropriate medical attention should always be sought for any ailments. Do not disregard professional medical advice or delay seeking medical treatment as a result of this report.

In so far as permitted by law BRC expressly disclaims any and all responsibility for any liability, loss, injury, damage, expense or risk which may be or is incurred as a consequence, directly or indirectly, of any use or application of this report.

**The Brain Resource Company**©

BRC Operations Pty Limited ABN 45 098 619 115

Email: info@brainresource.com URL: www.brainresource.com

Figure 6.

**Comments:** Whereas PHO and CSARCS-A measures were not revealing and in fact, contained findings that could be considered incompatible with a diagnosis of ADD (low neuroticism/subliminal reactivity; paradoxical relaxation response in the stress condition of the Serial 7s) this patient's neurocognitive test scores were replete with positive findings that could be considered supportive of a diagnosis of ADD. Mild to moderate significant performance deficits involving memory, attention and executive functioning are apparent in the above report.

In the context of the CP methodology "mere" positive clinical findings that are based on group norms or inter-group research findings are never sufficient to arrive at an unequivocal diagnosis. Such data can guide the diagnosis process, but ultimately, any diagnosis must be predominately based on intra-individual or individualized norms that are established on the basis of repeated measures (longitudinally) and especially in the context of performance or clinically relevant outcome measures that have a high degree of ecological validity. Thus, in this case, although indicators of ADD may be present one must ascertain to what extent they impact behavior, health and performance in the real world. In the case of this patient one must ask, do so-called deficit findings negatively influence his school work, social and interpersonal relationships and athletic performance? These questions will be answered in part as we move through the assessment and into the intervention process.

## 4. Quantitative EEG (qEEG, brain mapping): Case Study II

qEEG or brain mapping is an advanced and sophisticated procedure for establishing pre-intervention brain response tendencies and for concurrently validating "red-flag" findings from the initial neurocognitive test battery. It affords important insight into brain function in the assessment (pre-intervention diagnostic) phase or before beginning psychotherapy and provides a snap-shot in time that can be used later for comparative purposes (post therapy or intervention). It is an especially useful procedure for detecting subtle changes in brain function that transcend subjective clinical impressions. Event-related potentials (ERP; e.g., P300 ERP; see Andreassi, 1995) latencies that reflect psychological states, focusing tendencies, performance decrement as a function of age, as well as the effects of pharmacological treatment and mental training are emerging as illuminating predictor and outcome measures in the diagnostic and efficacy testing process (Carlstedt, 2008). This procedure is carried out in a special laboratory and should only be administered by applied neuroscience specialists in collaboration with neuropsychologists and specially trained psychologists. qEEG is also a precursor to neurofeedback (see interventions below) and is used to help determine the most effective brainwave biofeedback protocol as well as assess the effects of neurofeedback in treating specific disorders.

Since qEEG is a relatively expensive procedure it is usually only used when basic neurocognitive testing reveals major red flags or to guide neurofeedback. In the case of our athlete-patient a qEEG could not be performed due to financial reasons[5]. Hence, for illustrative purposes an additional case study of a patient who underwent a qEEG is briefly

[5] The qEEG procedure is not always reimbursed by insurance companies.

presented. Out takes from the case of a 55 year old former professional tennis player with mild depression are presented in Figure 7.

While it is beyond the scope of this chapter to extensively elucidate the intricacies of the qEEG procedure I will briefly comment on findings that were most relevant to this patient's depression and performance issues. The patient's qEEG was generated from the BRC paradigm that is rapidly becoming the gold standard for clinical and normative databases of brain functioning. It has been used in over 90 published studies and grant funded investigations including NIH sponsored research and pharmaceutical trials (see BrainNet, 2007).

**Comments:** What stood out most in this particular patient was a high level of delta activity in both the eyes open and closed conditions. Delta involves slow wave brain activity and is most associated with sleep states. In an "awake" condition it can be considered abnormal and even of neurological relevance and may be an EEG-concomittant of depression (ref.). However, since this patient is a highly functional and successful businessman and competitive athlete (he now plays senior tennis after a career as a world-class professional tennis player) one must be cautious when generalizing from group norms and their implications to a specific individual.

As a result of the qEEG and those from a few other athletes with similar findings a working hypothesis centering on delta wave activity and brain "idling" as a response to non-salient stimuli is being developed (Dietrich, 2004; Carlstedt, 2008). It proposes that in highly functioning individuals, to conserve finite amount of cortical metabolic resources (see Dietrich) that are available and needed to function at peak levels when it counts the most (e.g., when negotiating or planning as a businessman or when encountering a critical moment during a sport competition), downtime, or performance irrelevant epochs during one's day will result in an adaptive almost "slumber-like" state even if an individual is "awake." In such individuals, increased waking state delta, which to some practitioners might signal brain pathophysiology (and result in a diagnosis of ADD), may in fact, merely indicate that an individual has gone "offline." This hypothesis is currently being tested and is very relevant to our patient-athlete whose performance data lends preliminary support to this hypothesis. One caveat must be mentioned though; this former professional tennis player did complain of depression and pointed out that still playing competitive tennis took him back to a more happy and carefree time in his life. Since increased waking state delta activity has also been associated with depression (ref), this patient's qEEG delta findings may indeed reflect a predominant waking state that was alleviated whenever he played tennis or engaged in business activities that demanded a more alert cognitive state (as reflected in greater beta brainwave activity and faster P300 ERP latencies).

Again, this assessment procedure points to the clinical utility of qEEG and the need to go beyond mere clinical intuition and impressions when dealing with complex clinical cases.

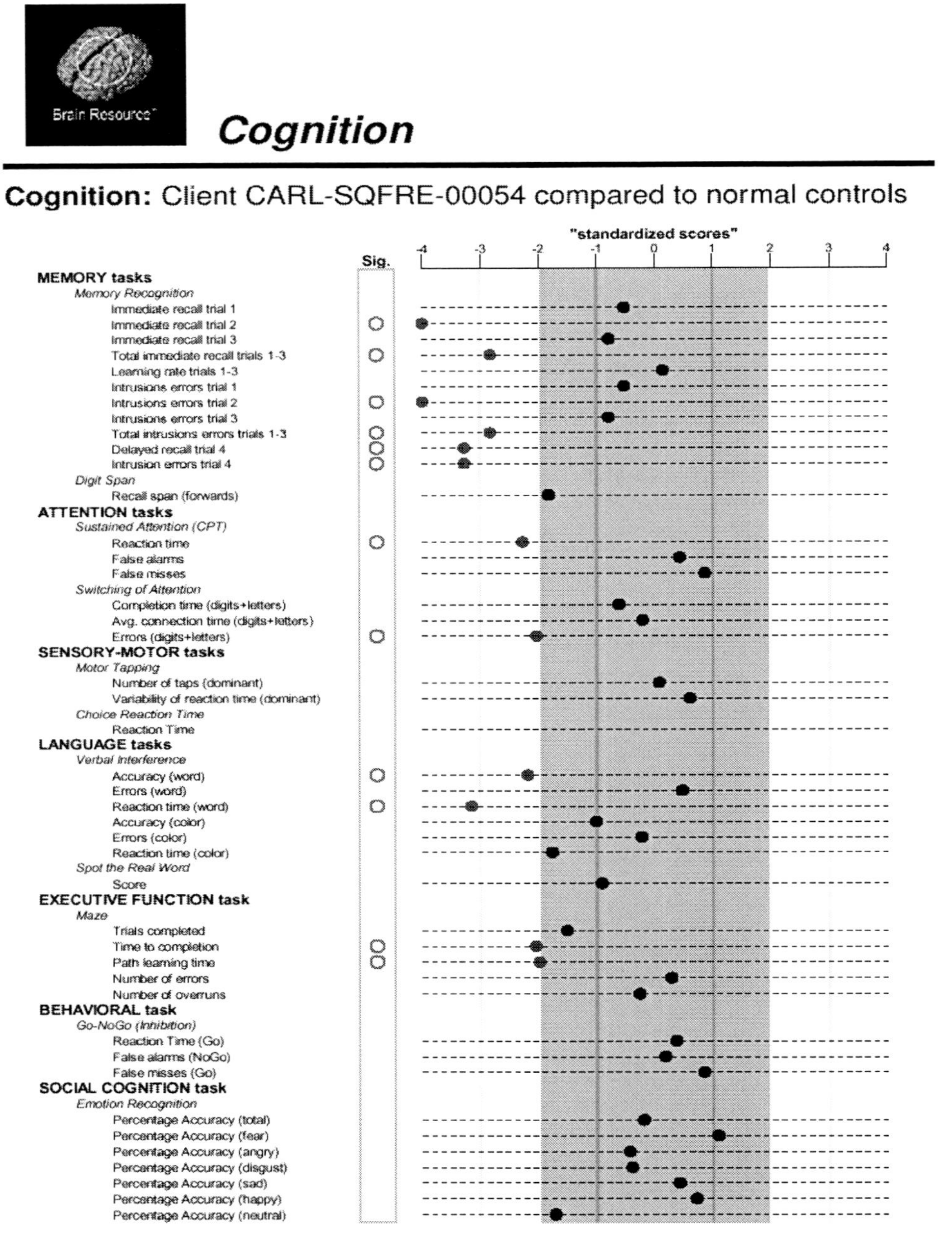


For convenience, the tasks are organized by broad cognitive groupings. The circles on the left indicate statistically significant differences compared with the normal control. The "standardized scores" on the right are normalized for age and gender, which means differences from zero reflect differences from 'average peer' (also known as z-scores). Positive "standardized scores" indicate above average scores, negative "standardized scores" are below average (Avg = average). "Standardized scores" beyond -2 to +2 are statistically significant. False alarms (respond when should not) = false positive; errors of commission. False misses (not respond when should) = false negatives; errors of omission. Intrusion = words not on the list. Specialist interpretation is required.

Figure 7.

## 3. Electrical Brain Function (EEG & ERP)

### 3.1 Statistical summary of the Electrical Brain Function scores

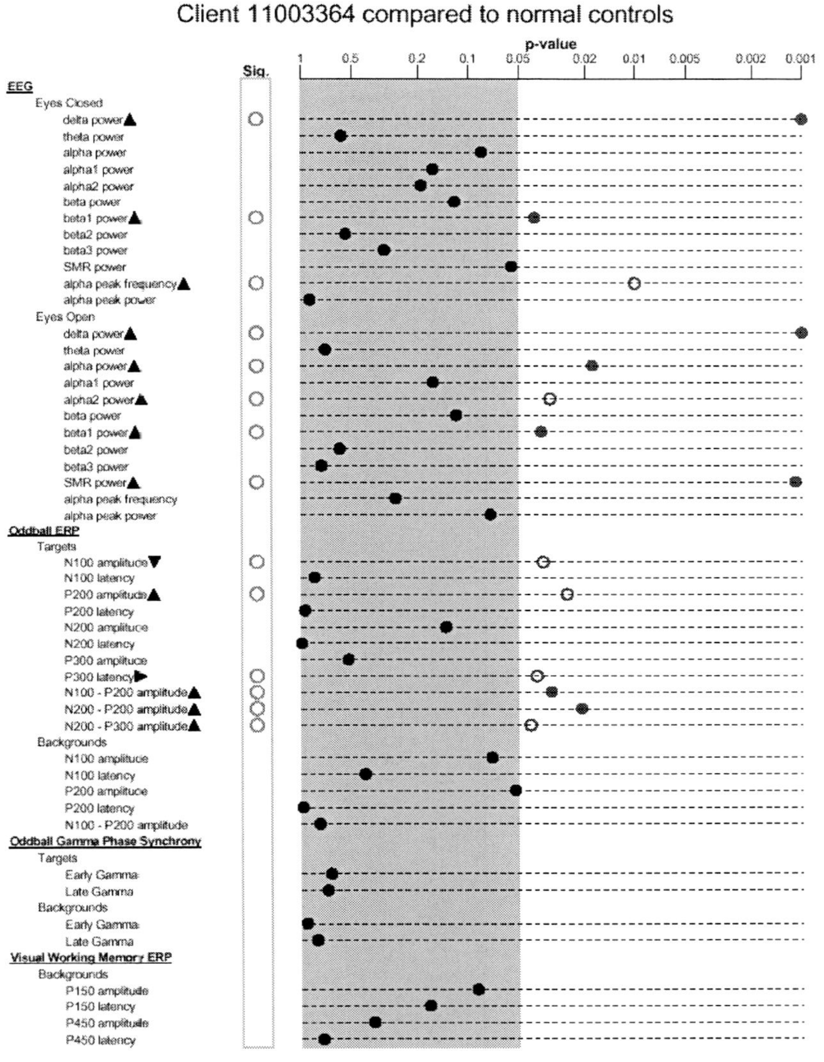

The open circles on the left indicate statistically significant differences compared with the normal controls (matched for age and sex). Triangles show the direction of change. The statistical analyses undertaken include: i) Solid circles reflect Mahalanobis differences for sites F3, Fz, F4, C3, Cz, C4, P3, Pz and P4. ii) Open circles reflect when Mahalanobis analysis across all sites was additionally significant. iii) Squares reflect t-test significance on the key site for that paradigm according to the scientific literature. Working memory is analysed using t-tests.

The direction and spatial distribution of selected key statistically significant finding is shown in the graphs on pages 28 to 30. The summary of factor analysis scores is shown on page 27.

Figure 8.

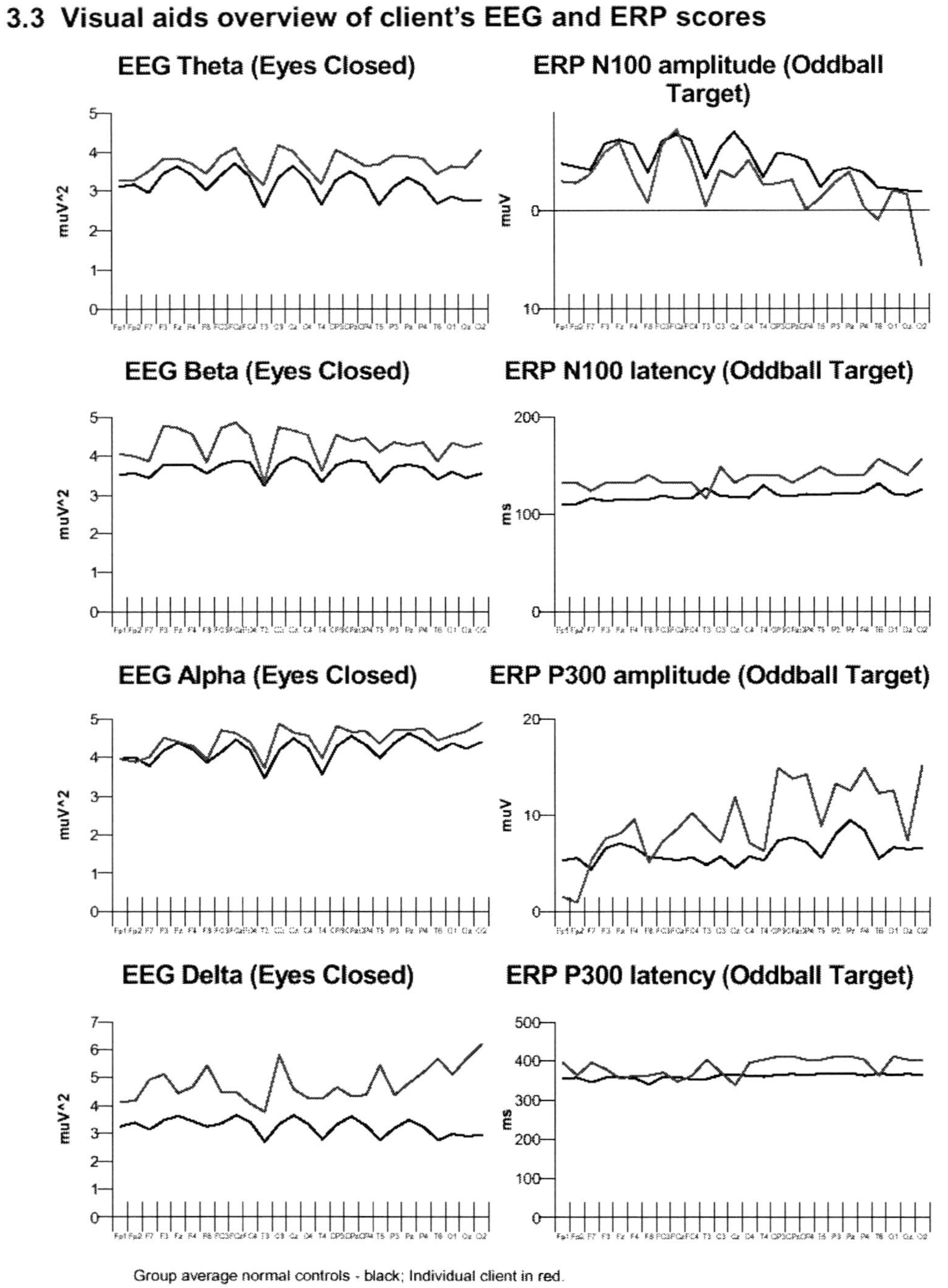
3.3 Visual aids overview of client's EEG and ERP scores
EEG Theta (Eyes Closed)
muV^2
ERP N100 amplitude (Oddball Target)
muV
EEG Beta (Eyes Closed)
muV^2
ERP N100 latency (Oddball Target)
ms
EEG Alpha (Eyes Closed)
muV^2
ERP P300 amplitude (Oddball Target)
muV
EEG Delta (Eyes Closed)
muV^2
ERP P300 latency (Oddball Target)
ms
Group average normal controls - black; Individual client in red.

Figure 9.

### 3.4 Visualization of THE most stastically significant result in each paradigm
(followed by all sites data)

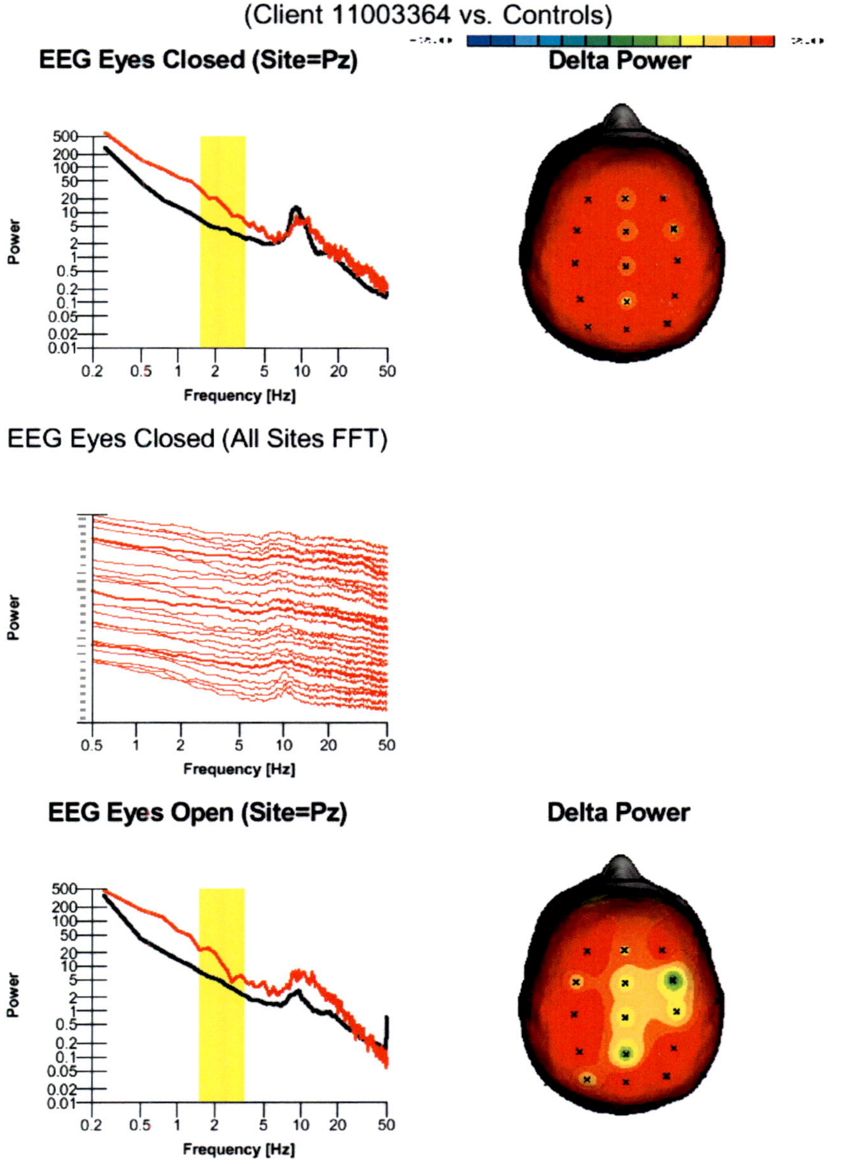


The waveforms across sites (Fz, Cz, Pz in bold) show the client's data for paradigms with statistically significant findings. The single site figures reflect the electrical brain function data in the subject (red) compared to their age and gender matched controls (black).

The head maps reflect the spatial distribution of the statistically significant findings as indicated by the yellow bars in the single site waveforms (increases are shown in red and decreases in blue). If the data is not applicable or missing at a site, that site is not shown.

Figure 10.

## 6. Assessment of Heart Rate Variability

Heart Rate Variability (HRV; not to be confused with mere heart rate) is emerging as a reliable indicator of both peak performance states and dysfunctional response tendencies (Lehrer et al., 2003; Carlstedt, 2008). It has been found to reflect psychological and emotional fluctuations to a variety of stimuli in numerous settings including psychotherapy (during which it is routinely monitored as part of CP diagnostic process). HRV is an autonomic nervous system (ANS) measure that reveals moment to moment changes in physiological reactivity (Malik & Camm, 1995). Excessive physiological reactivity at baseline is reflected in greater activation of the sympathetic branch of the ANS while lesser reactivity ranges on a continuum from focused alertness to being relaxed (parasympathetic responding). All patients are routinely assessed on HRV, not only to determine reactive tendencies to cognitive stress (as previously mentioned) but longitudinally over the course of psychotherapy and even outside the office to assess ANS responses to real world stressors and determine a patient's ability to engage in prescribed interventions that were learned in the office. For example, rather than merely teach a patient diaphragmatic breathing to achieve relaxation, in an evidence-based approach such as the CP, it would not be assumed that this method will have a positive effect or that the patient will transfer to the real world that which he or she learned in the office. Consequently, interventions are monitored in the field until a patient demonstrates the ability to utilize an intervention technique and attain benchmark goals for mind-body change that can be inferred from HRV reports that are obtained in the field.

**Comments:** Below you will find a sample autonomic assessment report of our patient-athlete. He was routinely assessed for HRV prior to every baseball game and at-bat for the course of the 2006 summer season. Especially, in the case of psychophysiological and cognitive disorders it is important to ascertain the impact of a patient's symptoms in the context of important life and performance areas. Since sports performance is a very important part of this patient's life it was necessary to determine to what extent the disorder affected performance on the basis of objective outcome measures that were obtained in ecologically valid contexts (actual competition). It is interesting to note, that consistent with an individual who is low in neuroticism or subliminal reactivity, the patient, although exhibiting high heart rate still manifested predominantly parasympathetic responding as reflected in a LF: HF ratio of 0.6 (6 times as much high frequency than low frequency activity). This finding highlights that frequently, but erroneously, a high heart rate at baseline, is interpreted to indicate nervousness, when in fact, a more sensitive indicator of ANS balance (LF: HF ratio) indicates otherwise. Thus, a complete spectrum analysis of HRV is preferred over more simple and oftentimes manually derived less sensitive measures like mere heart rate when attempting to assess physiological reactivity.

Additional pre-game baseline HRV analyses revealed consistent relative parasympathetic dominance in our patient, suggesting that baseball had a relaxing effect on him and could possibly, again, call into question the diagnosis of ADD.

Taken in concert, this patient's ANS-HRV response profile at baseline, during the *Serial 7s* stress test and prior to games can be considered paradoxical and/or inconsistent with the profile of an individual with "actual" ADD and again cautions practitioners not to arrive at a diagnosis of ADD without extensive longitudinal, ecological valid testing that incorporates objective performance outcome measures (more on this patient's outcome measures later). ADD may be nothing more than selective inattention and boredom that only manifests itself contextually and disappears when salient and motivating stimulation exists (e.g., playing baseball) and points to the need to go well beyond cursory diagnostics that oftentimes are made on the basis of simple symptom check-lists. This can be achieved by integrating user friendly instrumentation into the patient evaluation process.

## 8. Psychological Outcome Measures and Performance Statistics I.

In addition to more high-tech assessment and monitoring procedures the statistical analysis of psychological performance is also an important component in the evaluation of patients and athletes. Psychological performance statistics provide objective insight into behavioral tendencies during real world tasks including test taking, executive decision making, or carrying out a job related endeavor like driving a car or flying an airplane during which symptoms of a particular disorder (e.g., ADD, anxiety, depression) can negatively affect the ability to focus and perform. Patients who are given a diagnosis should be assessed in the context of what they do to determine the extent to which symptoms interfere with duties that may have safety implications or have an important impact on themselves and others (bottom line of a business in which team cooperation is critical). Relative to our case study, performance statistics from baseball were used as outcome measures (at baseline and post intervention) to measure the impact of ADD on his performance and the effects of interventions to his ameliorate symptoms and increase attention.

I have validated an assessment procedure in athletes that can also be applied to clinical patients in which the criticality of a competitive or life event is weighted to determine the effect of any number of clinical predictor variables (e.g., PHO factors, diagnosis, HRV and other psychophysiological) on these events (e.g., effect of a neurocognitive test score on job performance; Carlstedt, 2008).

Critical moments are competitive or performance events that elicit differential psychophysiological responses that can either facilitate or hinder performance. They range from 1-5 in magnitude with five being the highest level of criticality. Critical moment performance has been found to be strongly associated with numerous CP assessment measures including CSARCS-A *Athlete's Profile*, stress test response and pre-action HRD. For example, High or Low SA/HS-Low SR/N & High SC/RC; greater high frequency HRV shift between baseline & stress task; and greater magnitude pre-action HRD trends are associated with better critical moment performance; Carlstedt, 2004, 2008; Couture, 2007; Martin, 2007).

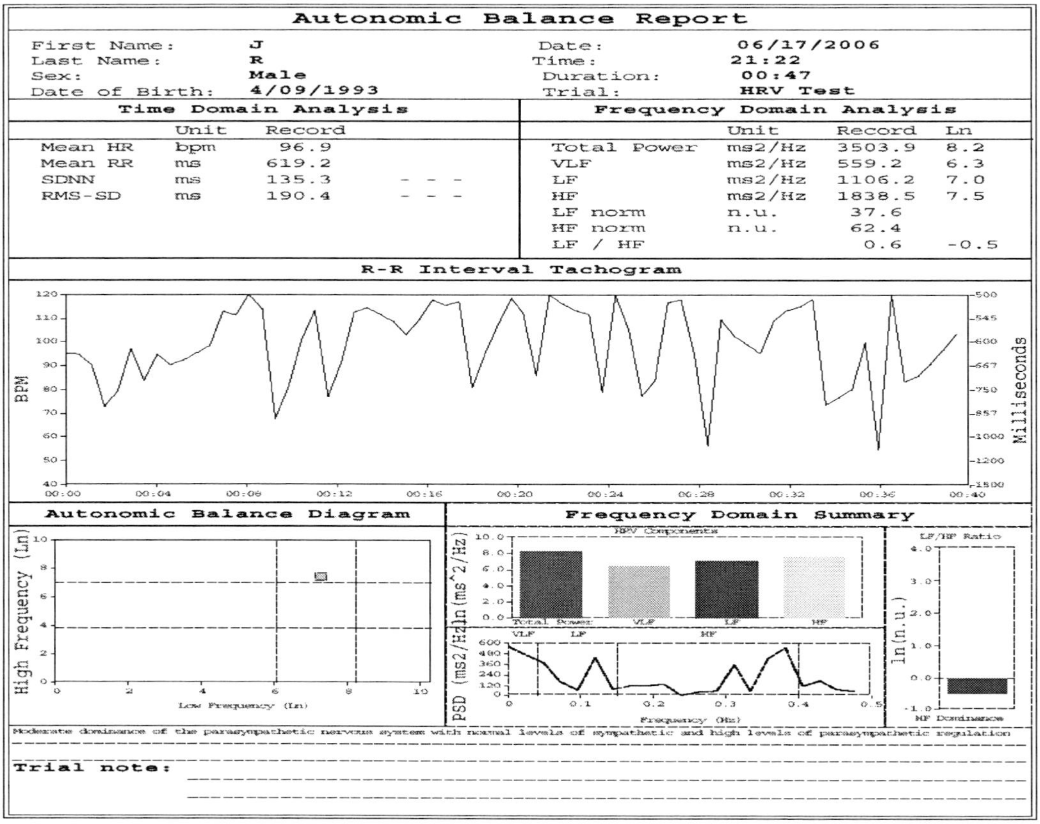

**Autonomic Balance Report**

| | | | |
|---|---|---|---|
| First Name: | J | Date: | 06/17/2006 |
| Last Name: | R | Time: | 21:22 |
| Sex: | Male | Duration: | 00:47 |
| Date of Birth: | 4/09/1993 | Trial: | HRV Test |

**Time Domain Analysis**

| | Unit | Record | |
|---|---|---|---|
| Mean HR | bpm | 96.9 | |
| Mean RR | ms | 619.2 | |
| SDNN | ms | 135.3 | - - - |
| RMS-SD | ms | 190.4 | - - - |

**Frequency Domain Analysis**

| | Unit | Record | Ln |
|---|---|---|---|
| Total Power | ms2/Hz | 3503.9 | 8.2 |
| VLF | ms2/Hz | 559.2 | 6.3 |
| LF | ms2/Hz | 1106.2 | 7.0 |
| HF | ms2/Hz | 1838.5 | 7.5 |
| LF norm | n.u. | 37.6 | |
| HF norm | n.u. | 62.4 | |
| LF / HF | | 0.6 | -0.5 |



Moderate dominance of the parasympathetic nervous system with normal levels of sympathetic and high levels of parasympathetic regulation

**Trial note:**

Figure 11

Critical moment analyses are designed to induce stress and increase demands on attention that can be negatively impacted by a particular disorder and allows practitioners to determine how well a symptomatic patient performs under pressure and to what extent symptoms like anxiety or lack of attention disrupt the seamless completion of a task. Critical moments analyses should be carried out in ecological settings and situations whenever possible or include reward and punishment elements if carried out in the laboratory or office. For example, in an anxiety patient a critical moment paradigm could be designed in which the patient is required to master, stepwise, a series of tasks having continually rising levels or amounts of stressors (ranging from 1-5). Mastery would be demonstrated on the basis of reaching and maintaining specified HRV parameters either passively (mentally) or through an active intervention like RSA biofeedback.

## 9. Psychological Performance Statistics II: Focus and Anxiety Control Threshold Analysis

This assessment procedure involves structuring specific performance tasks that test a patient's ability to maintain mind-body-technical control and successfully complete designated tasks (e.g., carry out a series of prescribed motor tasks [e.g., executive maze]).

Success to attempt ratios, are calculated to arrive at a *Psychological Proficiency Quotient* (PPP) for technical control and focus (concentration). Focus and anxiety thresholds are operationalized on the basis of task specific performance outcome and psychophysiological correlates of such performance including EEG or HRV and can be assessed at baseline (pre-intervention) and post intervention to determine gains that are made relative to actual improved task performance and on the basis of increased measures of attention and reduction of anxiety. One could extend on the critical moment paradigm (above) to incorporate the PPQ statistic.

Our athlete-patient's alleged ADD symptoms and their impact on his important life areas were assessed in the context of baseball performance. Since ADD is seen by some as an artificial or manufactured cluster of symptoms that is rarely diagnosed on the basis of gold standard diagnostic batteries and may be nothing more than selective boredom, engaging an individual who supposedly has this disorder in activities that he or she likes can provide additional direct and indirect clues into attentional processes (Desgranges, Desgranges & Kenneth, 1993). The rationale being, that if an individual professes to like an activity (like baseball in this case) or is even passionate about it they will want to focus and succeed, whereas if they hate school or their job, such an emotion will mediate ADD symptoms. Consequently, it was interesting to see if our patient-athlete would falter and exhibit poor attention or focus in an environment that he voluntarily wanted to be in. If our athlete, despite loving baseball and wanting to focus and ergo, succeed at a high level, exhibited ADD-like symptoms during competition even though he possessed the technical skills to do very well, then one could use such information as an additional layer of ecological evidence in support of a "real" diagnosis of ADD and intervene accordingly.

The following charts depict pre-intervention HRV and pre versus post mental training baseball performance statistics.

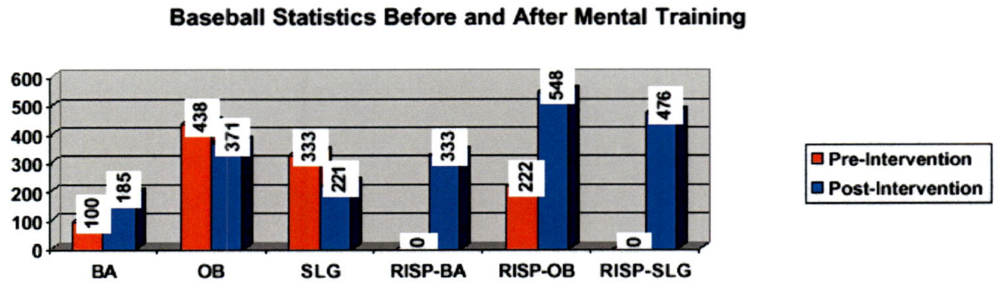


Figure 12

**Comments:** The athlete's pre-intervention performance as interpreted on the basis of objective longitudinal baseball statistical outcome measures could be seen as consistent with an individual with ADD (they were very poor). In addition, despite having excellent technical skills as a batter, the fact that he was not able to generate the number of "hits" necessary to be classified as a good hitter suggests that underlying psychological or psychophysiological issues may be interfering with his "hitting" the ball in a consistent manner.

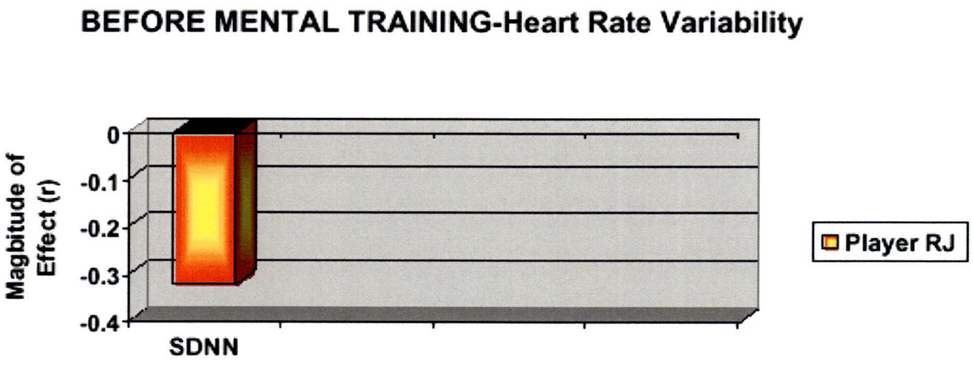


Figure 13

**Comments:** In addition to the performance statistics, this player (as were all players on the team) was monitored for HRV prior to every at-bat during official league games pre-intervention and during the intervention phases of the CP. What emerged were individual psychophysiological (HRV) profiles that were associated with select baseball outcome measures. In this player SDNN, the so-called HRV index was negatively correlated with performance. This finding can be explained in the context of what is known about the neurophysiology (EEG) of peak performance in which heart rate deceleration (HRD) has been found to be a concomitant of the left to right brain hemispheric shift that occurs as strategic planning (left-frontal lobe localized) shifts to more relative right-hemispheric activation (diffuse right hemispheric activation and quieting or idling of the frontal lobes) that is associated with attending to the task stimuli (e.g. the ball as it is pitched; visuoperceptual activity). Since HRD involves a more constant (less variable) linear slowing of the heart (in contrast to alternately increasing and decreasing heart cycles that marks greater HRV and more SDNN) it is hypothesized that when more SDNN or greater HRV is exhibited when batting the above mentioned brain-motor performance dynamics are more likely to be disrupted and negatively impact performance. Relative to an athlete with ADD, one would expect this dynamic to be more frequently disrupted, especially in sports or other settings in which longer periods of inactivity may test an individual's ability to remain focused during pauses in the action. As such, HRV and HRD should be incorporated into ADD assessment and performance batteries whenever patient relevant ecological tasks involve self-paced action or temporally isolated response demands that have a pre-action to action phase shift that must be seamlessly mastered (e.g., transition from flying a plane or driving a car to having to land or take evasive action, a scenario in which ADD could lead to accidents).The patient's diagnostic phase of the CP has now been completed.

While ADD may indeed be a valid diagnosis, how this athlete fares in the intervention phase may offer additional insight or evidence in support of the diagnosis or help rule it out.

## Interventions: Orientations and Perspectives

Practitioners are often quick to claim or believe that an intervention works. This is to be expected since the credibility of mental health practitioners is predicated on treatment methods that have symptom ameliorating effects. While positive group findings are frequently cited to support the continued use of a particular intervention, they do not necessarily generalize to the individual. In other words, just because a statistically significant majority of patients in a treatment group may appear to have benefited from an intervention does not mean that a large effect size has been demonstrated (i.e., high degree of inter and intra-subject potency). Group findings are based on mean differences between the treatment and control group. However, the responses of subjects in a group are only considered in the context of group-averages but fail to establish the amount of the variance an intervention contributes to explaining treatment outcome in each individual subject independently. Moreover, significance level (*p* value) is no longer considered the benchmark in efficacy testing, instead effect size and confidence intervals are deemed to be superior indicators of intervention efficacy in more rigorous outcome studies (Cohen, 1994). These methodological issues suggest that caution must be exercised when attempting to generalize group findings on intervention efficacy to individual patients. More importantly, psychotherapy and mental health interventions are mostly exercised at the level of the individual and as such, ultimately, efficacy must be demonstrated in each patient independently and irrespective of what group findings may suggest regarding treatment outcome success. This was clearly demonstrated in our study of baseball players that contained the athlete with ADD from the case study in this chapter in which although, as a team an intervention was associated with impressive statistical performance gains, at the intra-individual level treatment response and performance outcome was quite discrepant.

Rather than rely on claims of effectiveness the CP approach to interventions focuses on efficacy testing at the intra-individual level. Interventions are always applied in the context of efficacy-outcome research that is cognizant of following factors; 1) intervention amenability 2) intervention compliance 3) longitudinal staying power or time to achieve an effect 4) temporal gradients of an intervention (time of day when engaged in and amount of each session), 5) selection and operationalization of criterion/dependent outcome variables (e.g., intervention success = HRV changes or improvement in a performance outcome measure like increased focus threshold [e.g., Test of.Variables of Attention score; T.O.V.A., 2007), 6) ecological validity 7) individual as opposed to group outcome analyses (Carlstedt, 2004, 2008).

Clinical interventions must also be grounded conceptually and be shown to elicit neuropsychophysiological responses that can be observed, monitored and analyzed in real time and in the context of ecological situations, settings and tasks. The CP approach to intervention extends well beyond merely administering a treatment method that is presumed to work and brings accountability to the assessment and intervention process in the form of ongoing validation and efficacy testing. Rather than assume that a particular intervention works, be it progressive relaxation, cognitive-restructuring or any number of techniques in clinical psychology, ecological, longitudinal monitoring and efficacy testing is demanded at the intra-individual level. Anything less can be considered cursory and lacking and not in the best interest of patients.

## INTERVENTION AMENABILITY

The selection of the most appropriate intervention method(s) is to a large extent dependent on a patient's profile of hypnotic susceptibility-neuroticism-repressive coping since specific constellations of these measures have been found to influence intervention amenability, effectiveness and compliance (Carlstedt, 2004; Wickramasekera, 1988).

Individuals who are high in hypnotic susceptibility are most receptive to visually-based interventions whereas those who are how in this measure and concurrently high in repressive coping have a skeptical cognitive style and require much convincing to even see a practitioner let alone engage in psychological treatment, especially modalities that have more esoteric and visual elements (Wickramaskera, 1988). Wickramaskera (1988, 2003) describes a so-called "Trojan horse" method of getting this subset of patients into the office in the first place and then winning them over by exposing them to data-driven interventions that provide objective insight into mind-body dynamics that are associated with certain disorders that they have been oblivious to and how positive health facilitative methods like respiratory sinus arrhythmia (RSA) can be learned through biofeedback. It is beyond the scope of chapter to elucidate further on the intervention facilitating or hindering effects of various HRMTP constellations. Most important is to keep in mind that hypnotic susceptibility and repressive coping are strong predictors of intervention amenability and compliance (Wickramaskera, 1988, 2003).

## ON-GOING MONITORING

All interventions are monitored (psychophysiologically) and tested for efficacy in the context of statistical outcome measures (performance statistics [e.g., games won] and/or mind-body measures [e.g., HRV]) to determine if, when, why, to what extent and how they are working and in whom. For example, even in the case of psychodynamic-therapy or couples therapy patients/clients are monitored using HRV instrumentation to gain better insight into changes in physiological reactivity that may go undetected on the basis of verbal report or expressions to the therapist alone. Additional modalities can also be used, including electrodermal activity, EEG and assessment can now be undertaken in an ambulatory manner in the real world which is particularly revealing in patients with anxiety and other psychophysiological disorders.

## STANDARD CP INTERVENTION MODALITIES:

### Heart Rate Variability/Respiratoty Sinus Arrhythmia Biofeedback (HRV/RSA)

HRV/RSA biofeedback, when engaged in according to a strict protocol that documents a patient's or athlete's autonomic nervous system response tendencies in the context of real world stressors can be effective in helping achieve mind-body control and reduce symptoms associated with anxiety and related disorders. (Lehrer et al., 2003). In three longitudinal ecological studies of tennis and baseball players (including a subset of athletes with competitive anxiety) carried out during actual official competition, large statistical performance gains by players after they learned to manipulate HRV in the desired direction, as determined by their pre-intervention *IZOF* and *Athlete's* profiles[6]were revealed. In the baseball and one of the tennis studies players were monitored and engaged in HRV/RSA biofeedback prior to each at bat when on the bench or during changeovers in tennis (Carlstedt, et.al., 2007, 2008). This breathing-based intervention should not be confused with clinical relaxation procedures. When applied to sports, breathing rate and rhythm are *prescribed* on the basis of an athlete's *IZOF/Athlete's* profile. It is not about arbitrarily "taking a deep breath" to "relax" (the cliché approach); rather, manipulating psychophysiology in the direction that has been established as most performance facilitative on the basis of extensive monitoring and analysis of HRV prior to commencing mental training. HRV/RSA techniques can also be used to consciously induce the HRD that routinely occurs when competitive stress is absent, during times of duress. Successful HRV training is dependent on determining the rate and rhythm of an athlete's exhale cycle through the meticulous monitoring and analysis of this psychophysiological response over the course of many training sessions and actual competition (Carlstedt, 2004, 2007, 2008). While these studies were carried out in athletes with competitive anxiety (and the one ADD player whose case study has been presented throughout this chapter) what is important is that the ambulatory assessment methodology and intervention be applied in a similarly controlled manner in patients. This requires that patients with psychophysiological disorders be equipped with user friendly HRV monitoring devices that record data as programmed in advance or instructed both for the establishment of real world baselines of ANS/HRV responding and during interventions (e.g., RSA/HRV biofeedback to manage symptoms once they occur).

## NEUROFEEDBACK: CARLSTEDT FRONTAL LOBE PROTOCOL

Since all psychophysiological disorders originate centrally (e.g., hypothalamic-pituitary-adrenal axis; amygdala, frontal-lobe pathways) the manipulation brain wave activity (EEG) that is associated with the onset of stress and anxiety or occurs concomitant to attention deficits (in ADD), to restore homeostatic (asymptomatic) baseline levels of EEG may be one of the most direct means of symptom amelioration (Rossiter, 2004).

Indeed, scores of studies have demonstrated the shaping of brain wave activity through operant conditioning of EEG and neurofeedback's utility as an effective non-pharmacological alternative to the treatment of various psychophysiological disorders including depression, anxiety disorders and ADD (Hammond, 2005).

---

[6] It should be noted that competitive anxiety symptoms resemble those observed in clinical anxiety disorders and that studying ANS responses in athletes in vivo, during actual competition affords important insight into symptom generation, progression and amelioration on the basis of ongoing monitoring of psychophysiology. The "playing field" provides a laboratory and ecologically-based window into mind-body processes when individuals are under real-world stress that has clinical implications and also allows for the testing of ambulatory methodologies that can be applied to patient populations as well.

Although still considered experimental by some, neurofeedback or brain wave biofeedback is an intervention modality that is based on extensive research of the electrical activity of the brain in response to numerous task demands, stressors and experimental stimulus presentation-response paradigms. One species-wide finding that is relevant to performance and its disruption due to the onset of symptoms is that during routine pre-action phases leading up to task relevant motor responses a relative left to right brain hemispheric shift has been shown to occur (Hatfield, Landers & Ray, 1984). This shift is thought to reflect strategic planning occurring in the left frontal lobe and other left regions (to a lesser extent) of the brain giving way to the visuoperceptual and motor performance demands, a predominantly right hemispheric function. In the absence of stress, clinical or competitive anxiety, depression symptoms and cognitive disruptions associated with ADD, as well as mere intrusive thoughts, this left to right shift occurs routinely and performance or task demands are successfully mastered. However, when heightened stress or the self-perception of threat is encountered or subjectively experienced, vulnerable individuals are apt to experience negative intrusive thoughts that infiltrate and remain in the ruminative left frontal lobe region of the brain. This disrupts the left to right shift that is associated with the successful transition from strategic planning to action and helps explain inexplicable performance breakdowns in a wide variety of settings and situations ranging from sports to test taking to driving a car or making business or other decisions that require action responses (Carlstedt, 2004, Carlstedt, 2004b).

Neurofeedback allows patients to observe their brain waves on a computer screen and then consciously manipulate cortical EEG frequencies and amplitudes in the direction that is most associated with mind-body homeostasis or successful performance (e.g., the left to right shift). Over time, self-generated brain responses are shaped and reinforced to the extent that patients or athletes can be weaned off neurofeedback instrumentation. If successfully "programmed," a patient will then unconsciously exhibit the same brain baseline, adaptive or symptom reducing activity that was generated in the laboratory in response to real world stressors. While this may sound easy, one must be cautioned that such a process must be validated in each individual patient. There are no mass quick-fix solutions and neurofeedback protocols must be based on extensive monitoring, assessment and analysis of an individual's brain response tendencies in a variety of situations and settings that are most important to successfully dealing with stressors in one's life. This author is currently testing a *Frontal-Lobe Protocol* based on Dietrich's (2004) *Transient Hypofrontality Hypothesis*, proposing that the royal road to better brain regulation and subsequent amelioration of symptoms or the disruption of performance that is associated with central dysfunction (e.g., ADD, anxiety) lies in consciously or even subliminally being trained to induce frontal lobe idling in the face of stressors, symptoms and complex attentional and motor task demands via neurofeedback that targets this brain region (Carlstedt, 2007). Preliminary results have been encouraging.

Neurofeedback has been integrated into the CP universal clinical trials for practitioners in conjunction with the Brain Resource Company whose databases of normative and clinical databases of brain wave activity (qEEG) has resulted in numerous findings pertaining to ADD (see BRC).

## Cerebral Laterality Manipulation Training

The self-manipulation of cerebral laterality is a low-tech analogue to neurofeedback whereby patients are taught to consciously attempt to induce the previously discussed left to right cortical shift prior to action or when experiencing symptoms. This can be done by blocking the intake of stimuli through the eyes and ears in such a manner that the brain hemisphere that is contralateral to the blockade is stimulated/activated (e.g., blocking stimuli to the left visual field of each eye will result in greater activation of the left brain hemisphere; Schiffer, 1998; Carlstedt, 2001). Schiffer (1997) has reported on the amelioration of depression and PTSD symptoms in patients who used special goggles to manipulate cerebral laterality.

## Discussion

It is important that the above assessment and intervention procedures be applied in an integrative manner and not in isolation. Their use should be based on hierarchical-heuristic diagnostic logic that is multi-tiered and cognizant of a procedure's status in the evidence-chain. For example, if one is interested in a patient's brain processing tendencies it is not sufficient to assume that self-report tests will be 100% accurate in predicting them. Especially, when there is uncertainty or with red-flagged and borderline cases additional neurocognitive and EEG testing is usually indicated. Furthermore, findings are considered to have limited value if they are not empirically linked to actual clinical and performance outcome measures. A patient who exhibits excellent mind-body regulation when encountering real world stressors who happens to have negative mind-body markers on the basis of a self-report test would not be diagnosed as having an anxiety disorder if in reality he or she is indeed objectively shown to exhibited autonomic balance in ecologically valid stress situations. Moreover, interventions should always be tested for efficacy in the context of numerous performance and neuropsychophysiological outcome measures and modified according to the data. Interventions are not limited to those presented in this chapter. The ones that were used were highlighted because of their applicability to the presented case studies. Any intervention can be used within the context of the CP and UCT project, as can virtually any assessment instrument or testing modality. What is crucial, though, is the need to integrate validation, reliability and efficacy testing procedures into all clinical pursuits and interventions, which is mandated by the CP and UCT project. The cornerstone of assessment validation and efficacy testing procedures is HRV ambulatory monitoring and the study of derived ANS measures in relation to objective, ecological, longitudinal outcome measures, regardless of the intervention that is being used. Intervention type will be classified and data obtained from a specific treatment will be archived in its own database for comparative, analytic and efficacy testing purposes. Advances in HRV instrumentation and their user-friendly properties make it an ideal modality for obtaining information continually over the course of treatment, information that is lacking that may have important implications for better understanding the intervention process that extends well beyond clinical impressions or the anecdotal.

It should be noted that regardless of practitioners' credentials they must be trained in the CP to use it. The CP demands rigor and can only be applied in the context of strict procedural guidelines that stipulate who can do what. This is determined by a practitioner's level of education and training. The CP advances a multi-faceted delivery system in which levels of training and certification determines what procedures can be carried out by a practitioner.

## CONCLUSION

The Carlstedt Protocol is a validated, evidence-based approach to patient assessment and intervention. It is grounded in extensive field research that was carried out over the last ten years that continues to be replicated and extended. This line of inquiry has isolated key mind-body measures that have high predictive validity relative to patient's autonomic nervous system reactivity. The goal of the CP universal assessment and intervention project is to establish a worldwide network of practitioners that recognize the need to engage in standardized and validated methods of patient assessment, intervention, efficacy testing and databasing of mind-body responding. The model presented in this chapter is unprecedented in terms of its scope, methodological sophistication, procedures and the data that it has generated. It affords practitioners with an evidence-based template that form the basis of informed diagnostics, treatment and efficacy testing.

Practitioners in private practice or institutional settings who are interested in participating in the CP Universal Clinical Trials project are encouraged to contact the author of this chapter for more information (rcarlstedt@americanboardofsportpsychology.org).

## REFERENCES

Andeassi, J. L. (1995). *Psychophysiology: Human behavior and physiological responding.* Hillsdale, NJ: Lawrence Erlbaum Associates.

Borger, N., Van der Meere, J., Ronner, A., Alberts, E., Geuze, R. & Bogte, H. (1999).

Heart rate variability and sustained attention in ADHD children - attention deficit-hyperactivity disorder. *Journal of Abnormal Child Psychology.*

Biocom Technologies [Computer software] (2007). *Heart rate scanner and heart rate tracker.* Poulsbro, WA: Biocom Technologies.

Brain Net (2007). *Publications database and downloadable articles.* Sydney: Brain Research and Integrative Neuroscience Network.

Brain Resource Company (2007). *International brain database project.* Sydney: Brain Resource Company.

Carlstedt, R.A. (2001). *Line bisecting test reveals relative left brain hemispheric predominance in highly skilled athletes:Relationships among cerebral laterality, personality, and sport performance.* Doctoral dissertation, Saybrook Graduate School, San Francisco.

Carlstedt, R.A. (2004b). *Critical moments during competition: A mind-body model of sport performance when it counts the most.* NY: Psychology Press.

Carlstedt, R.A. (2007; in press). Integrative evidence-based tennis psychology: Perspectives, practices, and findings from a ten year validation investigation of the Carlstedt Protocol. *Proceedings of the International Tennis Federation 3rd Congress on Science and Technology.*

Carlstedt, R.A. (2008). *Evidence-based applied sport psychology: A manual for practitioners,researchers and students.* New York: Springer.

Cohen, J. (1994). The earth is round (p < .05). *American Psychologist, 49*, 997-1003.

Costa, P.T. & McRae, R.R. (1992). *Revised NEO personality inventory and NEO five-factor inventory: Professional manual.* Odessa, FL: Psychological Assessment Resources.

Couture, J. (2007). *Critical moment performance, Athlete's Profile assessment and pre and post heart rate variability-performance relationships in college baseball players: An investigation of theTheory of Critical Moments and Athlete's Profile Models.* Technical report. NY: American Board of Sport Psychology.

Crowne, D. P., & Marlowe, D. (1960). A new scale of social desirability independent of psychopathology. *Journal of Consulting Psychology, 24*, 349-354.

Desgranges, K., Desgranges, L. & Karsky, K. (1995). Attention deficit disorder: Problems with preconceived diagnosis. *Child and Adolescent Social Work Journal*, 12 (1), 3-17.

Dietrich, A. (2004). The transient hypofrontality hypothesis, In R.A. Carlstedt (Chair), *Integrative sport psychology.* Symposium conducted at the annual convention of the American Psychological Association, Honolulu, Hawaii.

Drake, R.E., Goldman, H.H., Leff, H.S., Lehman, A.F., Dixon, L., Mueser, K.T. & Torrey, W.C. (2001). Implementing evidence-based practices in routine mental health service settings. *Psychiatric Services*, 52(1), 45-50.

Dykman, R. A. & Ackerman, P. (1993). Behavioral subtypes of attention deficit disorder. *Exceptional Children*, 60 (2), 132-141.

Eysenck, H. J., & Eysenck, S. (1968). *Eysenck personality inventory: Manual.* San Diego: Educational and Industrial Testing Service.

Fahrenberg J. & Myrtek, M. (1996). *Ambulatory psychophysiology: computer assisted psychological and psychophysiological methods in monitoring and field studies.* Seattle, WA: Hogrefe & Huber.

Fortino, D. (2001). *Affect regulation, emotional intelligence and addiction: A five-factor personality model to predict treatment outcome, and efficacy in heroin abusers.* Doctoral dissertation. San Francisco: Saybrook Graduate School.

Hammond, D.C. (2005). Neurofeedback treatment of depression and anxiety. *Journal of Adult Development,* 12 (2-3), 131-137.

Hatfield, B. D., Landers, D.L., & Ray, W. J. (1984). Cognitive processes during self-paced motor performance: An electroencephalographic profile of skilled marksman. *Journal of Sport Psychology, 6*, 42-59.

Hilgard, J. R. (1968). Personality and hypnotizability: Inferences from case studies. In E. R. Hilgard (Author), *The experience of hypnosis.* (pp.269-300). New York: Harcourt, Brace, & Jovanovich.

Holtmann M & Stadler C. (2006). Electroencephalographic biofeedback for the treatment of attention-deficit hyperactivity disorder in childhood and adolescence.*Expert Review of Neurotherapeutics*, 6(4), 533-540. Jovanov E., Raskovic, D., Price, J., Chapman, J., Moore, A. & Krishnamurthy, A.(2001). *Patient monitoring using personal area networks of wireless intelligent sensors. Biomedical Science Instruments*, 37, 373-378.

Lehrer P.M., Vaschillo E., Vaschillo, B., Lu S.E., Eckberg, D.L., Edelberg, R., Shih, W.J., Lin, Y., Kuusela, T.A., Tahvanainen, K.U., Hamer, R.M. (2003). Heart rate variability biofeedback increases baroreflex gain and peak expiratory flow, *Psychosomatic Medicine*, 65(5):796-805.

Martin, A (2006). *Critical moment performance, Athlete's Profile assessment and pre and post heart rate variability-performance relationships in youth ice hockey players: An investigation of the Theory of Critical Moments and Athlete's Profile Models*. Technical report. NY: American Board of Sport Psychology.

Malik, M. & Camm, A.J. (1995). *Heart rate variability*. Armonk, NY: Futura Publishing.

Nolan, R.P., Kamath, M.V., Floras, J.S., Stanley, J., Pang, C., Picton, P. & Young, Q.R. (2005. Heart rate variability biofeedback as a behavioral neurocardiac intervention to enhance vagal heart rate contro. *American Heart Journal*, 149(6), 1137.

Rossiter, T. (2004). The effectiveness of neurofeedback and stimulant drugs in treating AD/HD: Part I. Review of methodological issues. *Applied Psychophysiology and Biofeedback*, 29(2), 95-112.

Tellegen, A., & Atkinson, G. (1974). Openness to absorbing and self-altering experiences ("absorption"), a trait related to hypnotic susceptibility. *Journal of Abnormal Psychology*, *83*, 268-277.

T.O.V.A. (2007). Test of variables of attention. (www.hometova.com).

Schiffer, F. (1997). Affect changes observed with right versus left lateral visual field stimulation in psychotherapy patients: Possible physiological, psychological and therapeutic implications. *Comprehensive Psychiatry, 38*, 289-295.

Schiffer, F. (1998). *Of two minds*. New York; The Free Press.

Slipp, S. (2000). Introduction to neuroscience and psychoanalysis. *Journal of American Academy of Psychoanalysis*, 28:191-201.

Verdoux, H. & Begaud, B. (2004). Pharmaco-epidemiology:what do (and don't) we know about utilization and impact of psychotropic medications in real-life conditions? *British Journal of Psychiatry*, 185-193.

Wickramaskera, I. E. (1988). *Clinical behavioral medicine.* New York: Plenum.

Wickramaskera, I. E. (1998). Secrets kept from the mind but not the body and behavior:The unsolved problems of identifying and treating somatization of trauma. *Advances in Mind-Body Medicine*, *14*, 1-18.

Wickramasekera, I.E. (2003). The high risk model of threat perception and the Trojan horse role induction: Somatization and psychophysiological disease. In D. Moss, A. McGrady, T.C. Davies, & I. Wickramasekera (Eds.), Handbook of mind-body medicine for primary care (pp. 19-42.). Thousands Oaks, CA: Sage Publications.

# SECTION IV. MISCELLANEOUS LABORATORY METHODS

In: Toward a Science of Clinical Psychology
Editor: Luciano L'Abate, pp. 263-281
ISBN: 978-1-60456-062-6


*Chapter XIV*

# Common and Unique Factors in Assessing African American Couples

*Anthony L. Chambers and Jay Lebow*

## Abstract

With the divorce rate hovering around 50% for first marriages, there is a great need for systemically trained, marital therapists. Although couples therapy is a part of the practice of most therapists (Orlinsky & Ronnestad, 2005) few clinical or counseling psychologists have actually received formal training in couples therapy (Fishel, 2000). Even fewer psychologists have received adequate training in conducting culturally sensitive therapy (Kaslow, Celano, & Dreelin, 1995). The task of conducting culturally sensitive couple therapy is extremely challenging with ethnic minorities because not only does the therapist have to change from an individual to an interactional paradigm, but the therapist has to incorporate the couple's cultural context into their assessment of the couple's functioning. To further complicate matters, therapists are faced with the challenge of figuring out what problems/difficulties are a function of normative processes that all couples have to negotiate versus what problems/difficulties are a function of sociocultural constraints that are unique to the couple's cultural background. Furthermore, research repeatedly finds that the heterogeneity that exists *within* ethnic minority populations is not only significant, but is equally important to the heterogeneity that exists *between* populations (Cauce, Coronado, & Watson, 1998). It is this proverbial dance between "sameness vs. uniqueness" that couple therapists are confronted with when working with ethnic minority couples.

This volume is structured around the notion of a science based in linking research conducted in laboratory settings and real world practice. In this chapter, we describe the complex issues that emerge within such a frame in assessing African American couples. How are couples best assessed and should the foci, techniques, and meaning of assessment vary with the culture of the clients in focus?

We begin with a general understanding of how African American and Caucasian couples are similar. A study conducted by Allen & Olson (2001) found five types of African-American marriages, which were very similar in number and characteristics to Caucasian marriages. However, the etiological and contextual influences and meaning of those various marital types may differ across contexts (Hardy & Laszloffy, 2002). Next, we describe the unique challenges that face African American couples by reviewing existing research. This summary will include an historical overview of African American marriages as well as discuss the current state of African American marriages. We then discuss the clinical manifestations and implications of these findings. The chapter concludes with a methodology we have developed for assessing all couples, with a special emphasis on delineating assessment issues germane to African American couples.

## Summary of Research on African American Couples

### Historical overview of African American marriages

In order to understand the current state of African American marriages, it is important to have a historical and developmental context (Hardy & Laszloffy, 2002). The academic zeitgeist up until the 1970's commonly assumed that slavery engendered unstable African American families (Frazier, 1939; Moynihan, 1965; & Taylor, 2000). However, in the 1970's, historians of African American family life documented African Americans were able to develop and maintain a meaningful family structure (Blassingame, 1972). In fact, through an examination of census data and marriage licenses, some historians believe that two-parent families were the dominant family structure among African American families in 1860 (Guttman, 1976). Moreover, during the period immediately following slavery it was found that matriarchal, single family households were just as common among African American families compared to Caucasian families (Gutman). This was further supported by research finding comparable prevalence rates of two parent homes between African American and Caucasian families, 75% and 73% respectively (Furstenbert, Hershbert, & Modell, 1975).

More recent historical research on African American families has documented more heterogeneity in terms of African American family structure during slavery than previously reported (Wilson, 2002). Although there were many two parent families during slavery, research has also found that many slaves did not have a nuclear family but rather relied on an extended family structure (Stevenson, 1995). In fact, the diversity and flexibility of African American family structure during slavery helped ensure the survival of African-Americans (Stevenson, 1995). This historical diversity of African American family structures, including intact nuclear and extended families, provides an important context for understanding contemporary family patterns.

## Current State of African American marriages

U.S. Census data (2000) and sociological research has consistently found that African Americans have the lowest rates of marriage and lower marital stability than all other ethnic groups. 41% of African American adults are married compared to 62% of whites and 60% of Hispanics. In fact, the marriage rate among African Americans has decreased by 20% over the past 50 years (Tucker & Mitchell-Kernan, 1995). This pattern is even more pronounced among sub-groups. In 1940, almost 40% of African American men between that ages of 20-24 had been married; this decreased to 11.6% in 1990 (James, 1998). There have been a number of explanations offered for the disproportionately low marriage rate among African Americans including one emphasizing the higher rates of unemployment and bleak economic prospects for African American men resulting in a decreased interest in marriage due to their inability to fulfill the provider role and makes them less attractive husbands to women (Tucker & Mitchell-Kernan, 1995). Consistent with this viewpoint, research has noted that it is not possible for every African American college graduate to find a mate with similar education, which has been found to explain the disproportionately low marriage rate (Lichter, Anderson, & Hayward, 1995).

An unbalanced sex ratio in the number of available men and women has been identified as another important possible explanation (Guttentag & Secord, 1983). There is a dearth of marriageable African American men due to their disproportionately high mortality, substance abuse, and incarceration rates (Darity & Myers, 1995; Pinderhughes, 2002; Kiecolt & Fossett, 1995; Wilson & Neckerman, 1986). Wilson & Nickerman (1986) found that there were 73 males to 100 females in the general population of African Americans compared to 93 males to 100 females in the general population of Caucasians. However, using employment status as a proxy for men being marriageable, Darity & Myers (1995) found there were only 43 males to 100 females among African Americans compared to 63 males to 100 females among Caucasians. The implications of this disproportionately unbalanced sex ratio among African Americans include, but not limited to, higher rates of divorce and infidelity, and less commitment among men in relationships (Guttentag & Secord, 1983).

The African American middle class family has received increased attention in recent years (Pattillo, 2005). A major finding from this literature is that African American's position in the middle class is significantly more tenuous than it is for Caucasian's in the middle class (Pattillo, 2005). For instance, the average middle class African American person resides in a neighborhood where the median household income is $35,306 compared to $51,459 for Caucasians (Pattillo, 2005). Of particular importance is a recent finding from a study that found middle class African Americans have 2.6 higher odds of having a poor sibling than middle class Caucasians, which results in an increased likelihood of middle class African American families sharing their financial resources (Heflin & Pattillo, 2006). This finding is consistent with research documenting the prevalence of three generation households among some African Americans due to socioeconomic strains (Wilson, 1989).

Another interesting finding is that African American women are slower than Caucasians to legally divorce their spouse following separation (Cherlin, 1996). For instance, only 55% of African American women legally divorced their spouse within three years of separation compared to 91% of Caucasian women (Sweet & Bumpass, 1987). Moreover, African Americans are significantly less likely to get remarried following a divorce compared to Caucasians (Glick, 1997; Staples & Johnson, 1993).

Cohabitation has been another well-studied factor among sociologists. Studies have generally found that the number of cohabitating couples has significantly increased (e.g., Jayakody & Cabrera, 2002; Skinner, Bahr, Crane, & Call; 2002; U.S. Census Bureau, 1999) and the number of first unions ending in divorce has significantly increased (Bumpass & Lu, 2000; Casper & Cohen, 2000). With the increase in cohabitating unions and in divorce, especially among minority couples, research has attempted to understand the etiology behind these observations (e.g., Stanley, Rhoades, & Markman, 2006).

Other researchers have investigated the role of values and attitudes among African-Americans regarding cohabitation, marriage, and family roles in order to understand the trends in family formation (Hatchett, 1991). Using data from the National Survey of Black Americans, Hatchett found that in terms of the value of conjugal living, men felt that conjugal living was important for socioemotional reasons (raising children, a good love life, and companionship) whereas women felt that conjugal living was important for instrumental reasons (financial security). In terms of the value of marriage, married and never married men and women valued marriage despite the high divorce rate, whereas previously married men and women believed marriage was not as important (Hatchett, 1991).

Recently, Manning (1993) conducted a study to examine the transition to marriage and cohabitation between African-Americans and Caucasians. She found that cohabitation appears to be a precursor to marriage for Caucasian women, whereas cohabitation appears to be an alternative to singlehood for African-American women in that pregnant cohabiting African American women were no more likely to marry before their child was born than were single women.

Research has found that there are significant racial differences between births among women living in cohabitation unions. For instance, approximately 40% of Hispanics and 70% of African-Americans have births that occur outside of marriage (McLanahan, Garfinkel, Reichman, Teitler, 2001). Moreover, 40% among Mexican Americans, 29% among non-Hispanic Whites, and 18% among African-Americans (Bumpass & Sweet, 1989) had non-marital births within cohabitating unions, and these rates appear to be rising (National Center for Health Statistics, 1990, 1993). Given these observed racial differences, Manning & Landale (1996) used that National Survey of Families and Households survey to examine the extent to which cohabitation influences the likelihood to enter into premarital motherhood has a function of race and ethnicity. They found that among the different racial and ethnic groups, African American women had the highest rate of premarital childbearing, with the majority of premarital first births occurring outside of cohabitating unions. Caucasian women were the least likely to conceive their first child before marriage as opposed to African-Americans. Furthermore, Caucasian women who become pregnant, while either single or cohabitating, were more likely to marry before the birth of their first child.

Although sociological, economic, and structural constraints have undoubtedly contributed to the difficulties facing African American marriages, there is virtually no understanding of how these constraints manifest themselves into interpersonal problems between men and women. Hence, it is important that clinicians understand these data in order to provide a context and to generate possible hypotheses about the nature of the shared and unique difficulties facing African American couples. Moreover, it is equally important to assess the couple's and each individual's level of resiliency (Littlejohn-Blake & Darling, 1993). It is easy for the therapist to focus on the couple's problems and forget to assess the couple's strength. In the late 80's and early 90's, family scholars began challenging the notion that African American families are pathological and began delineating the strengths and resiliency inherent within African American families (Wilson, Chambers, & Woods, 2005). Hence, it is incumbent of the therapist to be the holder of hope and the conveyer of strength when the couple is overwhelmed by their problems. Overall, this is a multidimensional problem that requires a multidimensional assessment.

## Common Factors

The starting point for understanding any ethnic minority couple is to first understand the similarities that cut across race and ethnicity. It is our contention that there are more common factors in terms of what constitutes successful relationships across diverse populations than there are differences in the core aspects of relating across groups; however, it is the differences that most need to be understood.

The need for affiliation, love, and attachment are fundamental human needs (Bowlby, 1983). It is these basic needs that marital therapists can use as a starting point for understanding and empathizing with the psychological and emotional pain that occurs when a couple is experiencing relationship difficulties. Communication difficulties are among the most commonly cited problems among married couples in distress (Stanley, Markman, & Whitton, 2002). One of the most researched forms of couple's therapy is Behavior Marital Therapy (Christensen, Doss, & Atkins, 2005; Holtzworth-Munroe & Jacobson, 1991), whose primary purpose is to interrupt maladaptive communication patterns. Similarly, dynamics of power within a couple's relationship is a central theme that cuts across race, ethnicity, and SES (Hardy & Laszoffy, 2002; Rampage, 1994). In fact, power struggles often become a focus of the couple's therapy (Rampage, 1994). Then there are other special problems that any couple regardless of race, ethnicity or SES may face including domestic violence (Chambers & Wilson, 2007; Holtzworth-Munroe & Stuart, 1994), sexual dysfunction (Laumann, Gagnon, Michael, & Michaels, 1994), affairs (Whisman, Dixon, & Johnson, 1997) substance abuse (O'Farraell & Birchler, 1987), and depression (Beach, Smith, & Finchmam, 1994).

Given the prevalence and interrelatedness of these factors, Karney & Bradbury (1995) have proposed an empirically and theoretically driven model for understanding marital development, which can provide a conceptual framework for understanding marital functioning. They describe three central domains that impact marital quality and stability: Enduring Vulnerability, described as the stable demographic, historical, personality, and experiential factors that individuals bring to the relationship; Stressful Events, described as external circumstances that affect a relationship such as the effects of stress and economic variables; and Adaptive Processes, described as the ways individuals and couples contend with differences of opinion and individual or relationship difficulties and transitions. Each component in the model is conceptualized as comprising of multiple variables. The strength of the model is that it acknowledges variations among individuals and couples in terms of how they handle stressful events, individual differences, and the life experiences they bring to the relationship (Bradbury, Cohan, & Karney, 1998). Hence, this model offers what can serve as a culturally sensitive framework for explaining the impact enduring vulnerabilities and stressful events have on relationship functioning, quality and stability.

It is essential for couple therapists to realize that there are both factors common to all couples and factors that are special or have special meaning within diverse populations. That is, consistent with a multicultural perspective, it is important that therapists incorporate a *both/and* rather than an *either/or* perspective when attempting to understand the unique experiences that face African Americans (Hardy & Laszloffy, 2002). Moreover, it is important to keep in mind that heterogeneity exists within any population (Wilson, Chambers, & Woods, 2005), and therefore it is important for the therapist to grasp the idiosyncratic manifestations of relationship problems that couples face.

## Psychological and Interpersonal Considerations

Although disturbing findings such as the declining marriage rate among African Americans can be partially explained by structural constraints such as decreased employment opportunities for African American males, it only accounts for a relatively small portion of the explained variance (Mare & Winship, 1991). Hence, it is important to consider the psychological and interpersonal manifestations of the above sociological findings. This is especially important because social policy cannot change what happens between couples behind closed-doors and can only have effects over the long run. Moreover, because, African Americans are more likely to experience stressful events (Karney & Bradbury 1995), it is important to understand potential adaptive processes as that is the area where clinicians can intervene.

There are several interpersonal manifestations unique to African American couples that affect their adaptive processes. One of the most important constraints confronting the young subgroup of African American couples is that many do not have a healthy model for how to have a healthy relationship as evidenced by the fact that 46% of African American families are headed by females (Darity & Myers, 1995; Tucker & Mitchell-Kernan, 1995). The central task of marriage is the management of differences. Managing differences requires couples to be flexible and to accept influence from the other, which is easier when couples have clearly identified gender roles. However, given the disproportionately high divorce rate and high rate of out of wedlock births (Tucker & Mitchell-Kernan, 1995) among African Americans, one or both members of the couple may have been reared by single parent and therefore lack a model for how to manage differences in a marital context.

Given the gender disparities and unbalanced sex ratio among African Americans, clearly delineating gender roles is particularly challenging. It has been well documented that the challenges often manifest themselves in terms of power struggles and conflict over leadership (i.e., Black, 1999; Boyd-Franklin, 2003; Boyd-Franklin & Franklin, 1998; Hatchett, Veroff, & Douvan, 1995; Pinderhughes, 1998; 2002 ). There are at least a couple of layers to this issue. First, the traditional male role as the provider becomes not only compromised but challenged or surpassed by the woman. Second, the woman often maintains the role as the primary caregiver of their children (Pinderhughes, 2002; Tucker & Mitchell-Kernan, 1995). Given her unique role of being the mother, she may also assume the role as "house manager". Researchers have documented that the gender role confusion can place a significant stress on the dyadic subsystem as the woman may understandably feel overwhelmed, and the man may understandably feel emasculated and feel as though he has little to no influence in decision making (Hatchett et al., 1995; McLloyd, Cauce, Tacheuchi, & Wilson, 2000). Moreover, the gender role confusion among African American couples can lead to leadership difficulties that marital therapists have documented as essential for healthy marriages (Breunlin, Schwartz, & Mac Kune-Karrer, 1997; Pinsof, 1995).

Another significant issue disproportionately affecting African American couples is that of boundaries and privacy. Specifically, this issue manifests itself as many African Americans try to balance obligations to their spouse and to biological family members. Research suggests that multiple allegiances often take the form of either giving financial assistance to or needing to receive financial assistance from family members (Heflin & Pattillo, 2006; Wilson, 1989). Either way, the co-financial dependence has the potential to result in marital conflict in terms of the appropriate amount of financial assistance to either give or receive. Moreover, there can be marital conflict around the appropriate amount of information to share with family members. Conflict around sharing information can be a significant barrier to the formation of an "us", which is a critical task during the transition to marriage, and if never met, can result in a chronic level of marital dissatisfaction. To be clear, we are not suggesting that couples not help out their families. In fact, we espouse a both/and versus an either/or paradigm when working with African American clients (Hardy & Laszloffy, 2002). That is, we try to help couples find a way to protect their marital subsystem while maintaining a mutually agreed upon relationship with their respective families of origin. However, it is important that the clinician understand the context under which privacy issues can occur.

Finally, it is important to understand the interpersonal context of cohabitation among African Americans. An interesting study by Manning & Landale (1996) highlighted a challenge when working with cohabitating African Americans, which, unlike Caucasians, is that cohabitation is often a substitute for marriage, which can create challenges for understanding commitment among these couples. Commitment is critical for relationships to thrive (e.g., Stanley & Markman, 1992), and when one or both members of the couple do not feel that level of commitment, it can jeopardize the relationship. Research has shown that premarital cohabitation is linked to less dedication among men (Brown, 2004). In addition, cohabitation without plans to marry is linked to lower levels of relationship satisfaction (Stanley, Whitton, & Markman, 2004). Hence, clinicians need to understand the decision making process around the decision to cohabitate as well as understand the constraints preventing couples from either terminating the relationship or progressing the relationship to marriage (Stanley, Rhoades, & Markman, 2006).

The unique and common external stressors facing African American couples begins to illuminate the important adaptive processes that clinicians need to be cognizant of in order to appropriately assess the constraints preventing a satisfying relationship.

## Methodology for Assessing African American and Caucasian Couples

In keeping with the scientist-practitioner model, we believe that it is important that clinicians utilize a systematic and systemic method when assessing couples. Systematic, however, does not mean rigid. Any clinician that has done couples or family therapy knows that the complexity significantly increases with the addition of each family member in the direct system. That complexity becomes even more salient when the clinician attempts to understand and tease apart what aspect of the couple's problems is generalizable to all couples and what problems are unique to the African American culture. Hence, we believe it is important and possible to have a culturally sensitive framework that can organize the clinician's thinking about a particular couple's problems while maintaining the integrity and richness of each couple's story.

The framework we espouse is a four session evaluation that includes an initial conjoint session where both members of the couple are present in order to understand the couple's relationship problems followed by separate sessions in order to understand each person's individual histories and potential enduring vulnerabilities. The evaluation concludes with the therapist providing feedback to the couple that is used to establish a working alliance. Although the notion of routinely meeting with each member of the couple separately as part of an evaluation is not new (e.g., Emery, 2002), it is rarely delineated in enough detail that the procedure could be replicated. However, there is a version of the model that has been delineated with sufficient detail (Fishel, 2000), that can be easily replicated and adapted to African American couples.

The goals for the first session with a couple are not too dissimilar from the goals of a first session with an individual. That is, the primary goal is to make the couple feel comfortable and heard in order to increase the probability of coming back for a second session (it should be noted that in our experience, explaining in the initial phone call that a four session evaluation will be conducted decreases the probability of the couple dropping out after the first session). The therapist also aims to understand and expand each couple member's definition of the problem. Prototypic areas to assess in this session include their relationship history, the development of their current problem, sexual functioning, general level of compatibility, if they have kids, to assess their functioning, and finally to obtain a clear statement about how they would know if couples therapy was a success.

We also have them complete the Systemic Therapy Inventory of Change at the time of the first session. This is a repeated measure used throughout therapy that assesses not only couple functioning, but also individual functioning, family functioning, child functioning in the family (if relevant), and experience in family of origin. The measures assesses demographic variables as well as expectations for treatment; that utilized after the first session also assesses the psychotherpauetic alliance utilizing the revised version of Pinsof's Therapeutic Alliance Scales (Pinsof, 1994) . The Systemic Inventory of Change is designed to assess change over the course of therapy in the individual, couple, family, and child domains as well as in the alliance.

Then, the therapist schedules two individual sessions in order to get to know each of them better. A delicate, yet important issue that therapists must be cognizant of when meeting with each member of the couple individually, is the issue of confidentiality. Individual sessions always carry the risk of disclosing "secret" information that their partner is not privy to. Therapists differ significantly in their comfort level of being the keeper of secrets while doing couples therapy, with some therapist understandably believing that the therapy can be enhanced when a skilled couples therapist knows all of the secret knowledge because it places him or her in a better position to be helpful (Emery, 2002). Although we recognize the benefits of such a position, it is our position that if the therapist is the keeper of secrets it can be particularly damaging to the alliance. Moreover, being the keeper of a secret potentially places the therapist in an ethically compromising position of attempting to be an equal advocate for both members of the couple while maintaining a secret. This is particularly problematic for African American couples, which we will discuss in further detail later. Hence, we explicitly tell the couple the parameters of confidentiality for the individual sessions.

During the individual sessions, the therapist aims to understand each person's level of commitment to their relationship, each person's psychiatric history including mood disorders, suicidality, anxiety, and other mental illness, each person's drug and alcohol usage (past and present), any health or medical problems, history of sexual abuse, and to evaluate any past and/or present domestic violence. In addition, we assess each person's family of origin history with an eye towards understanding how their parents' relationship may elucidate their current relationship problems. Given that one of the goals of couple's therapy is to promote flexibility, we have found that asking what values their parents instilled in them can be helpful for understanding potential constraints to their functioning as many individuals have strong allegiances to their parents' conception of "right and wrong", which are often at the root of power struggles.

Finally, there is the feedback session held with the couple. In the feedback session, the therapist should comment on the positive factors in their relationship, provide feedback about the level of severity of their problems, present their problems in a developmental context, offer a dyadic/systemic conceptualization of their relationship problems, and make recommendations for treatment.

Couples therapy is contraindicated when there is ongoing violence and the violent partner is unwilling or unable to negotiate a no-violence contract (Goldner, 1998), when only one member is committed to working on the relationship, when there have been repeated failed attempts at couples therapy, when there is a high degree of mistrust and a lack of any positive feelings towards their partner, when there is an ongoing affair that person is unwilling or conflicted about ending, and finally when one or both members of the couple have an individual disorder that requires specialized treatment such as bi-polar, posttraumatic stress disorder (PTSD) or severe drug/alcohol addiction.

## Case Illustration Using Systemic Therapy Inventory of Change (STIC) Data

The field of couple and family therapy lacks empirical understanding of how couples and families change in therapy and what kinds of therapist interventions are associated with these changes. If the field of couple and family therapy is ever to be based on a scientific foundation, an empirically grounded theory of how couples and families change must be developed that can guide and improve interventions. The Systemic Inventory of Change (STIC) was created to address this need. Participants in an outpatient psychotherapy clinic were invited to complete the STIC questionnaire. The STIC questionnaire assesses individual, relationship, and family functioning. Participants were invited to complete only the sections of the questionnaires that were relevant to them. Our research team is completing a paper that demonstrates the reliability and validity of the STIC as well as describes the scale construction (Pinsof et al., 2007). We have also normed the STIC with a non-therapy seeking, random sample of 2500 individuals representative of the U.S. population. These data are currently be analyzed for publication and will provide norms for each of the STIC scales for Caucasians, African Americans, and Latinos.

As we have noted throughout this chapter, there are many issues that couple therapists have to consider when assessing African American couples. One of the more salient issues germane to African American couples is related to gender disparity and the subsequent conflict around power struggles and leadership resulting in feelings of unfairness. Thus, we have chosen a case that uses preliminary STIC data to illustrate the salience of power and unfairness.

Jacob and Sarah is an African American couple in their early 40's. They both completed college and professional school at very prestigious universities in the Northeast and their household annual income was over $100,000. They have been married for 8 years and have two young children. Sarah's appearance was a bit disheveled and her face showed signs of visible stress. Jacob, on the other hand, looked like a "Pre-Madonna" as it was clear that looks are important to him. Their presenting problem was "communication problems". During the four session evaluation, Sarah disclosed that he resents Jacob for having a commission only job that is not sufficient for paying their bills and has resulted in "eating through her savings" to pay the bills. Her feelings of unfairness were palpable and enhanced when she reported disliking her job, but does not quit because it pays the bills. She also reports taking on a significant amount of the childcare. Jacob reports palpable feelings of not being appreciated. He was quick to report that he also does a fair share of the childcare and household chores and would do more but states that Sarah criticizes the way he completes childcare and household chores, which is why he has curtailed his involvement. He also is quick to report that he is working a lot of hours trying the best that he can to provide for his family, and he wished that she could see and appreciate his efforts. By the conclusion of the four session evaluation it was clear that there were mutual feelings of unfairness and that this couple had some prototypic gender difficulties around leadership, dependability, and fairness.

In order to get an assessment of how salient their issues of unfairness were relative to other couples, we examined Jacob's and Sarah's STIC scores on the Relationship With Partner (RWP) scale relative to the total sample of couples in our database. The total sample consisted of 298 heterosexual individuals in a committed relationship who were seeking therapy in an outpatient clinic and volunteered to complete the STIC instrument.

The RWP scale assesses domains relevant to couple functioning including Positivity, Trust, Commitment, Inequity, Anger, Sexual Satisfaction, and Violence. We conducted One-Sample T-tests to compare Jacob's and Sarah's scores to the total sample. The two scales that they both reported being more problematic relative to the total sample were the Inequity and Intimacy scales. The items that comprise the Inequity scale are "My partner often complains that I don't do my share of the work around the house." and "I am expected to do too much." The items that comprise the Intimacy scale are "Our relationship feels empty." and "We are each other's best friend." All items were scored so that a higher score is better (i.e., no problems). Sarah had statistically, significantly lower scores on the Inequity scale ($t=-24.97$, $p=.00$) and Intimacy scale ($t=-25.51$, $p=.00$). Jacob also had statistically, significantly lower scores on the Inequity scale ($t=-33.77$, $p=.00$) and Intimacy scale ($t=-25.51$, $p=.00$). That is, Jacob and Sarah reported more problems with inequity and intimacy compared to other individuals in therapy who are in committed relationships. These findings are consistent with the therapist's clinical judgment about Jacob's and Sarah's difficulties. The findings are also consistent with the literature documenting the disproportionate impact of gender role difficulties among African American couples, all of which suggest that this is an area for couple's therapist to pay particular attention to when assessing African American couples.

## Applicability of the four session evaluation strategy with African American couples & helpful tips for clinicians

We do believe that there many (if not more) common factors between couples of different races and ethnicities, particularly in the United States given that we all share a common American value system. However, it is our experience that couples therapists who do not recognize the critically important contextual and interpersonal nuisances that face African American couples, miss important constraints that impede treatment. Moreover, given the racial inequities in this country, it is also likely that some of the problems that face all couples, such as economic hardship, disproportionately affect historically disenfranchised populations such as African Americans. For instance, the research presented in the section above on Current state of African American marriages clearly indicates that African Americans experience a disproportionate number of external stressors.

Utilizing the four session model as we have described above has at least three advantages when working with African American couples. First, although not conclusive, research has generally found that African American clients terminate therapy significantly earlier than Caucasian clients, often times after the first session (e.g., Greenspan & Kulish, 1985; Sue, McKinney, & Allen, 1976; Sue, McKinney, Allen, & Hall, 1974). Explicating over the phone that you conduct a four session evaluation with every couple tends to increase the probability of the couple successfully entering treatment. Although we are sure there are couples who may dislike this approach, we have yet to find a couple complain about this format. Second, providing a four session evaluation communicates to the couple a sense of hope, caring, and understanding, which can potentially promote the trust necessary for developing a therapeutic alliance. The pervasive mistrust African Americans have toward the health care system, especially the mental health care system, is palpable (Parham, 1999). The origins for this mistrust are steeped in slavery and fostered with incidents like the Tuskegee Experiment (Freimuth et al, 2001). Moreover, as a result of frequently being marginalized in multiple facets of this society, African Americans are used to not being listened to. Hence, individual sessions with each member of the couple may be one of the few times they have felt listened to and felt that their complaints were taken seriously. Third, African Americans' sense of justice and fairness is also palpable (Freimuth et al, 2001). This structure promotes that sense and letting each member of the couple know that you will not be keeping secrets is not only reassuring but potentially therapeutic.

## Areas that Require Special Attention When Assessing African American Couples

### *Trust*

The importance of trust in a relationship is not breaking news. However, when it comes to the history of mistrust between African Americans and numerous facets of our society combined with normative challenges everyone faces when trust has been broken, it is no wonder that trust among African Americans is sometimes challenging to foster. In fact, research has cited that non-clinical paranoia is a cultural phenomenon stemming from a long history of racism and discrimination (Combs et al, 2006). Another recent study showed that African Americans score higher than Caucasians on subclinical measures of paranoia (Combs, Penn, & Fenigstein, 2002). The actual incident that creates the mistrust between African American couples usually does not differ from couples of any race or ethnicity (i.e., money, affairs, violence, etc...) (Allen & Olson, 2001), however, what is sometimes different is the process of forgiving. The process of forgiving and regaining trust is constrained by individual, familial, societal, and historical experiences of mistrust. That is, the unique history African Americans have with trust being broken provides an important context for understanding relationship difficulties germane to trust and forgiveness. In fact, research has found that African American women are less forgiving than Caucasian women when it comes to infidelity (Patterson, 1998). Hence, the therapist must assess and pay careful attention to each person's past experiences of forgiveness and each person's current level of resentment. The therapist would be advised to assess this mistrust from the vantage point of understanding the broader function of skepticism in order to enhance the therapeutic alliance.

### *Gender, leadership and power*

In light of the prevalent gender disparities among African Americans, ones that often run counter to those in the rest of American society, particularly with respects to education and income, it is important for the couple's therapist to understand each person's conceptualization of gender and to what extent does their relationship approximate their conceptualization. Similarly, African American couples where the woman is more educated and makes more money than the man often carry the added problem of unclear leadership, which research shows can lead to conflict (Hatchett et al., 1995; McLloyd et al., 2000). These couples often have difficulty making decisions and further confusion about their respective roles in the family. One of the more common manifestations of this difficulty is the man feeling he has no influence in the family because he is not fulfilling the role as the primary provider and at home he may feel that this spouse is overly critical of everything he does. Similarly, the woman may complain that he is participating enough around in the family and that she feels she has to do everything. This can result very tense power struggles because the man is feeling emasculated, the woman is feeling overstressed, and neither of them feel that the other is accepting influence from them. Hence, it is important that the therapist assess for this potential dynamic, realizing the larger contextual and systemic constraints facing African American women and men (see section above on current state of African American marriages).

### *Commitment*

The assessment of the couple's level of commitment is particularly salient for cohabitating African American couples in light of research showing that cohabitation is less likely to lead to marriage for African Americans than for any other racial or ethnic group (Manning & Landale, 1996). Paradoxically, we have found in our clinical experience that many cohabitating African American couples will state a relatively high level of commitment. Hence, it is important for the therapist to assess the couple's vision of a future, if any, as well as assess for constraints preventing them from deepening their relationship. Potential constraints include, but are not limited to financial strains, excessive conflict, high (possibly unrealistic) expectations about marriage and gender roles, and difficulty forming an "us" because they believe completing their individual goals and getting married are an either/or proposition instead of a both/and proposition.

### *Family of Origin/Extended Family*

A careful assessment of each person's family of origin is critical for understanding current relationship functioning in every family, but these factors are even more vital in African American families. First, given the disproportionately high divorce rate among African Americans (U.S. Census, 2000), many African Americans did not grow up with a healthy model of how a marriage should work (McLanahan, Garfinkel, Reichman, & Teitler, 1999). In these circumstances, it is important that the therapist get a sense of what type of marriage they envisioned, what is the etiology or source for that model, and how realistic is their model. Second, although the support and influence of the extended family among African Americans can be a source of strength (Wilson, 1989), it can also have a paradoxically constraining effect on the marriage as it can prevent the couple from forming an "us". The formation of an "us" is a critical task during the transition to marriage, which includes the ability to "separate" from their family of origin to form a new family. To be clear, we are not suggesting that the formation of an "us" and separating from family of origin is an either/or proposition but rather a both/and proposition. That is, the therapist is to assess whether or not the couple has created a set of guidelines around the type of information they will share with their families of origin and which they will keep private. The issue of privacy and the formation of an "us" can be particularly constrained if the household includes the couple's parents, siblings, and/or cousins are residing with the couple. In such circumstances, it is important for the therapist to assess the couple's decision making process around this issue to be sure that the decision was mutual. If the decision was mutual, then the assessment is around how the couple has established their own routine and managed the distribution of resources. However, if the decision was not mutual, then it is important for the therapist to assess the level of resentment as that can be a significant constraint to treatment unless it is addressed. Moreover, in light of research cited earlier on the spreading of financial resources among impoverished siblings (Heflin & Pattillo, 2006), the economic strain this potentially places on the middle class sibling who is in a relationship can present an allegiance struggle with feelings of being confused and torn between providing for his/her nuclear family and providing for his/her extended family. Again, this does not have to be an either/or decision, but it is something for the therapist to assess as a possible constraint for achieving relationship satisfaction. If this situation is present in the couple, then it is also important for the therapist to assess for mutual feelings of resentment, which can beget in these situations.

### *Uniqueness and Strength*

Although this chapter has presented general trends and issues facing African American couples, it is important that the therapist does not take this information and assume a "one size fits all" approach. For every African American couple you find facing this issue you will find at least one African American couple not facing that issue. Hence, the best way to be a culturally aware therapist is to employ the scientific method in the manner of the local clinical scientist as described by George Stricker (Stricker & Trierweiler, 1995), using this information to formulate hypotheses and then *test* the hypotheses to see if it is true rather than assume it is true! We believe this hypothesis testing approach fits nicely with the four session evaluation method we have described, which will allow you to be aware of the possible issues and constraints germane to a particular couple while allowing for the possibility of a couple not fitting a particular profile. That is the essence of a scientific approach.

Along those lines, research has begun to discover protective factors specific to African American marriages. For instance, Orbuch, Veroff, and Hunter (1998) found that in stable African American marriages, the wives more collaborative compared to Caucasian wives who were more compliant. This difference is reflective of African American men's and women's preference for an equal partner in decision making rather than a submissive partner given than their family survival is dependent on an active partnership and friendship (Carolan & Allen, 1999).

Despite all of the challenges African American individuals and families face, they have mostly preserved! That is, many African Americans have beat the odds and have gone on to obtain an education, a successful career, raise successful children, and maintain a sense of identity in the face of denigration. Hence, the therapist needs to explicitly look for the strengths and any obstacles they have overcome because it is that strength often goes unnoticed and ultimately a resource that goes untapped; yet it is precisely those strengths the therapist can use to galvanize the couple to reinvigorate the notion of hope and the ability to overcome their relationship struggles (Walsh, 2003).

## REFERENCES


Allen, W. D. & Olson, D. H. (2001). Five types of African-American marriages. *Journal of Marital and Family Therapy, 27(3),* 301-314.

Beach, S. R. H., Smith, D. A., & Finchmam, F. D. (1994). Marital interventions for depression: Empirical foundation and future prospects. *Applied and Preventative Psychology, 3*, 299-250.

Black, L. W. (1999). Therapy with African-Americans. In P. Papp (Ed.), *Couples on the fault line* (pp. 205 221). New York: Guilford Press.

Blassingame, J. (1972). *The slave community.* New York: Oxford University Press.

Bowlby, J. (1983). Attachment and loss: Retrospect and prospect. *Annual Progress in Child Psychiatry & Child Development*, 29-47.

Boyd-Franklin, N. (2003). *Black families in therapy: Understanding the African American experience (2nd ed.)*. New York, NY: Guilford Press.

Boyd-Franklin, N., & Franklin, A. J. (1998). African American couples in therapy. In M. McGoldrick (Ed.), *Re-visioning family therapy: Race, culture, and gender in clinical practice* (pp. 268-281). New York, NY: Guilford Press.

Bradbury, T.N., Cohan, C.L., & Karney, B.R. (1998). Optimizing longitudinal research for understanding and preventing marital dysfunction. In T.N. Bradbury (Ed.), *The developmental course of marital dysfunction* (pp. 279-311). New York: Cambridge University Press.

Breunlin, D. C., Schwartz, R. C., & Mac Kune-Karrer, B. (1997). *Metaframeworks: Transcending the models of family therapy.* San Francisco, CA, US: Jossey-Bass.

Brown, S. L. (2004). Moving from cohabitation to marriage: A comparison of relationship quality. *Social Science Research, 33(1),* 1-20.

Bumpass, L.L., & Lu, H. H. (2000). Trends in cohabitation and implications for children's family contexts in the United States. *Population Studies, 54,* 29-41.

Bumpass, L., & Sweet, J. (1989). National estimates of cohabitation. *Demography, 26,* 615-630.

Carolan, M., & Allen, K. (1999). Commitments and constraints to intimacy for African-American couples at midlife. *Journal of Family Issues, 20(1),* 5-24.

Casper, L. M., & Cohen, P. (2000). How does POSSLQ measure up? *Social Problems, 47,* 112-133.

Cauce, A.M, Coronado, N., & Watson, J. (1998). Conceptual and methdological issues in conducting culturally competent research. In M. Hernandez & R. Isaacs (Ed.), *Promoting Cultural Competence in Children's Mental Health Services.* N.J: Brookes.

Chambers, A. L., & Wilson, M. N. (2007). Assessing a Typology of Male Batterers with the Personality Assessment Inventory. *Journal of Personality Assessment 88(1),* 58-66.

Cheriln, A. (1996). *Public and private families.* New York: McGraw-Hill.

Christensen, A., Doss, B. D., & Atkins, D. C. (2005). A Science of Couple Therapy: For what Should We Seek Empirical Support?. In W. M. Pinsof, and J. Lebow (Eds.) *Family Psychology: The Art of the Science.* Oxford/New York: Oxford University Press.

Combs, D. R., Penn, D. L., & Fenigstein, A. (2002). Ethnic differences in subclinical paranoia: An Expansion of norms of the Paranoia Scale. *Cultural Diversity & Ethnic Minority Psychology, 8(3),* 248-256.

Combs, D. R., Penn, D. L., Cassisi, J., Michael, C., Wood, T., Wanner, J., Adams, S. (2006). Perceived racism as a predictor of paranoia among African Americans. *Journal of Black Psychology, 32(1),* 87-104.

Darity, W. A., Jr., & Myers, S. L., Jr. (1995). Family structure and the marginalization of Black men: Policy implications. In M. B. Tucker & C. Mitchell-Kernan (Eds.), *The decline in marriage among African Americans* (pp. 263-308). New York: Russell sage Foundation.

Emery, R. E., & Sbarra, D. (2002). Addressing separation and divorce during and after couple therapy. In A. S. Gurman and N. S. Jacobson (Eds.), *Clinical handbook of couple therapy, 3rd Ed.* (pp569-593). New York: The Guilford Press.

Fishel, A. (2000). "Couples therapy" In Psychiatry: Update and board preparation, ed. by Theodore A. Stern and John B. Herman, New York: McGraw Hill.

Frazier, F. E. (1939). *The Negro family in the United States.* Chicago, IL: University of Chicago Press.

Freimuth, V., S., Quinn, S. C., Thomas, S. B., Cole, G., Zook, E., & Duncan, T. (2001). African American's views on research and the Tuskegee syphilis study. *Social Science & Medicine, 52(5),* 797-808.

Furstenberg, F., Hershberg, T., & Modell, J. (1975). The origins of the female-headed black familiy: The impact of the urban experience. *Journal of Interdisciplinary History, 6,* 211-233.

Glick, P. (1997). Demographic pictures of African American families. In H. McAdoo (Ed.), *Black families* (3rd ed., pp. 118-138). Thousand Oaks, CA: Sage.

Greenspan, M., & Kulish, N. M. (1985). Factors in premature termination in long term therapy. *Psychotherapy, 22,* 75-82.

Goldner, V. (1998). The treatment of violence and victimization in intimate relationships. *Family Process, 37,* 263-286.

Guttentag, M. & Secord, P. F. (1983). *Too many women: The sex ratio question.* Beverly Hills: Sage Publications.

Guttman, H. (1976). *The black family in slavery and freedom, 1750-1925.* New York: Pantheon.

Hardy, K. V., Laszloffy, T. A. (2002). Couple therapy using a multicultural perspective. In A. S. Gurman and N. S. Jacobson (Eds.), *Clinical handbook of couple therapy, 3rd Ed.* (pp569-593). New York: The Guilford Press.

Hatchett, S. J. (1991). Women and men. In J. S. Jackson (Ed.), *Life In Black America* (pp. 84-104). Newbury Park, CA: Sage Publications.

Hatchett, S., Veroff, J., & Douvan, E. (1995). Marital stability and marriage among black and white couples in early marriage. In M. B. Tucker & C. Mitchell-Kernan (Eds.), *The decline in marriage among African Americans* (pp. 177-211). New York: Russell sage Foundation.

Heflin, C. M., & Pattillo, M. (2006). Poverty in the family: Race, siblings and socioeconomic heterogeneity. *Social Science Research, 35*, 804-822.

Holtzworth-Munroe, A., & Jacobson, N. S. (1991). Behavioral marital therapy. In A. S. Gurman & D. P. Kniskern (Eds.), *Handbook of family therapy, Vol 2* (pp. 96-133). Philadelphia, PA: Brunner/Mazel, Inc.

Holtzworth-Munroe, A. & Stuart, G. L. (1994). Typologies of male batterers: Three subtypes and the differences among them. *Psychological Bulletin, 116*, 476-497.

James, A. D. (1998). What's love got to do with it?: Economic viability and the likelihood of marriage among African American men. *Journal of Comparative Family Studies, 29(2),* 1-13.

Karney, B.R., & Bradbury, T.N. (1995). The longitudinal course of marriage and marital instability: A review of theory, method, and research. *Psychological Bulletin, 118*, 3-34.

Kaslow, N. J., Celano, M., & Dreelin, E. D. (1995). A cultural perspective on family theory and therapy. *Psychiatric Clinics of North America, 18*(3), 621-633.

Kiecolt, K., & Fossett, M. (1995). Mate availability and marriage among African Americans: Aggregate and individual-level analysis. In M. B. Tucker & C. Mitchell-Kernan (Eds.), *The decline in marriage among African Americans* (pp. 121-135). New York: Russell sage Foundation.

Laumann, E. O., Gagnon, J. H., Micheal, R. T., & Michaels, S. (1994). *The social organization of sexuality: Sexual practices in the United States.* Chicago: University of Chicago Press.

Lichter, D. T., Anderson, R. N., & Hayward, M. D. (1995). Marriage markets and marital choice. *Journal of Family Issues, 16(4),* 412-431.

Littlejohn-Blake, S. M., & Darling, C. A. (1993). Understanding the strengths of African American families. *Journal of Black Studies, 23(4),* 460-471.

Manning, W. M. (1993). Marriage and cohabitation following premarital conception. *Journal of Marriage and the Family, 55* (4), 839-850.

Manning, W. D., & Landale, N. S. (1996). Racial and ethnic differences in the role of ohabitation in premarital childbearing. *Journal of Marriage and the Family, 58* (1), 63-77.

Mare, R., & Winship, C. (1991). Socioeconomic change and the decline of marriage for blacks and whites. In C. Jencks & P. E. Peterson (Eds.), *The urban underclass* (pp. 175-204). Washington, DC: Brookings Institute.

McLanahan, S., Garfinkel, I., Reichman, N., & Teitler, J. (1999). Unwed parents or fragile families? Implications for welfare and child support policy. Working Paper #00-04. Princeton, NJ: Bendheim-Thoman Center for Research on Child Well-being, Princeton University.

McLloyd, V., Cauce, A., Tacheuchi, D., & Wilson,m L. (2000). Marital processes and parental socialization in families of color: A decade review of research. *Journal of Marriage and the Family, 62*, 1-27

Moynihan, D. P. (1965). *The Negro family: The case for national action.* Washington, D.C.: U.S. Government Printing Office.

National Center for Health Statistics. (1990). *Vital statistics of the United States, 1988.* Washington, DC: U.S. Government Printing Office.

National Center for Health Statistics. (1993). Advance report of final natality statistics ,
1990. *Monthly Vital Statistics Report, 41.* Washington DC: U.S. Government Printing Office.

O'Farrell, T. J., & Birchler, G. R. (1987). Marital relationships of alcoholic, conflicted, and nonconflicted couples. *Journal of Marital and Family Therapy, 13*, 259-274.

Orbuch, T. L., Veroff, J., & Hunter, A. (1999). Black couples, white couples: The early years of marriage. In E. M. Hetherington (Ed.), *Coping with divorce, single parenting, and remarriage: A risk and resiliency perspective* (23-43). *Ma*hwah NJ: Lawrence Erlbaum Associates.

Orlinsky, D. E., & Ronnestad, M. H. (2005). *How psychotherapists develop: A study of therapeutic work and professional growth.* Washington, DC: American Psychological Association.

Parham, T. A. (1999). Invisibility syndrome in African descent people: Understanding cultural manifestations of the struggle for self-affirmation. Counseling Psychologist, 27(6), 794-801

Patterson, O. (1998). Rituals of blood: Consequences of slavery in two American centuries. New York: Basic Books.

Pattillo, M. (2005). Black middle-class neighborhoods. Annual Review of Sociology 31,305-

329.

Pinderhughes, E. B. (1988). Treatment with middle class black families: A systemic perspective. In J. Coner-Edwards & J. Spurlock (Eds.). Black families in crisis (pp. 215-236). New York: Brunner-Mazel.

Pinderhughes, E. B. (2002). African American marriage in the 20th century. Family Process 41, 269-282. Pinsof, W. M. (1995). Integrative problem-centered therapy: A synthesis of family, individual, and biological therapies. New York, NY, US: Basic Books.

Pinsof, W. M. (1994a). An integrative systems perspective on the therapeutic alliance: Theoretical, clinical, and research implications. In A. O. Horvath & L. S. Greenberg (Eds.), The working alliance: Theory, research, and practice Wiley series on personality processes (pp. 173-195). Oxford, England: John Wiley & Sons.

Pinsof, W. M. (1994b). An integrative systems perspective on the therapeutic alliance: Theoretical, clinical, and research implications. In The working alliance: Theory, research, and practice (pp. 173-195). Oxford, England: John Wiley & Sons.

Pinsof, W. M., Lebow, J., Zinbarg, R., Knobloch-Fedders, L. M., Chambers, A. L., & Karam, E. (2007).

Reliability and validity data of the Systemic Therapy Inventory of Change. Manuscript in preparation.

Rampage, C. (1994). Power, gender, and marital intimacy. *Journal of Family Therapy, 16(1)*, 125-137.

Skinner, K. B., Bahr, S. J., Crane, D. R., & Call, V. R. A. (2002). Cohabitation, marriage, and remarriage. Journal of Family Issues, 23 (1), 74-90.

Stanley, S. M., & Markman, H. J. (1992). Assessing commitment in personal relationships. Journal of Marriage and Family, 54, 595-608.

Stanley, S. M., Markman, H. J., & Whitton, S. W. (2002). Communication, conflict and commitment: Insights on the foundations of relationship success from a national survey. Family Process, 41(4), 659-675.

Stanley, S. M., Rhoades, G. K., & Markman, H. J. (2006). Sliding versus deciding: Inertia and the premarital cohabitation effect. Family Relations, 55, 499-509.

Stanley, S. M., Whitton, S. W., Markman, H. J. (2004). Maybe I do: Interpersonal commitment levels and premarital or non-marital cohabitation. Journal of Family Issues, 25, 496-519.

Staples, R., & Johnson, L. B. (1993). Black families at the crossroads. San Francisco: Jossey-Bass.

Stevenson, B. (1995). Black family structure in colonial and antebellum Virginia: Amending the revisionist perspective. In M. B. Tucker & C. Mitchell-Kernan (Eds.), The decline in marriage among African Americans (pp. 27-56). New York: Russell Sage Foundation.

Stricker, G., & Trierweiler, S. J. (1995). The local clinical scientist: A bridge between science and practice. American Psychologist, 50(12), 995-1002.

Sue, S., McKinney, H. L., & Allen, D. B. (1976). Predictors of the duration of therapy for clients in the community mental health system. Community Mental Health Journal, 12, 365-375.

Sue, S., McKinney, H. L., Allen, D. B., & Hall, J. (1974). Delivery of community mental health services to black and white clients. Journal of Consulting and Clinical Psychology,

42, 794-801.

Sweet, J., & Bumpass, L. (1987). American families and households. New York: Russell Sage Foundation.

Taylor, R. L. (2000). Diversity within African American families. In D. H. Demo, K. R.Allen, and M. A. Fine,(Eds). (2000). Handbook of family diversity. (pp. 232-251). Oxford University Press: New York, NY.

Tucker, M. B., & Mitchell-Kernan, C. (1995). Trends in African American familyformation: A theoretical and statistical overview. In M. B. Tucker & C. Mitchell-Kernan (Eds.), The decline in marriage among African Americans (pp. 3-26). New York: Russell sage Foundation.

U.S. Census Bureau. (1999). *Statistical abstract of the United States: 1999* (119th ed.).Washington, DC: Bernan.

Walsh, F. (2003). Family resilience: Strengths forced through adversity. [References]. In F. Walsh (Ed.), *Normal family processes: Growing diversity and complexity (3rd ed )* (pp. 399-423). New York, NY: Guilford Press.

Whisman, M. A., Dixon, A. E., & Johnson, B. (1997). Therapists' perspectives of couple problems and treatment issues in couple therapy. *Journal of Family Psychology, 11,* 361-366.

Wilson, J. Q. (2002). *The marriage problem.* New York: HarperCollins Publishers.

Wilson, M. N. (1989). Child development in the context of the Black extended family. *American Psychologist, 44(2)*, 380-385

Wilson, M. N., Chambers, A. L., & Woods, L. (2005). Fathers in Minorities Families: The Importance of Social and Cultural Context. In W. M. Pinsof, and J. Lebow (Eds.) *Family Psychology: The Art of the Science.* Oxford/New York: Oxford University Press.

Wilson, W. J., & Neckerman, K. (1986). Poverty and family structure: The widening gapbetween evidence and public policy issues. In S. Danziger & D. Weinberg (Eds.), *Fighting poverty: What works and what doesn't* (pp. 232-259). Cambridge, MA: Harvard University Press.

In: Toward a Science of Clinical Psychology
Editor: Luciano L'Abate, pp. 283-305

ISBN: 978-1-60456-062-6


*Chapter XV*

# An Evidence-Based Approach to Psychiatric Rehabilitation

***Patrick W. Corrigan[1], Abigail K. Wassel and Jennifer D. Rafacz***

Many people with serious mental illnesses such as schizophrenia, bipolar disorder, major depression, and anxiety are unable to achieve the kinds of life goals befitting adults in our culture; they fail to obtain a meaningful career, pleasant home, intimate relationship, and good health. Disabilities derive from psychiatric disorders and lead to failure to achieve these goals. Psychiatric rehabilitation is meant to help people overcome their disabilities so they can accomplish personal ambitions. Over the past 20 years, service providers, consumers of care, and researchers have sought evidence-base practices (EBPs) that have been found effective for remediating disabilities. This chapter summarizes six of these EBPs and ends with consideration of future directions in evidence-based practices of psychiatric rehabilitation. We first describe fundamental constructs of rehabilitation and criteria for evidence before segueing into this information.

## Overview of Psychiatric Rehabilitation

Psychiatric rehabilitation is in its renaissance (Corrigan, Mueser et al., 2007). It is marked by an affirmative approach to the human condition, that change is possible and all goals within reach. This evolution is the product not only of clinical and services researchers, but of the consumers who receive these interventions. People with disabilities have come to understand what they want out of life and what role rehabilitation should play in accomplishing these goals. In the process, several key constructs have emerged that set the benchmarks for successful rehabilitation. Prominent among these is recovery from mental illness.

[1] Professor of Psychology, Illinois Institute of Technology, 3424 S State Street, Chicago, IL 60616 voice 312 567-6751, fax 312 567-6753, Corrigan@iit.edu

## Recovery from Mental Illness

Clinical psychologists and other professionals were not so long ago taught that the course of serious mental illnesses such as schizophrenia is poor and unremitting (Kraepelin, 1923), degrading into an inevitable dementia and massive loss of functions. This perspective robbed people with psychiatric disabilities of any ambitions about attaining life goals or hope that living will have meaning. Recovery as a construct and a goal has emerged to replace the poor prognosis of previous views. Nor is recovery just a pipe dream, it is a reality (Calabrese & Corrigan, 2005; Harding et al., 1988; Harrison et al., 2001). Long term follow-up research on schizophrenia, for example, supports a recovery rule of thirds. About one third of research participants seemed to have moved beyond the mental health system entirely and was pursuing life in what might be construed as "normal": competitive jobs, independent housing, and long term relationships. About one third of the sample achieved a semblance of these goals with the support of a competent mental health system. About one third of the sample seemed to show a continued undulating course marked by periods of symptoms and significant disabilities interspersed among periods of relative remission. Note that only a third of this last third (or one ninth of the entire sample) needed regular hospitalization or similar comprehensive services to manage their illness.

These data lead to two models of recovery: as outcome and as process. In terms of outcome, careful diagnosis of the breadth and depth of a disorder, and corresponding prescription of treatments and services that target identified symptoms and disabilities, will produce recovery. Liberman and Kopelowicz (2005) defined criteria that specified outcomes or endpoints of recovery. These included (1) *Psychotic symptoms:* ratings of moderate severity or below on scales reflecting positive and negative symptoms; (2) *Independence:* whether living alone or with others, recovery represents reliable adherence and self-management of medications; budgeting of one's funds for housing and food; and taking care of personal possessions and apartment; and (3) *Work or School:* at least half time employment or education in a normal, not sheltered, setting. Constructs like these suggest measurable benchmarks that can be tracked to measure recovery.

One of the purposes of recovery as a movement that emerged from consumers, survivors, and ex-patients was to re-inject hope into the lives of people diagnosed with these disorders. As a result, recovery from this perspective is less concerned about outcomes -- whether the person achieves some kind of symptom and disability free endpoint -- and more about processes. What actions and activities foster an environment where a person's search for a meaningful life can be supported? The wisdom of leaders in the consumer movement illustrates points about a meaningful life:

> "Recovery is a process, a way of life, an attitude, and a way of approaching the day's challenges. It is not a perfectly linear process. At times, our course is erratic and we falter, slide back, regroup, and start again. The need is to meet the challenge of the disability and to re-establish a new and valued sense of integrity and purpose within and beyond the limits of the disability; the aspiration is to live, work, and love in a community in which one makes a significant contribution." (Deegan, 1988).

> "Having some hope is crucial to recovery; none of us would strive if we believed it a futile effort…I believe that if we confront our illnesses with courage and struggle with our symptoms persistently, we can overcome our handicaps to live independently, learn skills, and contribute to society, the society that has traditionally abandoned us." (Chamberlin, 1997).

Although recovery as process deals with relatively more nebulous issues of purpose and vision, this perspective does not mean that assertions like these escape research evaluation. Ralph (2000, 2005) has reviewed more than a dozen studies that have examined some components of the process involved in recovery. Two points are important here. First, consumers and others who embrace recovery as a process still recognize the value of empirical research of this construct. Only with these kinds of analyses can we separate validated aspects of the processes from biased perceptions. Second, investigations of recovery as process offer some significant methodological problems. Note, however, that our presentation of recovery as outcome also highlighted methodological conundra in studying these concepts. We do not believe that the presence of barriers in using more "traditional" research methods highlights a failure of the theory as much as a challenge for researchers to develop strategies for testing the models.

## THE EVIDENCE-BASE FOR PSYCHIATRIC REHABILITATION

The six evidence-based practices that are the backbone of this paper represent the confluence of energies from several prominent sources: the National Institute of Mental Health, the Substance Abuse and Mental Health Services Administration and the Johnson and Johnson division of corporate contributions; professional groups like the American Psychiatric Association and the American Psychological Association; the Patient Outcomes Research Team; and leading researchers from Dartmouth University, the University of Maryland, and similar other groups. Their work was augmented with feedback by important consumer and advocacy groups including the National Alliance on Mental Illness and the National Mental Health Association. Two principles guided the work of this group; on values and the nature of the evidence (Drake, Goldman et al., 2001; Drake, Becker et al., 2006). These principles overlap considerably with the other chapters of this book. There are values that precede the definition and evaluation of serious mental illness and its rehabilitation. Recovery and empowerment are the embodiment of these values. Research is not needed to support these standards. On the contrary, evidence-based practices must incorporate consensual values and legal standards embodied by values like these. The nature of evidence is also complex and broad in scope. Defining the evidence and practices it supports is an ongoing dynamic process that needs to be conducted with a critical eye. Understanding practices will evolve under the scrutiny of the evidence. Mining the evidence is also a human process; understanding psychological epistemologies is necessary for a complete picture of the task of identifying the evidence base. One way this is done is through a consensus process of stakeholders informed about the data.

**Table 1: Current evidence-based practices**

| | |
|---|---|
| Illness Management and Recovery (IMR) | Individuals are taught how to effectively manage their illness and associated problems. This involves various behavior therapies and skills training strategies. This allows individuals to be better able to achieve their personal goals. The approach teaches a variety of skills so that the person is more effective when hampered by their illness. |
| Medication Management | Psychotropic medication is important for many individuals to control their illness and make therapy more effective. Clinical algorithms have been developed to guide practitioners in decisions about medication and dose, administration schedules, and titration of medications when the person's symptoms and other mental statuses occur. |
| Supported Employment Program (SEP) | This treatment helps people obtain competitive employment. There are a variety of services that are offered including job development, coaching, and counseling. Individuals receive services until they are comfortable with their jobs and no longer want a coach. |
| Assertive Community Treatment (ACT) | This case management program involves a multi-disciplinary team. A treatment plan is created that is individualized, comprehensive, flexible, and supportive in natural settings. This approach provides tools to obtain and maintain housing, employment, relationships, and relief from symptoms. |
| Family Therapies | This approach focuses on the needs of the families who care for individuals with psychiatric disabilities. Research has shown that many individuals live with their families and get various types of supports from them. This approach tries to facilitate support and resources for the person and their relatives, in the process making family interactions better. |
| Integrated Dual-diagnosis | This is an approach for individuals who suffer with a psychiatric disability and with problems of substance abuse. The course of psychiatric disability and outcomes are worse with co-morbid substance abuse. The approach integrates ways to provide care for mental illness and substance. |

### Six Evidence-Based Practices

Consensus efforts of various stakeholder groups under the two principles have yielded six evidence-based practices (EBPs); these are summarized in Table 1. We review the components of these practices as well as the evidence that support it.

## Illness Management and Recovery

Illness management and recovery (IMR) is an evidence-based approach that helps individuals achieve recovery and personal goals by increasing their ability to manage their psychiatric disability. The goal is to aid individuals so that they may work in collaboration with professionals and family members. IMR involves a combination of motivational, educational, and cognitive-behavioral strategies that expand the knowledge of individuals with psychiatric disabilities so that they progress toward their personal goals. Individuals with psychiatric disabilities learn about the nature and treatment of their psychiatric disability, how to identify and prevent relapses and hospitalizations, and how to cope more effectively with their symptoms (Mueser & Mackain, 2006).

Illness management involves providing information as well as strategies for adhering to treatment recommendations and medication, minimizing symptoms, and reducing the occurrences of relapse. Recovery-related goals include symptom relief in the present plus social and personal success in the long term (Deegan, 1988; Fisher, 1992; Leete, 1989). The process of reaching personal goals is achieved by increasing personal enjoyment in the world, a sense of self, hope, and optimism (Carpinello, Knight, Markowitz, & Pease, 2000; Corrigan et al., 1999). IMR encourages individuals with psychiatric disabilities to create an identity as being more than an individual with a psychiatric disability. This identity is built by facilitating self-efficacy, self-esteem, coping skills, and other skills needed to achieve personal goals.

IMR is based on three fundamental intervention components, which involve five specific evidence-based practices. The three intervention components are skills group training, nonpharmacological treatment for cognitive disabilities, and relapse prevention. The five evidence-based practices included in IMR are coping skills, social skills, psychoeducation, behavioral tailoring, and relapse prevention (Mueser et al., 2006; Mueser & Mackain, 2006).

The purpose of the skills training program is to help individuals with psychiatric disabilities to accept and live with their illness and to achieve personal life goals. Skills training helps individuals learn behaviors to overcome real-world obstacles to personal life goals (Mueser et al., 2002; Penn & Mueser, 1996). Skills are taught using social learning strategies, which include modeling, role playing, and other generalizable skills (Bellack, Mueser, Gingerich, & Agresta, 1997). Psychoeducation is one important part of skills training. Psychoeducation programs alone do not change the status of the individuals' functioning, but are useful in increasing knowledge that can enhance individuals' ability to make informed decisions (Goldman & Quinn, 1988). Psychoeducation provides information about their illness, its' course, its' causes, and ways to treat it.

Skill areas addressed by skills training groups include goal setting, problem solving, medication management, stress management, and coping skills (Atkinson, Coia, Gilmour, & Harper, 1996; Hogarty et al., 1997). Personal goal setting is a critical part of IMR; these goals are monitored throughout the course of the IMR program. Goals can include: improving role functioning, bettering social relationships, improving leisure time, and enhancing health. There is a step-by-step problem solving method where specific coping skills are learned. Medication management provides information about the role of medications and how they help individuals achieve personal and recovery goals. During stress management, individual are taught to recognize types of stress and their physical and emotional sequelae. Some stress management strategies include relaxation skills and imagery (Gingerich & Mueser, 1999). Coping skills increase the individuals' ability to manage symptoms and stress. These programs have been shown to reduce symptom severity (Leclerc, Lesage, Ricard, Lecomte, & Cyr, 2000; Lecomte et al., 1999).

Some cognitive dysfunctions that results from mental illness do not fade away even if prescribed medications are used correctly (Green, 1999). As a result, there are common cognitive strategies used for these cognitive disabilities. One strategy from cognitive therapy involves challenging dysfunctional cognitions. Additionally, cognitive rehabilitation programs remedy problems resulting from faulty information processing. Cognitive exercises are used to improve deficits. Approaches such as behavioral tailoring help individuals remember to take their medications. This involves finding ways to incorporate reminders into their daily routines so medications are incorporated into everyday life (Corrigan & Yudofsky, 1996; Mueser & Mackain, 2006; Velligan et al., 2002). Research has shown that behavioral tailoring increases adherence to prescribed medications (Boczkowski, Zeichner, & DeSanto, 1985; Cramer & Rosenheck, 1999).

Relapse prevention is an important component of IMR because relapse is common in people with psychiatric disabilities. Relapse can decrease the individuals' sense of well-being (Ralph, 2000; Miller, 1990). Relapse prevention programs have been shown to be more effective in keeping individuals out of the hospital than standard care procedures (Herz et al., 2000; Perry, Tarrier, Morriss, McCarthy, & Limb, 1999). This component focuses on teaching ways to cope with relapse while the individuals' are not overtaken by their psychiatric disability. Individuals with psychiatric disabilities learn in relapse prevention programs how to identify environmental triggers and early warning signs. The last part of relapse programs involves teaching the individuals to pair clues of relapse with behavioral responses to help prevent the occurrence of relapse (Herz et al., 2000; Perry et al., 1999). In addition, some programs teach family members how to identify early warning signs of relapse because individuals may not always be aware of the warning signs (Amador, Strauss, Yale, & Gorman, 1991).

## Medication Management

Medication management is important to help manage symptoms of psychiatric disabilities. Unfortunately, it is hindered by failure to follow prescriptions as drafted (Janick, Davis, Preskorn, & Ayd, 1997). Nor is failure to take medicine as prescribed endemic of psychiatric disorders alone. Noncompliance of prescribed medication is a problem for other medical illnesses including epilepsy (Jones, Butler, Thomas, Peveler, & Prevett, 2006), osteoporosis (Weycker, Macarios, Edelsber, & Oster, 2006), or asthma (DiMarten, 2004). Some non-compliant decisions about medication --e.g., not taking medication as prescribed -- can lead to relapse and increased medical costs (Davis & Andriukaitis, 1986; Kissling, 1991; Weiden et al., 1994). Noncompliance rates can range from 40% to 60% in individuals with schizophrenia (Kane & Borenstein, 1985; Lacro, Dunn, Dolder, Leckband, & Jeste, 2002; Novak-Grubic &Tavcar, 2002; Serban &Thomas, 1974; Weiden et al., 1994). Failure to take medication as prescribed occurs for a variety of reasons, including a dislike for the side effects of neuroleptics, a lack of insight by the individual, and severe psychotic symptoms.

Research has found that relapse prevention is the most common motivation to adhere to medication regimes (Yamada et al., 2006). Medication noncompliance is associated with poor clinical outcomes, decreases in quality of life, increased rates of relapses, and increased rates of hospitalization (Awad, 1993; Awad, Voruganti, & Heslegrace, 1995; Fenton, Blyler, & Heinssen, 1997). Other reasons for adherence include fear of rehospitalization, fulfillment of life goals, positive relations with prescribing clinician, perceived daily benefits, and positive family beliefs. Research has also found that most individuals are noncompliant due to distress by side effects (Yamada et al., 2006). Other reasons for noncompliance include problems related to access to treatment and embarrassment or stigma over medication or illness (Yamada et al., 2006). A review of articles since 1980 (Larco, Dunn, Dolder, Leckbank, & Leste, 2002) found that the factors that are consistently associated with noncompliance include poor insight, negative attitudes towards medication, previous occasions of noncompliance, substance abuse, inadequate aftercare, and poor therapeutic alliance. It was also found that factors such as age, gender, ethnicity, education level, severity of symptoms, and family involvement were not consistently associated with noncompliance (Larco et al., 2002),

The Texas Medication Algorithm Project (TMAP) was created to develop, implement, and evaluate medication algorithms (Gilbert et al., 1998; Rush et al., 1999). An algorithm is a computable set of steps for solving a problem and achieving a solution. Examples of algorithms in medicine include a moving circular slide to calculate medication doses or calculation of body mass index by knowing size and weight of the individual. Algorithms are more than guidelines; they provide a step-by-step process to identify treatment alternatives at key points in time. TMAP is an algorithm-driven treatment philosophy meant to for adult psychiatric disorders, mainly schizophrenia, major depression, and bipolar disorder. TMAP aims to improve quality of care and achieve the best possible outcomes for each dollar spent. TMAP is a treatment philosophy for medication management using medication algorithms to assist clinicians to more effectively work with the person with psychiatric disabilities as an active partner. Their research has found that individuals with schizophrenia and bipolar disorder experience better outcomes without high costs, while individuals with major depressive disorder experience better and more sustained outcomes, but at higher costs to the mental health system (Kashner et al., 2006).

Another evidence-based algorithm is the Case Management Adherence Guidelines (CMAG) (Aliotta, Vlasnik, & Delor, 2004). Individuals with psychiatric disabilities are assessed for medical knowledge and readiness to change. After the assessments, individuals are placed into one of four quadrants, high and low knowledge versus high and low motivation, and specific guidelines are used to help patients become and remain compliant to medication. This program is designed to identify individuals with low motivation and knowledge, which may prevent noncompliance. To be effective in using the guidelines an algorithm requires close attention to the individuals' illness, living situation, treatment, and a variety of other factors that may affect the individual (Aliotta, Vlasnik, & Delor, 2004).

## SUPPORTED EMPLOYMENT PROGRAMS

Supported employment is an evidence-based practice designed to help individuals with a severe psychiatric disability who want to work. According to the federal definition, supported employment is "competitive work in integrated work settings...consistent with the strengths, resources, priorities, concerns, abilities, capabilities, interests, and informed choice of the individual, for individuals with the most significant disabilities for whom competitive employment has not traditionally occurred; or for whom competitive employment has been interrupted or intermittent as a result of a significant disability" (Rehabilitation Act Amendments of 1998). While it was originally developed for individuals with developmental disabilities (Wehman, 1986), it also is effective for individuals with severe psychiatric disability (Cook et al., 2005; Mueser et al., 2004), increasing the vocational outcomes dramatically. Supported employment may also improve psychiatric symptoms and self-esteem. Evidence suggests it has effects on satisfaction with vocational services, leisure, and finances (Bond, Resnick, et al., 2001), though the findings in this area are mixed (Drake, Becker, Clark & Mueser, 1999). There are no apparently negative consequences as compared to traditional day treatment programs (Drake et al., 1999).

The most standardized and studied form of supported employment is the Individualized Support and Placement (IPS) model (Drake et al., 1999). This model has significantly better employment outcomes for individuals with severe psychiatric disability than a psychosocial rehabilitation program or standard services (Mueser et al., 2004) and brokered prevocational skills training (Drake, McHugo, Becker, Anthony, & Clark, 1996). A study by Drake and colleagues (1994) compared employment outcomes of a day treatment center in New Hampshire with a nearby community mental health treatment center that converted to an IPS program. The competitive employment rate at the converted site increased dramatically, while it remained significantly lower at the day treatment site. Other quasi-experiments found similar results, as have randomized controlled experiments in other cities (Bond, Resnick, et al., 2001) as well as in Canada (Latimer et al., 2006).

Six critical components influence the effectiveness of supported employment services. First, supported employment services are committed to competitive employment. Supported employment programs also help the person rapidly search job options and help clients obtain jobs directly, rather than providing lengthy preemployment assessment, training, and counseling. Individualized job placements are directed according to client preferences, strengths, and work experiences. Follow-along supports are maintained indefinitely. Mental health and vocational service teams are closely integrated in a supported employment program. Finally, any person who wants to participate in the program is eligible for services (Bond, 2004).

Fidelity of a program to these criteria is the best predictor of positive competitive employment outcomes (Becker, Smith, Tanzman, Drake, & Tremblay, 2001; Becker, Xie, McHugo, Halliday, & Martinez, 2006). In order to ensure that a program has high fidelity, several scales have been developed, including the Individual Placement and Support fidelity scale (Bond, Becker, Drake, & Vogler, 1997) and the Quality of Supported Employment Implementation Scale (McGrew & Griss, 2005). While fidelity is an important factor in how successful a supported employment program is, other factors should also be looked at, including practitioner skills (Drake, Bond, & Rapp, 2006), local employment rate and staff-to-client ratio (Becker et al., 2006), social inclusion of the workplace (Fillary & Pernice, 2006), and clients' felt need for employment (Casper & Carloni, 2006). Supplementary social skills training need to be investigated, although it appears it may not have an effect on employment outcomes (Mueser et al., 2005).

While supported employment appears to be successful and cost-effective (Drake et al., 1999), there are some limitations. It is effective for individuals in African-American and Latino populations, but it is not clear if supported employment is appropriate for all ethnic groups (Bond, Becker, et al., 2001). Also, job maintenance rates are not very good, although this may be due more to clients' job dissatisfaction and lack of interest (Mak, Tsang, & Cheung, 2006). Other community and program factors also require more research to understand how to produce better outcomes (Bond, Becker, et al., 2001).

## ASSERTIVE COMMUNITY TREATMENT

Assertive community treatment (ACT) is an effective treatment for individuals most severely impaired by psychiatric disability. First developed by Stein and Test (1980), ACT consists of a team of professionals from psychiatry, nursing, social work, and other areas that work together to provide a variety of services for clients every day of the week. Services are provided in systems most convenient and relevant to the person with disabilities; e.g., their home, work place, or setting in which the person recreates. The team usually consists of ten to twelve staff members, and each member is cross-trained in peers' areas of expertise. Services offered include family involvement, rehabilitative approach to daily living skills, work opportunities, entitlements, health promotion, medication support, housing assistance, financial management, and counseling (Phillips et al., 2001).

Seven principles are basic to ACT programs. All of the services are provided directly by the ACT team rather than brokering them to an independent service provider. The range of treatment and services is comprehensive and flexible. Team members share responsibility for all of the individuals served by the team. Also, the staff-to-consumer ratio should be small (not more than one team member for ten consumers). Interventions are carried out at the most convenient settings. Support is maintained indefinitely, with service available at any hour. The team actively engages individuals in treatment (Corrigan, 2006).

Several positive outcomes are associated with ACT. It is cost-effective, costing no more than standard treatment while decreasing the number of days of hospitalization (Essock, Frisman, & Kontos, 1998; Latimer 2005). The income of consumers also increases (Horiuchi et al., 2006). ACT consumers seem better engaged and report more satisfaction with services (Killaspy et al., 2006). ACT also increases trust in providers, which makes consumers more open to encouragement and motivated to improve (Leiphart & Barnes, 2005).

ACT may not be effective for all individuals, however. The impact of ACT on individuals with dual-disorders is mixed (Calsyn, Yonker, Lemming, Morse, & Klinkenberg, 2005; Drake et al., 1998; Essock et al., 2006). ACT also does not seem to be any more effective than standard treatment for individuals with intellectual disability (Martin et al.,

2005; Oliver et al., 2005). There are often methodological issues in studying ACT, which may explain some of the negative findings (McHugo et al., 1998).

As mentioned earlier, program fidelity is a valuable predictor of the effectiveness of an evidence-based practice. The most widely used scale to measure program fidelity for ACT is the Dartmouth ACT Scale (Teague, Bond, & Drake, 1998). While the program fidelity as measured by this scale has shown mixed results (Bond & Salyers, 2004; McHugo, Drake, Teague, & Xie, 1999), it appears to be a valid and useful scale.

Many issues must be considered when implementing ACT. There should be enough ACT teams in a community to serve 50 percent of the individuals with severe psychiatric disability, which is about .06 of their adult population (Cuddeback, Morrissey, & Meyer, 2006). ACT team members need to especially monitor consumers closely during the first nine months of the program, when individuals are most likely to be admitted to the hospital (Joannette, Lawson, Eastabrook, & Krupa, 2005). Also, since many consumers of ACT have at least one active medical condition, team members need to have knowledge of the most common conditions and ensure that consumers have access to medical treatment (Ceilley, Cruz & Denko, 2006). ACT may need to be tailored to ethnic minorities (Yang et al., 2005) and rural areas (Gold et al., 2006).

## Family Therapies

The goal of family psychoeducation is to provide relatives education and support so that they may feel less burdened and more effective at helping their family members with mental illness manage their disability and avoid relapse. Research has shown that families are impacted by psychiatric disorders and that they feel increased levels of burden (Caqueo-Urizar & Guiterrez-Maldonado, 2006; Pillings et al., 2002). A majority of adults with psychiatric disabilities live with their families, who support these individuals emotionally, financially, and with issues related to treatment (Dixon, Adams, & Lucksted, 2000; Solomon & Draine, 1995). Family psychoeducation groups can come in a variety of different models. Most are illness specific, have a focus on treatment outcomes, and focus their attention to the well-being of the family. Family psychoeducation can be for anyone who is supporting the individual in their recovery: parents, brothers or sisters, other relatives, close friends, or even neighbors.

The advantage of this approach is that it focuses on the reality that the psychiatric illness is challenging on everyone involved. It also provides family members information so that they know how to help the individual and understand their illness. Family psychoeducation allows the individual to recover with the right type of help from their families. Family psychoeducation has been shown to be helpful for individuals with schizophrenia (Tomaras et al., 2000), bipolar illness (Rea et al., 2003), major depression (Emanuels-Zuurvenn & Emmelkamp, 1997), and borderline personality disorder (Gunderson, Berkowitz, & Ruizsancho, 1997).

Benefits of family psychoeducation for individuals with psychiatric disabilities include fewer symptoms, fewer relapses, and better relationships (Falloon et al., 1985; Miklowitz Simoneau et al., 2000; Simoneua, Miklowitz, Richards, Saleem & Georige, 1999). Everyone works together to help the individual solve problems related to finding and keeping a job, taking part in social activities, decreasing family stress, resolving disagreements about medication, increasing energy, and resolving problems with drugs and alcohol (SAMHSA, 2003).

Families are taught to help relatives reach their goals. While working on recovery, individuals with psychiatric disabilities learn the difference between their illness and who they are as a person. Therapists talk to the family about hopes for the future, family problems, relative's symptoms, and medication management. There are educational workshops where individuals and their families learn about mental illness and ways to aid recovery. Problem-solving groups help the individuals and their families identify and deal with the problems that mental illness puts in the way of recovery and life.

Family psychoeducation adheres to fifteen principles when working with the families and individuals with a psychiatric disability. The principles related to how therapy is provided include coordinating all elements of treatment to ensure everyone is working collaboratively, paying attention to social and clinical needs of the individual, providing medication management, addressing feelings of loss, providing explicit crisis plans, being flexible, and providing family access to other professionals. The principles that specifically focus on the family include the need to listen to families concerns and treat them as equal partners, explore family expectations for the program and individual, assess strengths and limitations of the families ability to support the individual, help resolve family conflict, provide relevant information for individual and family at proper times, improve communication in the family, training family in problem-solving techniques, and encourage family to expand social supports (Corrigan, 2006; Dixon et al., 2001).

There have been several family-based interventions that have been researched. Behavioral family management involves illness education, training in problem solving, and training in effective family communication (Falloon, Boyd, & McGill, 1984). Individuals in the behavioral family management program experience significantly less clinical relapse, fewer days of hospitalization, and lower depression rates (Fallon & Penderson, 1985). One family psychoeducation model developed by Anderson and colleagues (1986) focuses on connecting the family, illness education, ongoing support, and crisis intervention. Studies indicate that this program is effective in reducing relapse and enhancing vocational rehabilitation (Hogarty et al., 1986; Hogarty et al., 1991). The Schizophrenia Patient Outcomes Research Team includes family psychoeducation as a treatment recommendation for individuals with schizophrenia. They recommend family members be offered family psychosocial intervention for at least nine months, as well as education about the illness, family support, crisis intervention, and problem solving skills (Lehman & Steinwachs, 1998).

## INTEGRATED DUAL DIAGNOSIS

Substance use disorders are extremely common among people with severe psychiatric disability. Co-occurring substance problems are prevalent in many illnesses, especially in individuals with bipolar disorder (Levin & Hennessy, 2004) and schizophrenia (Cantor-Graae, Nordström, & McNeil, 2001). Substance abuse problems are also common in other mood disorders, anxiety disorders, posttraumatic stress disorder, and borderline personality disorder (McGovern, Xie, Segal, Siembab, & Drake, 2006). It also appears that individuals with antisocial personality disorder, especially if it is late-onset, have a high risk of substance use (Mueser et al., 2006).

While many treatments have been developed to treat severe psychiatric disabilities and substance use disorders separately, the most effective method to treat individuals with dual diagnoses is integrated treatment (Brunette, Mueser, & Drake, 2004; Drake et al., 2001). Other than integration of treatment, there are six critical components to provide the most effective treatment to individuals with dual disorders. First, it is important that case managers actively seek out clients where they live and provide treatment outside the office. Second, motivational interviewing is necessary to ensure clients are eager to pursue treatment. Third, social support needs to be provided, since large support systems are linked to recovery. Fourth, service providers should be prepared for long-term treatment. Fifth, treatment needs to address all aspects of a client's life. Finally, service providers need to be culturally competent (Corrigan, 2006). It also appears that stage-wise treatment, engagement interventions, and relapse prevention interventions may be important as well (Drake, Mueser, Brunette, & McHugo, 2004).

While it is important that treatments include these components, other treatments may also be utilized. Supported employment programs can help individuals with dual disorders find employment, which can be important for recovery (Becker, Drake, & Naughton, 2005). Assertive community treatment is also effective for client satisfaction and helping homeless clients stay in stable housing (Morse et al., 2006) as well as reducing substance use, increasing remission rates, increasing treatment retention rates, and decreasing hospital admissions (McHugo, Drake, Teague, & Xie, 1999). Behavioral therapies also hold promise for treating individuals with dual disorders (Carroll, 2004). Medication is an important tool in treating dual disorders as well. Clozapine may prevent substance abuse relapse in individuals with schizophrenia and substance abuse (Brunette, Drake, Xie, McHugo, & Green, 2006). Naltrexone and disulfiram appear to be effective in decreasing alcohol use in clients with psychotic spectrum disorders and substance abuse disorders (Petrakis, Nich, & Ralevski, 2006). Specialized interventions also have positive outcomes for women with dual disorders and a history of violence (Domino et al., 2005; Morrissey et al., 2005) and for individuals with dual disorders who are frequently imprisoned (Chandler & Spicer, 2006).

Service providers need to be aware of several aspects of their clients in order to provide treatment successfully. Psychosocial aspects of substance use in individuals with severe psychiatric impairment are very important, and need to be taken into consideration for treatment (Drake, Wallach, Alverson, & Mueser, 2002). Relapse is very common, and is most likely to happen in men, those with less than a high school education, living independently, and not continuing treatment (Xie, McHugo, Fox, & Drake, 2005). Relapse prevention needs to include several key components, such as reducing exposure to substances, fostering motivation for abstinence, self-monitoring, recognizing and coping with cravings and negative affect, identifying thought processes with relapse potential, and deploying a crisis plan if necessary (McGovern, Wrisley, & Drake, 2005). Also, service providers should be aware of the increased risk of certain medical disorders (Dickey, Normand, Weiss, Drake, & Azeni, 2002).

While treatment for individuals with dual disorders is very complex, long term outcomes appear to be positive. Individuals with schizophrenia and substance abuse improved steadily for 10 years after receiving treatment in many areas of life, including symptoms, substance abuse, institutionalization, functional status, and quality of life (Drake, McHugo, et al., 2006).

**Table 2: Developing evidence-based practices**

| | |
|---|---|
| Consumer Operated Services (COS) | This practice is developed by and provided to individuals with the psychiatric disabilities. At the heart of this program is self-empowerment that guides peer-directed recovery. Preliminary evidence suggests that these programs improve symptoms, increase social networks, and enhance the quality of life. |
| Supported Education (SEd) | This focuses on helping adults achieve higher education by providing counseling and support services to those attending post-secondary education. The programs help individuals be successful in their educational goals by providing transportation to school, helping with the application process, tutoring, and tuition assistance. Services like these are provided by education specialists in the school setting. |
| Faith-Based Interventions | These interventions are based on research that shows that aspects of religion affect individuals' mental health and well being. This approach focuses on the spiritual health of the individual. |

## Practices Still Awaiting an Evidence Base

The six practices mentioned here are only the seeds of a comprehensive mental health service system. Listed in Table 2 are examples of other practices prominent in the mental health services research literature that still await convincing findings that support an evidence base. Consumer operated services have more than a 40 year history; these are largely peer support programs developed by people with mental illness for people with mental illness (Clay, 2005; Campbell, 2005). Supported education provides skills training, resources, and support for people with psychiatric disabilities seeking academic goals (Mowbray, Collins, et al., 2005; Mowbray, Moxley, & Brown, 1993). The research literature is rich with qualitative investigations demonstrating the impact of consumer operated services and supported education. Quasi-experimental studies also document the evidence that supports it. Mostly absent from the literature is more rigorously obtained findings that support an evidence-based claim. Faith-based interventions are unique because they provide support through religious observation. This practice may be effective since spirituality is a commonly endorsed coping method for those experiencing psychiatric disabilities (Tepper, Rogers, Coleman, & Malony,

2001). The purpose of presenting these practices here is not to assert a place for them at the research table but instead note that additional practices are in development and will probably be added to the list of EBPs over time.

Some advocates have noted that the criteria for classifying a service as effective and worthwhile -- an empirical evidence-base-- reflects the priorities of the research community, but not necessarily the community of consumers, survivors, and ex-patients (Fisher & Ahern, 2002; Frese, Stanley, Kress, & Vogel-Scibilia, 2001). In particular, traditional empirical research does not necessarily include the kinds of epistemologies that led to the development of such important ideas of the consumer movement as empowerment and recovery (Corrigan, 2004; Van Tosh, Ralph, & Campbell, 2000). Moreover, empirical research approaches do not easily crosswalk with more ethereal constructs such as spirituality (Plante & Sherman, 2001), a concept that has a central role in many consumer conceptions of recovery. Cautions like these are meant to be guides, not barriers. Rehabilitation services will only continue to develop as stakeholders examine the evidence.

## References


Aliotta, S.L., Vlasnik, J.J., & Delor, B.D. (2004). Enhancing Adherence to long-term medication therapy: A new approach to assessing and treating patients. *Advances In Therapy, 21(4), 214-231.*

Amador, X.F., Strauss, D.H., Yale, S.A., & Gorman J.M. (1991). Awareness of illness in schizophrenia. *Schizophrenia Bulletin, 17*, 113-132.

Anderson, C.M., Reiss, D.J., & Hogarty, G.E. (1986). *Schizophrenia and the Family.* New York: Guilford Press.

Atkinson, J.M., Coia, D.A., Gilmour, W.H., & Harper, J.P. (1996). The impact of education groups for people with schizophrenia on social functioning and quality of life. *British Journal of Psychiatry, 168,* 199-204.

Awad A.G. (1993): Subjective Response to Neuroleptics in Schizophrenia. *Schizophrenia Bulletin, 19,* 609-618.

Awad, A.G., Hogan, T.P., Voruganti, L.N.P., & Heslegrave, R.J. (1995). Patients Subjective Experiences on Antipsychotic Medications: Implications for Outcome and Quality of Life. *Int. Clin. Psychopharmacology 1995, 10 (Suppl. 3),* 123-133.

Becker, D. R., Drake, R. E., & Naughton, W. J. (2005). Supported employment for people with co-occurring disorders. *Psychiatric Rehabilitation Journal, 28(4),* 332-338.

Becker, D. R., Smith, J., Tanzman, B., Drake, R. E., & Tremblay, T. (2001). Fidelity of supported employment programs and employment outcomes. *Psychiatric Services, 52(6),* 834-836.

Becker, D. R., Xie, H., McHugo, G. J., Halliday, J., & Martinez, R. A. (2006). What predicts supported employment program outcomes? *Community Mental Health, 42(3),* 303-313.

Bellack, A.S., Mueser, K.T., Gingerich, S., & Agresta, J. (1997). *Skills training for schizophrenia a step-by step guide.* New York: Guilford Press.

Boczkowski, J., Zeichner, A., & DeSanto, N. (1985). Neuroleptic compliance among chronic schizophrenic outpatients: An intervention outcome report. *Journal of Consulting and*

*Clinical Psychology, 53,* 349-355.

Bond, G. R. (2004). Supported employment: Evidence for an evidence-based practice. *Psychiatric Rehabilitation Journal, 27(4),* 345-359.

Bond, G. R., Becker, D. R., Drake, R. E., Rapp, C. A., Meisler, N., Lehman, A. F., et al. (2001). Implementing supported employment as an evidence-based practice. *Psychiatric Services, 52(3),* 313-322.

Bond, G. R., Becker, D. R., Drake, R. E., & Vogler, K. M. (1997). A fidelity scale for the individual placement and support model of supported employment. *Rehabilitation Counseling Bulletin, 40(4),* 265-284.

Bond, G. R., Resnick, S. G., Drake, R. E., Xie, H., McHugo, G .J., & Bebout, R. R. (2001). Does competitive employment improve nonvocational outcomes for people with severe mental illness? *Journal of Counseling and Clinical Psychology, 69(3),* 489-501.

Bond, G. R., & Salyers, M. P. (2004). Prediction of outcome from the Dartmouth assertive community treatment fidelity scale. *CNS Spectrums, 9(12),* 937-942.

Brunette, M. F., Drake, R. E., Xie, H., McHugo, G. J., & Green, A. I. (2006). Clozapine use and relapses of substance use disorder among patients with co-occurring schizophrenia and substance use disorders. *Schizophrenia Bulletin, 32(4),* 637-643.

Brunette, M. F., Mueser, K. T., & Drake, R. E. (2004). A review of research on residential programs for people with severe mental illness and co-occurring substance use disorders. *Drug and Alcohol Review, 23,* 471-481.

Calabrese, J.D., & Corrigan, P.W. (2005). Beyond dementia praecox: Findings from long term-follow-up studies of schizophrenia. In R.O. Ralph and P.W.Corrigan (Eds.), *Recovery in Mental Illness: Broadening Our Understanding of Wellness* (63-84). Washington D.C., American Psychological Association

Calsyn, R. J., Yonker, R. D., Lemming, M. R., Morse, G. A., & Klinkenberg, W. D. (2005). Impact of assertive community treatment and client characteristics on criminal justice outcomes in dual disorder homeless individuals. *Criminal Behaviour & Mental Health, 15(4),* 236-248.

Campbell, J. (2005). Effectiveness findings of the COSP Multisite Research Initiative. *Grading the evidence for consumer-driven services*, UIC NRTC Webcast, Chicago, IL.

Cantor-Graae, E., Nordström, L. G., & McNeil, T. F. (2001). Substance abuse in Schizophrenia: A review of the literature and a study of correlates in Sweden. *Schizophrenia Research, 48,* 69-82.

Caqueo-Urizar, A. & Guiterrez-Maldonado, J. (2006). Burden of care in families of patients with schizophrenia. *Quality of Life Research, 15,* 719-724.

Carpinello, S.E., Knight, E.L., Markowitz, F.E., & Pease, E.A. (2000). The development of the mental health confidence sale: A measure of self-efficacy in individuals diagnosed with mental disorders. *Psychiatric Rehabilitation Journal, 23,* 236-242.

Carroll, K. M. (2004). Behavioral therapies for co-occurring substance use and mood disorders. *Biological Psychiatry, 56,* 778-784.

Casper, E. S., & Carloni, C. (2006). Increasing the utilization of supported employment services with the need for change scale. *Psychiatric Services, 57(10),* 1430-1434.

Ceilley, J. W., Cruz, M., & Denko, T. (2006). Active medical conditions among patients on an assertive community treatment team. *Community Mental Health Journal, 42(2)* 205-

211.

Chandler, D. W., & Spicer, G. (2006). Integrated treatment for jail recidivists with co-occurring psychiatric and substance use disorders. *Community Mental Health Journal, 42(4),* 405-425.

Chamberlin, J. (1997). Confessions of a non-compliant patient. *National Empowerment Center Newsletter.* Lawrence, MA: National Empowerment Center.

Clay, S. (2005). *On Our Own, Together Peer Programs for People with Mental Illness.* Vanderbilt University Press

Cook, J. A., Leff, S., Blyler, C. R., Gold, P. B., Goldberg, R. W., Mueser, K. T., et al. (2005). Results of a multisite randomized trial of supported employment interventions for individuals with severe mental illness. *Archives of General Psychiatry, 62*, 505-512.

Corrigan, P.W. (2004). Guidelines for enhancing personal empowerment ofpeople with psychiatric disabilities. *American Rehabilitation, Autumn*,10-21.

Corrigan, P. W. (2006). Recovery from schizophrenia and the role of evidence-based psychosocial interventions. *Expert Review of Neurotherapeutics, 6(7),* 993-1004.

Corrigan, P.W., Giffort, D., Rashid, F., Leary, M., Okeke, I., & Lickey, S. (1999). Recovery as a Psychological Construct. *Community Mental Health Journal, 35(3),* 231-239.

Corrigan, P.W., Mueser, K.T., Bond, G.R., Drake, R.E., & Solomon, P.(2007). *The principles and practice of psychiatric rehabilitation: An empirical approach.* New York: Guilford Press.

Corrigan, P.W., & Yudofsky, S.C. (1996). *Cognitive rehabilitation for neuropsychiatric disorders.* American Psychiatric Association.

Cramer, J.A., & Rosenheck, R. (1999). Enhancing medication compliance for people with serious mental illness. *The Journal of Nervous and Mental Disease, 187,* 53-55.

Cuddeback, G. S., Morrissey, J. P., & Meyer, P. S. (2006). How many assertive community treatment teams do we need? *Psychiatric Services, 57(12),* 1803-1806.

Davis, J. M., & Andriukaitis, S. (1986) The natural course of schizophrenia and effective maintenance drug treatment. *Journal of Clinical Psychopharmacology, 6*, 2S-10S.

Deegan, P.E. (1988). Recovery: The lived experience of rehabilitation. *Psychosocial Rehabilitation Journal, 11(4),* 11-19.

Dickey, B., Normand, S. T., Weiss, R. D., Drake, R. E.. & Azeni, H. (2002). Medical morbidity, mental illness, and substance use disorders. *Psychiatric Services, 53(7),* 861-867.

DiMarten, M.R. (2004). Varients in patients' adherence to medical recommendations: A quantitative review of 50 years of research. *Medical Care, 42,* 200-209.

Dixon, L., Adams, C., & Lucksted, A. (2000). Update on Family Psychoeducation for Schizophrenia. *Schizophrenia Bulletin, 26,* 5-20

Dixon, L., McFarlane, W.R., Lefley, H., Luckstead, A., Cohen, M., Falloon, I., et al. (2001). Evidence-based practices for services to families of people with psychiatric disabilities. *Psychiatric Services, 52(7),* 903-910.

Domino, M. E., Morrissey, J. P., Chung, S., Huntington, N., Larson, M. J., & Russell, L. A. (2005). Service use and costs for women with co-occurring mental and substance use disorders and a history of violence. *Psychiatric Services, 56(10),*1223-1232.

Drake, R. E., Becker, D. R., Biesanz, J. C., Torrey, W. C., McHugo, G. J., & Wyzik, P. F.

(1994). Rehabilitation day treatment vs. supported employment: I. vocational outcomes. *Community Mental Health Journal, 30(5),* 519-532.

Drake, R. E., Becker, D. R., Clark, R. E., & Mueser, K. T. (1999). Research on the individual placement and support model of supported employment. *Psychiatric Quarterly, 70(4),* 289-301.

Drake, R.E., Becker, D.R., Goldman, H.H., & Martinez, R.A. (2006). The Johnson & Johnson - Dartmouth community mental health program: Disseminating evidence-based practice. *Psychiatric Services,* 57, 302-304.

Drake, R. E., Bond, G. R., & Rapp, C. (2006). Explaining the variance within supported employment programs: Comment on "What predicts supported employment outcomes?" *Community Mental Health Journal, 42(3),* 315-318.

Drake, R. E., Essock, S. M., Shaner, A., Carey, K. B., Minkoff, K., Kola, L., et al. (2001). Implementing dual diagnosis services for clients with severe mental illness. *Psychiatric Services, 52(4),* 469-476.

Drake, R.E., Goldman, H.H., Stephen Leff, H., Lehman, A.F., Dixon, L., Mueser, K.T., et al. (2001). Implementing evidence-based practices in routine mental health service settings. *Psychiatric Services, 52(2),* 179-182.

Drake, R. E., McHugo, G. J., Becker, D. R., Anthony, W. A., & Clark, R. E. (1996). The New Hampshire study of supported employment for people with severe mental illness. *Journal of Counseling and Clinical Psychology, 64(2),* 391-399.

Drake, R. E., McHugo, G. J., Clark, R. E., Teague, G. B., Xie, H., Miles, K. et al. (1998). Assertive community treatment for patients with co-occurring severe mental illness and substance use disorder: A clinical trial. *American Journal of Orthopsychiatry, 68(2),* 201-215.

Drake, R. E., McHugo, G. J., Xie, H., Fox, M., Packard, J., & Helmstetter, B. (2006). Ten-year recovery outcomes for clients with co-occurring schizophrenia and substance use disorders. *Schizophrenia Bulletin, 32(3),* 464-473.

Drake, R. E., Mueser, K. T., Brunette, M. F., & McHugo, G. J. (2004). A review of treatments for people with severe mental illnesses and co-occurring substance use disorders. *Psychiatric Rehabilitation Journal, 27(4),* 360-374.

Drake, R. E., Wallach, M. A., Alverson, H. S., & Mueser, K. T. (2002). Psychosocial aspects of substance abuse by clients with severe mental illness. *The Journal of Nervous and Mental Disease, 190(2),* 100-106.

Emanuels-Zuurvenn, L. & Emmelkamp, P. (1997). Spouse-aided therapy with depressed consumers. *Behavior Modification, 21,* 62-77.

Essock, S. M., Frisman, L. K., & Kontos, N. J. (1998). Cost-effectiveness of assertive community treatment teams. *American Journal of Orthopsychiatry, 68(2),* 179-190.

Essock, S. M., Mueser, K. T., Drake, R. E., Covell, N. H., McHugo, G. J., Frisman, L. K., et al. (2006). Comparison of ACT and standard case management for delivering integrated treatment for co-occurring disorders. *Psychiatric Services, 57(2),* 185-196.

Falloon, I.R.H., Boyd, J.L., & McGill, C.W. (1984). *Family Care of Schizophrenia: A Problem-Solving Approach to the Treatment of Mental Illness.* New York: Guildford Press.

Falloon, I.R.H., Boyd, J.L., McGill, C.W., Williamson, M., Razni, J., Moss, H.B., et al.

(1985). Family management in the prevention of morbidity of schizophrenia. *Atchives of General Psychiatry, 42,* 886-896.

Fallon, I.R.H. & Penderson, J. (1985). Family management in the prevention of morbidity of schizophrenia: The adjustment of the family unit. *British Journal of Psychiatry, 147,* 156-163.

Fenton, W. S., Blyler, C. R., & Heinssen, R. K. (1997). Determinants of medication compliance in schizophrenia: Empirical and clinical findings. *Schizophrenia Bulletin, 23,* 637-651.

Fillary, R., & Pernice, R. (2006). Social inclusion in workplaces where people with intellectual disabilities are employed: Implications for supported employment professionals. *International Journal of Rehabilitation Research, 29(1),* 31-36.

Fisher, D.B. (1992). Humanizing the recovery process. *Resources, 4,* 5-6.

Fisher, D.B. & Ahern, L. (2002). Evidence-Based Practices and Recovery. *Psychiatry Services, 53,* 632-633

Frese, F.J., Stanley, J., Kress, K. & Vogel-Scibilia, S. (2001). Integrating Evidence-Based Practices and the Recovery Model. *Psychiatric Services, 52,* 1462-1468.

Gilbert, D.A., Altshuyler, K.Z., Rago, W.V., Shon, S.P., Crismon, M.L., Toprac, M.G., et al. (1998). Texas Medication Algorithm Project: Definitions, rationale, andmethods to develop medication algorithms. *Journal of Clinical Psychiatry, 59,* 345-351.

Gingerich, S., & Mueser, K.T. (1999). Illness Management and Recovery. In R.E. Drake, M.R. Merrens, & D.W. Lynde (Eds.), *Evidence-based mental health practice* (395-424). New York: W.W. Norton & Company.

Gold, P. B., Meisler, N., Santos, A. B., Carnemolla, M. A., Williams, O. H., & Keleher, J. (2006). Randomized trial of supported employment integrated with assertive community treatment for rural adults with severe mental illness. *Schizophrenia Bulletin, 32(2),* 378-395.

Goldman, C.R., & Quinn, F.L. (1988). Effects of a patient education program in the treatment of schizophrenia. *Hospital and Community Psychiatry, 39(3),* 282-6.

Green, M.F. (1999). Interventions for neurocognitive deficits. *Schizophrenia Bulletin, 25,* 197-200.

Gunderson, J.G., Berkowitz, C., & Ruizsancho, A. (1997). Families of borderline consumers: A psychoeducational approach. *Bulletin of the Menniger Clinic, 61,* 446-457.

Harding, C.M, Brooks G.W., Ashikaga, T., Strauss, J.S., & Breier, A. (1987). The Vermont longitudinal study of persons with severe mentalillness, II. Long-term outcome of subjects who retrospectively metDSM-III criteria for schizophrenia. *American Journal of Psychiatry, 144,* 727-735.

Harrison, G., Hopper, K., Craig, T., Laska, E., Siegel, C., Wanderling, J., et al. (2001). Recovery from psychotic illness: a 15- and 25-year international follow-up study. *The British Journal of Psychiatry*, 178, 506-517.

Herz, M.I., Lamberti, J.S., Minz, J., Scott, R., O'Dell, S.P., McCartan, L., et al. (2000). A program for relapse prevention in schizophrenia: a controlled study. *Archives of General Psychiatry, 57,* 277-283.

Hogarty, G. Anderson, C.M., Reiss, D.J. Kornblit, S.J., Greenwald D.P., Javna C.D., et al. (1986). Family psychoeducation, social skills training, and maintenance chemotherapy in the aftercare treatment of schizophrenia I: One-year effects of a controlled study on relapse and expressed emotion. *Archives of General Psychiatry, 43,* 633-642.

Hogarty, G. Anderson,C.M., Reiss,D.J., Kornblith,S.J., Greenwald, D.P., Ulrich, R.F., et al. (1991). Family psychoeducation, social skills training, and maintenance chemotherapy in the aftercare treatment of schizophrenia II : Two-year effects of a controlled study on relapse and expressed emotion. Environmental-Personal Indicator in the Course of Schizophrenia (EPICS) Research Group. *Archives of General Psychiatry, 48,* 340-347.

Hogarty, G., Greenwald, D., Ulrich, R., Kornblith, S., DiBarry, A., Cooley, S., et al. (1997). Three year trials of personal therapy among schizophrenic patients living with or independent of family, II: Effects on adjustment of patients. *American Journal of Psychiatry, 154(11),* 1514-1524.

Horiuchi, K., Nisihio, M., Oshima, I., Ito, J., Matsuoka, H., & Tsukada, K. (2006). The quality of life among persons with severe mental illness enrolled in an assertive community treatment program in Japan: 1-year follow-up and analyses. *Clinical Practice & Epidemiology in Mental Health, 2(18).* Retrieved February 12, 2007, from http://www.cpementalhealth.com/content/2/1/18.

Janicak, P. G., Davis, J. M., Preskorn, S. H., & Ayd, F. J. (1997). *Principles and practice of psychopharmacotherapy* (2nd ed.). Baltimore: Williams & Wilkins.

Joannette, J. A., Lawson, J. S., Eastabrook, S. J., & Krupa, T. (2005). Community tenure of people with serious mental illness in assertive community treatment in Canada. *Psychiatric Services, 56(11),* 1387-1393.

Jones, R.M. Butler, J.A., Thomas, V.A., Peveler, R.C., & Prevett, M. (2006). Adherence to treatment in patients with epilepsy: Associations with seizure control and illness beliefs. *Seizure, 15,* 504-508.

Kane, J.M., & Borenstein, M. (1985). Compliance in the long-term treatment of schizophrenia. *Psychopharmacology Bulletin 21,* 23–27.

Kashner, T.M., Rush, A.J., Crismon, M.L., Toprac, M., Carmody, T.J., Miller, A.L., et al. (2006). An empirical Analysis of costs outcomes of the Texas medication algorithm project. *Psychiatric Services, 57(5), 648-659.*

Killaspy, H., Bebbington, P., Blizard, R., Johnson, S., Nolan, F., Pilling, S., et al. (2006). The REACT study: Randomised evaluation of assertive community treatment in north London. *British Medical Journal, 332,* 815-820.

Kissling, W. (1991). The current unsatisfactory state of relapse prevention in schizophrenic psychoses - Suggestions for improvement. *Clinical Neuropharmacology, 14 (SUPPL. 2),* S33-S44.

Kraepelin , E. (1923). *Psychiatrie* ( Vol. 3, Ed. 8.). Leipzig: Johann Ambrosius Barth

Lacro J.P., Dunn L.B., Dolder C.R., Leckband, S.G., Jeste, D.V. (2002). Prevalence of and risk factors for medication nonadherence in patients with schizophrenia: a comprehensive review of recent literature. *Journal of Clinical Psychiatry, 63(10),*892-909.

Latimer, E. (2005). Economic considerations associated with assertive community treatment and supported employment for people with severe mental illness. *Journal of Psychiatry & Neuroscience, 30(5),* 355-359.

Latimer, E. A., Lecomte, T., Becker, D. R., Drake, R. E., Duclos, I., Piat, M., et al. (2006). Generalisability of the individual placement and support model of supported employment: Results of a Canadian randomised controlled trial. *The British Journal of Psychiatry, 189*, 65-73.

Lehman, A.F. & Steinwachs, D.M. (1998). At issue: Translation research into practice: The Schizophrenia Patient Outcomes Research Team (PORT) treatment recommendations. *Schizophrenia Bulletin, 24,* 1-9.

Leclerc, C., Lesage, A.D., Ricard, N., Lecomte, T., & Cyr, M. (2000). Assessment of a new rehabilitative coping skills module for persons with schizophrenia. *American Journal of Orthopsychiatry, 70,* 380-388.

Lecomte, T., Cyr, M., Lesage, A.D. Wilde J., Leclerc C., & Ricard N. (1999). Efficacy of a self-esteem module in the empowerment of individuals with schizophrenia. *Journal of Nervous and Mental Disease, 187*, 406-413.

Leete, E. (1989). How I perceive and manage my illness. *Schizophrenia Bulletin, 8*, 605–609.

Leiphart, L. R., & Barnes, M. G. (2005). The client experience of assertive community treatment: A qualitative study. *Psychiatric Rehabilitation Journal, 28(4),* 395-397.

Levin, F. R., & Hennessy, G. (2004). Bipolar disorder and substance abuse. *Biological Psychiatry, 56,* 738-748.

Liberman, R.P., & Kopelowicz, A. (2005*).* Recovery from schizophrenia: A concept in search of research. *Psychiatry Services, 56,* 735-742.

Mak, D. C. S., Tsang, H. W. H., & Cheung, L. C. C. (2006). Job termination among individuals with severe mental illness participating in a supported employment program. *Psychiatry, 69(3),* 239-248.

Martin, G., Costello, H., Leese, M., Slade, M., Bouras, N., Higgins, S., et al. (2005). An exploratory study of assertive community treatment for people with intellectual disability and psychiatric disorders: Conceptual, clinical, and service issues. *Journal of Intellectual Disability Research, 49(7),* 516-524.

McGrew, J. H., & Griss, M. E. (2005). Concurrent and predictive validity of two scales to assess the fidelity of implementation of supported employment. *Psychiatric Rehabilitation Journal, 29(1),* 41-47.

McGovern, M. P., Wrisley, B. R., & Drake, R. E. (2005). Relapse of substance use disorder and its prevention among persons with co-occurring disorders. *Psychiatric Services, 56(10),* 1270-1273.

McGovern, M. P., Xie, H., Segal, S. R., Siembab, L., & Drake, R. E. (2006). Addiction treatment services and co-occurring disorders: Prevalence estimates, treatment practices, and barriers. *Journal of Substance Abuse Treatment, 31,* 267-275.

McHugo, G. J., Drake, R. E., Teague, G. B., & Xie, H. (1999). Fidelity to assertive community treatment and client outcomes in the New Hampshire dual disorders study. *Psychiatric Services, 50(6),* 818-824.

McHugo, G. J., Hargreaves, W., Drake, R. E., Clark, R. E., Xie, H., Bond, G. R., et al. (1998). Methodological issues in assertive community treatment studies. *American Journal of Orthopsychiatry, 68(2),* 246-260.

Miklowitz, D.J., Simoneau, T.L., George, E.I., Richards, J.A., Kalbag, A., Sach-Ericsson, N., et al. (2000). Family-focused treatment of bipolar disorder: One-year effects of a psychoeducation program in conjunction with pharmacotherapy, *Biological Psychiatry, 48,* 582-592.

Miller, J.S. (1990). Mental illness and spiritual crisis: Implications for psychiatric rehabilitation. *Psychosocial Rehabilitation Journal, 14,* 29-45.

Morrissey, J. P., Jackson, E. W., Ellis, A. R., Amaro, H., Brown, V. B., & Najavits, L. M. (2005). Twelve-month outcomes of trauma-informed interventions for women with co-occurring disorders. *Psychiatric Services, 56(10),* 1213-1222.

Morse, G. A., Calsyn, R. J., Klinkenberg, W. D., Helminiak, T. W., Wolff, N., Drake, R., et al. (2006). Treating homeless clients with severe mental illness and substance use disorders: Costs and outcomes. *Community Mental Health Journal, 42(4),* 377-404.

Mowbray, C.T., Collins, M.E., Bellamy, C.D., Megivern, D.A., Bybee, D., & Szilvagyi, S. (2005). Supported education for adults with psychiatric disabilities: an innovation for social work and psychosocial rehabilitation practice. *Social Work, 50(1),* 7-20.

Moxley, D.P., Mowbray, C.T., & Brown, K.S. (1993). Supported education. In P.W. Flexer, & P. Solomon (Eds.), Psychiatric rehabilitation in practice (pp. 137-153). Boston: Andover Medical Publishers.

Mueser, K. T., Aalto, S., Becker, D. R., Ogden, J. S., Wolfe, R. S., Schiavo, D., et al. (2005). The effectiveness of skills training for improving outcomes in supported employment. *Psychiatric Services, 56(10),* 1254-1260.

Mueser, K. T., Clark, R. E., Haines, M., Drake, R. E., McHugo, G. J., Bond, G. R., et al. (2004). The Hartford study of supported employment for persons with severe mental illness. *Journal of Counseling and Clinical Psychology, 7(3),* 479-490.

Mueser, K.T., Corrigan, P.W., Hilton, D.W., Tanzman, B., Schaub, A., Gingerich, S., et al. (2002). Illness management and recover: A review of the research. *Psychiatric Services, 53(10),* 1272-1284.

Mueser, K. T., Crocker, A. G., Frisman, L. B., Drake, R. E., Covell, N. H., & Essock, S. M. (2006). Conduct disorder and antisocial personality disorder in persons with severe psychiatric and substance use disorders. *Schizophrenia Bulletin, 32(4),* 626-636.

Mueser, K.T., & Mackain, S. (2006). Illness management and recover. *The National GAINS Center for Systemix Change for Justice-involved people with mental illness.*

Novak-Grubic,V. & Tavcar, R. (2002) Predictors of noncompliance in males with first-episode first-episode schizophrenia, schizophreniform and schizoaffective disorder. *European Psychiatry, 17,* 148 –154

Oliver, P. C., Piachaud, J., Tyrer, P., Regan, A., Dack, M., Alexander, R., et al. (2005). Randomized controlled trial of assertive community treatment in intellectual disability: The TACTILD study. *Journal of Intellectual Disability Research, 49(7),* 507-515.

Penn, D.L. & Mueser, K.T. (1996). Research updates on the psychosocial treatment of schizophrenia. *American Journal of Psychiatry, 153(5),* 607-617.

Perry, A., Tarrier, N., Morriss, R., McCarthy, E., & Limb, K. (1999). Randomized controlled trial of efficacy of teaching patients with bipolar disorder to identify early symptoms of relapse and obtain treatment. *British Medical Journal, 318,* 149-153.

Petrakis, I. L., Nich, C., & Ralevski, E. (2006). Psychotic spectrum disorders and alcohol abuse: A review of pharmacotherapeutic strategies and a report on the effectiveness of naltrexone and disulfiram. *Schizophrenia Bulletin, 32(4),* 644-654.

Phillips, S. D., Burns, B. J., Edgar, E. R., Mueser, K. T., Linkins, K. W., Rosenheck, R., et al. (2001). Moving assertive community treatment into standard practice. *Psychiatric*

*Services, 52(6),* 771-779.

Pillings, S. Bebbington, P. Kuipers, E., Garety, P., Geddes J., Martindale, B., et al. (2002). Psychological treatments in schizophrenia: Meta-analysis of family intervention and cognitive behavior therapy. *Psychological Medicine, 32(5),* 763-782.

Plante, T. G., & Sherman, A. S. (2001). *Faith and Health: Psychological Perspectives.* New York: Guilford.

Ralph, R. O. (2000). Recovery: contribution to the Surgeon General's report on mental health. *Psychiatric Rehabilitation Skills, 4,* 480-517.

Ralph, R.O. (2005). Verbal definitions and visual models of recovery: Focus on the recovery model. In R.O. Ralph and P.W. Corrigan (Eds.), *Recoveryin Mental Illness: Broadening Our Understanding of Wellness* (131-145). Washington D.C., American Psychological Association

Rea, M.M., Tompson, M.C., Miklowitz, D.J., Goldstein, M.J., Hwang, S., & Mintz, J. (2003). Family-focused treatment versus individual treatment for bipolar disorder: results of a randomized clinical trial. *Journal of Consulting and Clinical Psychology, 71(3),* 482-492.

Rehabilitation Act Amendments of 1998: Title IV of the Workforce Investment Act of 1998, Pub Law 105-220, 112 Stat 936.

Rush, A.J., Rago, W.V., Crismon, M.L., Toprac, M.G., Shon, S.P., Suppes, T., et al. (1999). Medication treatment for the severely and presistantly mentally ill: The Texas Medication Algorthm Program. *Journal of Clinical Psychiatry, 60,* 284-291.

SAMSHA, Center of Mental Health Services. (2003*). Family pscyhoeducation: Implementation resource kit.* Retrieved February 02, 2007, from http://download.ncadi.samhsa.gov/ken/pdf/toolkits/family/04.FamPsy_InfoCons.pdf.

Serban, G.A., & Thomas, A. (1974). Attitudes and behaviors of acute and chronic schizophrenic patients regarding ambulatory treatment. *American Journal of Psychiatry, 136,* 991-995.

Simoneau, T. L., Miklowitz, D. J., Richards, J. A., Saleem, R., & George, L. (1999). Bipolar disorder and family communication: The effects of a psychoeducational treatment program. *Journal of Abnormal Psychology, 108,* 588-597.

Solomon, P. & Draine, J. (1995). Subjective burden among family members of mentally ill adults. *American Journal of Orthopsychiatry, 65,* 419-427.

Stein, L. I., & Test, M. A. (1980). Alternative to mental hospital treatment: I. conceptual model, treatment program, and clinical evaluation. *Archives of General Psychiatry, 37,* 400-405.

Teague, G. B., Bond, G. R., & Drake, R. E. (1998). Program fidelity in assertive community treatment: Development and use of a measure. *American Journal of Orthopsychiatry, 68(2),* 216-232.

Tepper, L., Rogers, S.A., Coleman, E.M., & Malony, H.N. (2001). The Prevalence of Religious Coping Among Persons With Persistent Mental Illness. Psychiatric Services, 52, 660-665.

Tomaras, V., Mavreas, V., Economou, M., Ioannovich,E., Karydi, V., & Stefanis, C. (2000). The effect of family intervention on chronic schizophrenics under individual psychosocial treatment: a 3-year study. *Social Psychiatry Psychiatric Epidemiology, 35(11),* 487-493.

Velligan, D.I., Prihoda, T.J. Ritch, J.L. Maples, N., Bow-Thomas, C.C., & Dassori, A. (2002). A randomized single-blind pilot study of compensatory strategies in schizophrenia outpatients. *Schizophrenia bulletin, 28(2)*, 283-292.

Van Tosh, L., Ralph, R.O., Campbell, J. (2000). The rise of consumerism. *Psychiatric Rehabilitation Skills, 4(3),* 383-409.

Wehman, P. (1986). Supported competitive employment for persons with severe disabilities. *Journal of Applied Rehabilitation Counseling, 17,* 24-29.

Weiden, P., Rapkin, B., Mott, T., Zygmunt, A., Goldman, D., Horvitz-Lennon, M., et al. (1994). Rating of Medication Influences (ROMI) scale in schizophrenia. *Schizophrenia Bulletin 20,* 297– 310.

Weycker, D., Macarios, D., Edelsberg, J., & Oster, G. (2006). Compliance with drug therapy for postmenopausal osteoporosis. *Osteoporosis International, 17(11),* 1645-1652.

Xie, H., McHugo, G. J., Fox, M. B., & Drake, R. E. (2005). Substance abuse relapse in a ten-year prospective follow-up of clients with mental and substance use disorders. *Psychiatric Services, 56(10),* 1282-1287.

Yamada, K. Watanabe, K., Nemoto, N., Fujita, H., Chikaraishi, C., Yamauchi, K., et al. (2006). Prediction of medication noncompliance in outpatients with schizophrenia: 2-year follow-up study. *Psychiatry Research, 41(1),* 61-69.

Yang, J., Law, S., Chow, W., Andermann, L., Steinberg, R., & Sadavoy, J. (2005). Assertive community treatment for persons with severe and persistent mental illness in ethnic minority groups. *Psychiatric Services, 56(9),* 1053-1055.

In: Toward a Science of Clinical Psychology
Editor: Luciano L'Abate, pp. 307-320
ISBN: 978-1-60456-062-6


*Chapter XVI*

# VIRTUAL REALITY THERAPY: A VISION FOR A NEW PARADIGM

*Max M. North, Sarah M. North and Chad B. Burwick*

## ABSTRACT

Reality, like beauty, is in the eye of the beholder. This is not to be taken as a cynical statement about the human condition; instead, this is a fact of life. Virtual reality research explores just how far this statement travels in a scientific setting (North & North, 1994; Krijn et al., 2004). This ground-breaking field develops applications created as a consequence of the mind's ability to deceive itself, from training, to entertainment, to medical surgery. While there are many definitions of virtual reality, the most useful for the topic of this chapter is the human-computer interaction definition put forth by Sheridan (1992): a virtual reality exists when a user becomes an active participant in a computer-generated, three-dimensional world. Virtual reality provides a complete 360-degree visual display and other sensory inputs to users in order to create a simulation of a real-life situation that feels completely authentic and, in fact, produces many of the same psychological effects that a user might experience in a similar real-life scenario.

There are currently two major types of systems used in the generation of virtual reality: the head-mounted display (HMD) and the computer automatic virtual environment (CAVE) (North et al., 1996b). An HMD system transmits images to small screens directly in front of the user's eyes; motion trackers embedded in the headgear then determine the position of the user's gaze, and the computer displays the appropriate perspective, allowing the user to look around the virtual world just as he would in a real setting. In a CAVE system, users walk into a cube of large projection screens; three-dimensional effects are accomplished by wearing stereoscopic shutter glasses, which track the movement of the user's head and filter out the correct portions of light. While only one user may control the movement of the virtual world in the CAVE, a number of participants may enter and become fully immersed at the same time. In both types of systems, users are provided with a complete 360-degree field of vision, becoming totally immersed in the virtual world. This environment can be supplemented, to impressive effect, with sound, tactile stimuli (North, North & Coble, 1996c) and even scent (Varner, 1993), all controlled through a computer.

By far the most common application of virtual reality is professional training. A fully immersive simulation allows astronauts, fire-fighters (Tate et al., 1997), and even surgeons (Hoffman and Vu, 1997) to experience activities that would be unsafe or costly to reproduce during real-life training. However, virtual reality technology has caught the eye of a growing number of researchers in the field of clinical psychology. Over the past decade, dedicated researchers have used the immersive powers of virtual reality alongside the healing powers of behavioral psychology to offer very encouraging alternatives to existing psychotherapies (North, North & Coble, 1996a). We call this approach Virtual Reality Therapy (VRT, or VR therapy). In VRT, immersive virtual realities are used to aid a trained psychiatrist in the therapy of a client, most often by recreating a cognitive-behavioral exposure therapy approach within a virtual setting.

Virtual Reality Therapy exposes patients to virtual situations of increasing intensity and duration, seeking to provoke anxiety and then tear away that anxiety response through repetition, as in a typical exposure therapy. The advantage of VRT over the more common in-vivo approaches is the control it can give to the therapist. Because situations of exposure are simulated by a computer, therapists can choose precisely the intensity and duration of these experiences (North & North, 1994). Our vision for VRT in the future is that as virtual reality technology becomes more powerful and less expensive, therapists will have far more control in their therapeutic practice as well as a much wider range of alternative therapies. Clients (patients) will share in these benefits.

The actual treatment process varies, but it typically includes 15- to 45-minute sessions administered weekly for at least 8 weeks. In a desensitization process, the therapist sequences virtual scenes from least threatening to most, and the subject controls the advancement of scenes. Researchers of VRT collect data from subjects most often in survey form, using measures such as the Subjective Units of Discomfort/Distress Scale (SUDs) periodically during treatment. Treatment is often succeeded by a follow-up, which evaluates the effectiveness of a study in the long-term (North et al., 1995a, 1996a). Because the technology involved in this therapy is still relatively new, the costs involved can be prohibitive. However, as research evolves and as therapeutic practice sees more and more success, these costs will fall as the benefits rise.

The primary goal of this chapter is describe the VRT vision. This vision has behind it the weight of over a decade of solid research and fascinating new trends in technology and psychology. To walk the reader through this vision, this chapter will begin with a brief overview of the driving issues behind VRT study. With these issues in mind, we will examine both the seminal and most recent works in the field of VRT in an effort to trace the growth of the field and to understand its direction. Finally, this chapter will speculate on what we believe to be the next generation of VRT, outlining the therapies, theories, and technologies that will begin to realize VRT's ultimate promise an essential psychiatric tool.

## Dominant Issues

Before encountering the major studies, it is important to understand the underpinnings of research in Virtual Reality Therapy. Three central considerations mold the study of VRT: the type of therapy employed; the level of "presence," or the perception of reality; and safety. In this field, researchers must act as part psychologist and part computer scientist, and it is in these capacities that every study is concerned with therapeutic practices, presence, and safety.

## THERAPEUTICS

As mentioned above, the dominant psychological philosophy behind current VRT study is that of cognitive-behavioral therapy. VRT has thus far most often taken the form of exposure therapy because it is perhaps the most intuitive application of virtual reality technology. Furthermore, it is particularly suited to the practice of systematic desensitization therapy because of the high level of control it affords the therapist. The reviews of studies in this chapter are designed to elaborate on the existing methodology and philosophy behind VRT research.

However, researchers and clinicians should be encouraged to branch out, and indeed they are: forays into other therapeutic methods, as well as research on the synergistic potential of VRT, have yielded fruitful results (Krijn et al., 2004, Wiederhold et al., 1998). VRT research draws on traditional therapy techniques, a fact of which researchers are continually mindful; those involved in the study of VRT must at the very beginning concern themselves with a specific psychological approach and the myriad factors involved in its implementation, just as in traditional forms of therapy. The challenges particular to VRT, however, place an additional strain on researchers; the implementation of virtual reality to a therapeutic practice requires that we tackle problems of technology as well as those of psychology (North et al., 1996b). Furthermore, it is our personal belief that VRT merits its own unique treatment techniques; finding the therapies of the future is yet another challenge for researchers. In VRT, the treatment approach concerns not only existing therapy techniques, but also the exciting possibilities that only virtual reality can unlock. We are involved in a very creative enterprise.

## PRESENCE

Both Naiman (1992) and Loomis (1992; 1993) have argued that the normal human experience is not of the physical world but of our perceptions of the physical world. Presence is the term used in the study of virtual reality to denote the level of immersion; it is the qualitative measure of just how real a virtual experience feels to the subject. Because presence is such a subjective quality, it is difficult for the researcher to properly quantify. Held and Durlach (1992) discuss specifically the need to define the sensorimotor and cognitive factors that contribute to presence. Three measurable physical variables, proposed by Sheridan (1992), include the extent of sensory information, the control of relationship of sensors to the environment, and the ability to modify the physical environment. Other objective measures of presence include heart rate and body posture, but, as Krijn et al. (2004) point out, it is especially difficult in VRT to interpret these measurements, as anxiety induced in the normal course of exposure therapy leads to similar physical effects.

There has unfortunately not been enough research specifically on the problem of measuring presence or on the qualitative elements of a virtual setting that might affect presence. Some research suggests that the inclusion of the sense of touch, and the sense of smell may actually be more effective than visual and auditory treatments in creating sense of presence. However, future studies will require more conclusive and explicit details about the variables that determine the creation of presence. The future depends on making such variables more quantifiable and tractable.

## SAFETY

Safety is of course an important concern in any medical practice. There are some safety concerns associated with VRT. First, virtual exposure therapy carries health concerns because it provokes anxiety in the subject. Stanney (1995) identifies the subjects most at risk as those who suffer from panic attacks, those with heart disease or epilepsy, and those taking drugs with major physiological or psychological effects. These concerns must be, and are, addressed by the screening process. Additionally, some people experience symptoms ranging from headache to epileptic seizure when exposed to visual stimuli which flicker in the 8- to 12-Hz range. The general feeling in the field is that continued advances in technology will abate some of these dangers. Practitioners, of course, will always need to be mindful of these issues, just as in any medical procedure.

## RESEARCH

This section provides a very brief review of the existing research in VRT. In order to look forward, we must look behind us and identify those areas of VRT that are most promising and those that need more research. We must also recognize the salient issues that direct our study and those issues that we must resolve moving forward. VRT is used in the treatment of a variety of psychological disorders; while agoraphobia is certainly the most prevalent area of VRT study, there is also substantial prior research concerning the potential for VRT use in treating autism, obsessive-compulsive disorders, attention deficit/hyperactivity disorder, and post traumatic stress disorder. This section includes a brief look at each of these research areas.

## PHOBIAS

The first use of Virtual Reality Therapy was in the treatment of phobias. In 1994, we conducted the seminal study in VRT, one designed to combat the fear of flying (North et al., 1994). Since that time, no less than nine more studies have shown positive results in treating the fear of flying (North et al., 1995, 1996a, 1996d, 1997a; Hodges et al., 1996; Wiederhold et al., 1998; Klein, 2000; Kahan, Tanzer, Darvin, and Borer, 2000; Rothbaum et al., 2000, 2002; Mühlberger et al., 2001, 2003; Maltby et al., 2002). Countless more have been successful in treating fear of heights (acrophobia), fear of closed spaces (claustrophobia), fear of spiders (arachnophobia), fear of public speaking, and various other phobias. Our own research, and that of many others, has concentrated on such disorders, primarily because virtual reality lends itself so readily to exposure and desensitization therapies, the most successful therapies in the treatment of phobic disorders.

As mentioned in the previous section, direct control over the setting and parameters of exposure therapy is one tremendous advantage of VRT. This control allows for excellent treatment of agoraphobia with panic disorder. In a series of studies, our team exposed subjects to very specific and detailed agoraphobic situations (a few of which were a dark barn, a covered bridge, and the presence of black cats) to determine the efficacy of VRT in the treatment of this disorder (North et al. 1995a; 1995b; 1996a; 1996c).

Control over the virtual scenario is just one advantage of VRT. Other important benefits include cost and safety. These concerns were what prompted our studies on the fear of flying; because exposing a patient to air travel in vivo is an exorbitant process, VRT provides not only a more controlled and safer alternative to in vivo flight exposure, but also one that is far less expensive. VRT allows the client to experience flight more often, more cheaply, and with far fewer health concerns.

Fear of public speaking is another phobia whose treatment using VRT could remove the monetary and logistic troubles that exposure therapy commonly faces. Authors of this chapter initiated the first known study examining the ability of VRT to treat this disorder in 1997 (North et al., 1997). This study involved sixteen participants selected by a two-stage screening process; participants were assigned to either a VRT group or a control. The VRT group was subjected to five 10- to 15-minute sessions. Real world follow-ups showed a significant reduction in anxiety symptoms. Although the sample size of this study was small, the results were consistent with other studies in VRT for phobia, and further studies on VRT treatment of the fear of speaking have shown similar success. Anderson, Rothbaum, and Hodges (2003) reported on two case studies in which VRT was used to treat social phobia. The two patients were treated with a mixture of one or two in vivo and at least four virtual reality exposures. This combination of exposure led to a significant reduction in anxiety in both patients. Finally, Harris, Kemmerling, and North (2002) performed a study of 14 students with public speaking anxiety; this study is promising because of the wide range of testing rubrics, including ATPS, HR, LSAS, and PRCS. Because of the limited number of studies and the sample size of these studies, VRT's effectiveness in treating fear of public speaking is not yet conclusive. However, preliminary results have been promising and significant. Furthermore, therapists using VRT would gain a tremendous advantage in the treatment of this disorder: as in the treatment of fear of flying, VRT provides an alternative to in vivo exposure that is far more customizable and far less costly.

Just as safety is one of the appeals of choosing VRT for treatment of the fear of flying, it is also the primary concern of researchers in the treatment of acrophobia. Virtual Reality Therapy can perform the systematic desensitization process on an acrophobic patient in complete safety. An eight-story building rooftop in virtual space poses no more physical danger to the patient than the carpeted floor of a psychiatrist's office. No less than eight studies have explored this therapeutic advantage. The first known study of VRT implementation in acrophobia treatment took place in 1995 (Rothbanm, Hodges, et al., 1995a; 1995b). This study involved 20 subjects exhibiting acrophobia; 12 subjects were placed in Virtual Reality Therapy, while the other 8 were placed on the waiting list. Results showed that VRT was significantly more effective than no treatment; indeed, the results were on par with anxiety reduction given by Cohen's in vivo exposure study done in 1977 (Rothbanm, Hodges, et al., 1995a; 1995b). Following the success of this study, authors of this chapter performed a case study over the following year (North, North, & Coble, 1996a; 1996b; 1996c). This study involved a single subject over eight VR sessions. The improvement was striking; posttest follow-ups showed the treatment significantly reduced anxiety and avoidance behavior in the subject. Since then, many others have expanded on this research (Emmelkamp et al., 2001; 2002; Choi et al., 2001; Kamphuis et al., 2002; Krijn et al., 2004). The future in using VRT to treat acrophobia must focus primarily on strengthening the research; this means incorporating more subjects in group studies as well as conducting further in-depth case studies.

Other classes of phobia that have been treated by VRT include claustrophobia (Botella et al., 1998, 2000); fear of driving (Schare et al., 1999; Wald & Taylor, 2000), and arachnophobia (Carlin et al., 1997; Garcia-Palacios et al., 2002). Results have paralleled the success of other agoraphobias, but these fields require much more research. Future studies must do more than simply provide more data and larger sample sizes. They must also address the significant issue of presence which is particularly predominant in the research of phobias. Presence is the term we give to the general feeling of immersion participants feel in virtual environments. If the sense of presence is not sufficiently complete, then no anxiety is produced, and the principle behind most VRT research—the principle of exposure and desensitization—fails to materialize. Dropout rates have been particularly high in two of the acrophobia VRT studies (Emmelkamp et al., 2002; Krijn et al., 2004); the researchers cited a lack of presence in the experiences of some subjects.

The future in phobia treatment using VRT relies firstly on further increasing the cost incentive by employing new technologies. It will also be necessary for researchers to gain a better understanding of the unique effects of virtual reality on patients, both to increase effectiveness and to further minimize potential health risks.

## Anxiety in the Classroom: OCD, ADD, and Test-Anxiety

In 2000, we conducted a case study on a student suffering from obsessive-compulsive disorder (North et al., 2000). Virtual reality sessions consisted of a simulated book-bag with various school supplies. The Subject reported significant reduction in anxiety; follow-ups indicated continued comfort levels. Because OCD has a significant anxiety component attached to it, exposure therapy is often used in practice to help patients with the disorder (Valente, 2002). Suitably studied and advanced, VRT could help therapists hone in on the most anxiety-provoking activities for a subject and to observe these activities in real time in the comfort of the office.

We have also begun work very recently on test- and math-anxiety. In the first in-depth case study of the effectiveness of VRT as a treatment for Math Anxiety, we worked with a 28-year-old male whose anxiety and avoidance behavior was disrupting normal academic activities. In six sessions of increasing intensity, the subject was exposed to a virtual test-taking experience in both a virtual classroom and a virtual auditorium. SUDS suggested that the anxiety provoked by these sessions was every bit as real as anxiety felt during live test taking situations and included physical symptoms such as increased heart rate, mild dizziness, and headaches. Our results strongly suggest that VRT can be an effective treatment method for reducing anxiety and improving the performance of subjects who suffer from Math Anxiety.

Rizzo et al. (2000) performed a study examining VRT's feasibility in treating Attention-Deficit/Hyperactivity Disorder (ADHD). Their study concluded that Virtual Reality Therapy could offer a valuable alternative to traditional treatment by giving therapists excellent control over the exposure environments and by providing patients with sufficient time to respond appropriately. Future research in the area could yield very successful results.

The challenge of future studies will be to validate and expand on this groundwork. These fields in VRT are strongly tied to the VRT studies in phobias because of their behavioral approach: treat the anxiety to treat the disorder. However, these disorders are significantly different from the family of phobias. Furthermore, OCD, ADD, and Test Anxiety are all common in students and of particular interest to the study of childhood disorders. Most VRT research has concentrated solely on the adult population; the future of these studies could be a bridge to the treatment of younger populations.

## Other Applications

The possible applications for Virtual Reality Therapy are legion, and there has been significant research in some of these applications. Post-traumatic stress disorder, eating disorders, and autism have all been the subject of VRT study. As early as 1996, researchers were exploring the possibility of the treatment of autism through VRT (Strickland, 1996). Riva (1997a; 1997b) constructed a virtual environment designed for body treatment image modification and tested it on a group of 60 subjects; this therapy has great potential in the treatment of eating disorders. Hodges et al. (1999) treated Vietnam War veterans for post-traumatic stress disorder (PTSD) using virtual environments that simulated the traumatic experiences; the clinician reported a 34% decrease in symptoms, while the patients themselves reported a 45% decrease. Although studies in these areas are still in the earliest stages, results are promising, and everything indicates that future technology—specifically the ability to provide client-created environments on demand—will create a powerful synergy with these treatments to make them extremely effective.

Other applications that do not directly deal with any specific psychological disorders include image or visualization therapy, in which patients are prompted to picture objects and even people. Glantz et al. (1997) proposed the development of virtual personae with whom patients can interact during therapy involving relationships or conflict resolution.

## VRT: The Next Generation

What should we look forward to as we move into the next phase of Virtual Reality Therapy? Naturally, the end goal is to see its common use in clinical practice. Toward that end, we hope to see trends that introduce new forms of treatment, new methods of delivery, and increasingly advanced technology.

## New Treatments

The future of Virtual Reality Therapy from the therapeutic perspective lies in finding innovative new treatments that can leverage the advantages of VRT to the fullest. This leverage will lie not only in applying existing therapy techniques to virtual reality technologies but also in exploring the synergistic possibilities of the technology as well as entirely new therapies unique to VRT. We hope to see in future studies a movement in two directions: toward clinical trials where existing research has already shown promise and toward new areas of therapy. Thus, in using VRT for the treatment of phobias, we expect much larger studies including clinical settings; in disorders that have proven especially difficult to diagnose and treat, such as ADHD, PTSD, and Autism, we expect to see VRT applied in exciting, innovative ways.

There is also a push to migrate other traditional treatment approaches into VRT implementations. An unpublished preliminary investigation at the authors' VRT laboratory explored the use of virtual environments in empty-chair therapy, a technique which operates by asking clients to visualize and confront a person with whom he is in conflict. This is a wonderfully simple technique, so why would anyone want to complicate it by incorporating a virtual environment? There are significant advantages to moving the empty chair into a virtual setting. The therapist can manipulate environmental effects, such as lighting, that can provide a more controlled setting. It may soon be possible to *fill* the empty chair. Several years ago, Glantz et al. (1997) proposed the use of three-dimensional virtual avatars that could visually represent the antagonist. Merely a shadow or outline of a figure is sufficient to elicit appropriate responses from the client; however, advances in technology will provide us the option of reconstructing almost flawlessly the features of a father, friend, relative, or whomever the therapist decides the client should confront in this virtual world. This type of therapy would be useful in general conflict resolution as well as in confronting fears of emotional and sexual intimacy.

Rehabilitation is another very important field of therapy that will soon see VRT in use. Holden & Todorov (2002) published a study exploring VRT's ability to facilitate motor learning in the process of physical rehabilitation. In another study, VRT was used in cognitive nervous system (CNS) dysfunction treatment (Rizzo et al., 2002). Merians et al. (2002) suggest the use of virtual reality in the rehabilitation of stroke patients. These recent studies are among the first to exhibit VRT's potential beyond the realm of anxiety disorders, and further research on this vein should be encouraged.

## New Theories

At this time, there is no concrete or empirically based evidence to explain why and how VRT works. There is a great need for researchers to investigate the psychological mechanics of VRT. As stated before, the idea of presence is a concept neither fully developed nor understood by researchers. This is just one of the theoretical aspects of VRT that will be fleshed out in the course of future research.

Furthermore, as the psychological processes that explain how humans experience virtual environments become more understood, we expect to see a more mature generation of VRT study in which researchers possess the luxury of a "unified theory of VR", to borrow a concept from the world of physics. Finer control over a patient's anxiety response will yield more effective therapy. One avenue toward this future may lie in the work of Frances Shapiro (1995). Just one decade ago, Shapiro introduced an exciting new paradigm in cognitive-behavioral theory called accelerated integrative information processing. One consequence of this theory states that the physical activities of the body, most especially eye movements, are integral to the processing of information by the mind. In a behavioral approach, modification of this physical activity leads to a modification of mental state. The treatment now in practice that has resulted from Shapiro's work is called Eye Movement Desensitization Reprocessing (EMDR). What is exciting about this development within the scope of Virtual Reality Therapy is that observation implies that some process very similar to EMDR has taken place in virtual settings during therapy. While virtual environments provide a strong sense of immersion, our own observations lead us to believe that advanced graphics seem to distract and overload human perception, causing interference in processes essential to problem solving and information reprocessing. This may mean that the success of VRT may have a good deal to do with Shapiro's information processing theory and its related therapies; this is certainly an avenue that will be explored in future research. Instead of the current practice of EMDR therapy, in which the therapist physically manipulates or distracts the client, this desensitization reprocessing could be performed within the virtual environment itself, possibly with a greater degree of control and precision.

The theories of Frances Shapiro and other psychological theories not yet fully explored by researchers of Virtual Reality Therapy will be just as important to the future success of this field as the explosive improvements in technology. Alongside large clinical studies in previously explored VRT treatments, theoretical research into virtual reality's operative effects on the human mind will continue to move VRT toward general practice among the psychiatric community.

## Introducing the Internet

The World Wide Web and Virtual Reality Therapy have grown up together; our team was performing the first known VRT study in 1994, just one year before the foundation of Yahoo! in 1995. As both technologies have grown in scope, so too have they grown in application. Because VRT and internet share somewhat of a common history, we hope that they may also share a common future. Already, virtual reality environments have been produced and streamed over the internet to distant points—this practice is prevalent in training simulators. The next leap is to employ VRT via an internet connection. This would remove the physical limitation that requires a therapist, his client, and the VR equipment to be in the same place at the same time. A therapist could provide therapy in real time from his Atlanta office to a patient in London, England. The client would only need a VR display connected to his computer. Through the use of his own VR equipment, the therapist could communicate with the patient and control the virtual experience. The only boundary standing in the way of this form of therapy is economics. It is unfortunately not economically feasible at this time to provide most clients with the necessary equipment. However, authors of this chapter are currently experimenting with an inexpensive device designed to work with a regular computer display that could provide appropriate levels of immersion. There is also a work-around alternative to requiring that the client possess any equipment. In several U.S. cities, there could be facilities connected by satellite to provide VR stations to users. A client would seek out the facility in his own city and set up a session with a therapist in another part of the world. Though internet-provided VRT is likely some years away, valuable research can and should start right away.

## VR on Demand: Client Controlled Environments

As noted earlier in this paper, detailed control over every aspect of the virtual experience is one of the greatest strengths of the Virtual Reality Therapy paradigm. This level of control comes much easier to the virtual medium than it does to practice in real life, but it is nevertheless not without its costs. Developing general scenarios for use in a study of agoraphobia is easy enough; such scenarios are often suitable for use in every case. However, the creation of a virtual environment on a case-by-case basis can be time consuming. The next leap in VRT is to provide a level of customization that will enable therapists to instantly design, create, and implement virtual environments for use with individual patients.

The bottleneck here is simply in the software. While there are many viable software suites for the development of virtual environments, general and widespread therapeutic practice will require something more tailor-made. It is not much of a stretch to imagine a system that can build itself in real-time to the needs of the client. Pilot studies by the authors have investigated the possibility of employing speech recognition software and a speech generation interface to build virtual environments. In a scene reminiscent of Star Trek, a therapist immersed in a virtual world could issue simple commands: "Computer, raise the lighting. Create a chair. A desk. Create a tree. Make the tree larger." In this manner, the therapist could immediately customize the environment for use in therapy.

Another potential consequence of this amazing level of control would be the utilization of psychotherapy techniques to allow the client to visually trace his memory in real-time using nothing but his voice. This has tremendous implications for regression therapy, the legitimate use of which is used to treat disorders resulting from traumatic experience.

## Summary and Recommendation

What this chapter has outlined is merely a fraction of what we hope will become the future of Virtual Reality Therapy. The new applications and theories suggested here represent only what we believe to be feasible in the very near future. Some decades from today, we can perhaps imagine virtual environments that are all but indistinguishable from reality. We can imagine entire therapy sessions taking place in virtual settings over the internet while the respective parties remain in the comfort of home or office. VRT may some day provide help for disorders that traditional therapy simply cannot provide. However, it is not the objective of this chapter to speculate, but instead to make the communities interested in our work aware of the tangible benefits VRT offers as well as the challenges that must be overcome to realize those rewards.

VRT should not be considered merely an enhancement to traditional methods of psychotherapy. Synergy with existing treatment is of course an important avenue of study, but the potential of VRT lies beyond, offering alternatives to medication and behavioral therapy. While the use of VRT in exposure therapy reproduces traditional desensitization therapy, it has its own unique effects as well as the potential for unlimited customization. Unlocking this potential will require prolonged, innovative, and collaborative research that focuses on multiple aspects of VRT. We must explore the psychological mechanics of the virtual experience including the sense of presence, and at the same time we must explore new therapeutic avenues with an emphasis on preparing VRT for general practice.

## Acknowledgement

The research projects described in this chapter were sponsored by several grants from Boeing Computer Services (Virtual Systems Department), U.S. Army Research Laboratory under contract DAAL03-92-6-0377, and supported by the Emory University and Georgia Institute of Technology Biomedical Technology Research Center (for the collaborative research of the fear of heights). The views contained in this document are those of the authors and should not be interpreted as representing the official policies of the U.S. government, either expressed or implied.

## References

Anderson, P., Rothbaum, B.O., & Hodges, L.F. (2003). Virtual reality exposure in the treatment of social anxiety. *Cognitive and Behavioral Practice*, *10*, 240-247.

Botella, C., Baños, R.M., Perpiñá, C., Villa, H, Alcañiz, M. & Rey, A. (1998). Virtual reality treatment of claustrophobia: A case report. *Behaviour Research and Therapy.*

Botella, C., Baños, R.M., Villa, H., Perpiña, C., & Garcia-Palacios, A. (2000). Virtual reality in the treatment of claustrophobic fear: A controlled, multiple-baseline design. *Behavior Therapy*, *31*, 583-595.

Carlin, A.S., Hoffman, H.G., & Weghorst, S. (1997). Virtual reality and tactile augmentation in the treatment of spider phobia: A case report. *Behaviour Research and Therapy*, *35*, 153-158.

Choi, Y.H., Jang, D.P., Ku, J.H., Shin, M.B., & Kim, S.I. (2001). Short-term treatment of acrophobia with virtual reality therapy (VRT): A case report. *Cyberpsychology and Behavior*, *4*, 349-454.

Emmelkamp, P.M.G., Bruynzeel, M., Drost, L., & van der Mast, C.A.P.G. (2001). Virtual reality treatment in acrophobia: A comparison with exposure in vivo. *Cyberpsychology and Behavior*, *4*, 335-339.

Emmelkamp, P.M.G., Krijn, M., Hulsbosch, A.M., de Vries, S., Schuemie, M. J., & van der Mast, C.A.P.G. (2002). Virtual reality treatment versus exposure in vivo: A comparative evaluation in acrophobia. *Behaviour Research and Therapy*, *40*, 509-516.

Garcia-Palacios, A., Hoffman, H., Carlin, A., Furness III, T.A., & Botella, C. (2002). Virtual reality in the treatment of spider phobia: A controlled study. *Behaviour Research and Therapy*, *40*, 983-993.

Glantz, K. Durlach, N.I., Barnett. R.C., Aviles, W.A. (1997). Virtual reality (VR) and psychotherapy: Opportunities and Challenges. *PRESENCE, Teleoperators and Virtual Environments. 6*(1).

Harris, S.R., Kemmerling, R.L., & North, M.M. (2002). Brief virtual reality therapy for public speaking anxiety. *Cyberpsychology and Behavior*, *5*, 543-550.

Held, R.M. and Durlach, N.I. (1992) Presence. *PRESENCE, Teleoperators and Virtual Environments*, 1(1), 109-112.

Hodges, L.F., Rothbaum, B.O., Alarcon, R., Ready, D., Shahar, F., Graap, K., Pair, J., Herbert, P., Gotz, D., Wills, D., & Baltzell., D. (1999). Virtual Vietnam: a virtual environment for the treatment of Vietnam war veterans with post-traumatic stress disorder, CyberPsychology & Behavior 2(1).

Hodges, L.A., Rothbaum, B.O., Watson, B.A., Kessler G.D., and Opdyke, D. (1996). Virtually conquering fear of flying. IEEE Computer Graphics & Applications, 16(6), 42-49.

Hoffman, H., and Vu, D. Virtual reality: teaching tool of the 21st Century? Academic Medicine. 1997; 72:1076-1081.

Holden, M.K., Todorov, E. (2002). Use of virtual environments in motor learning and rehabilitation. In Stanney, K.M. (Ed.), *Handbook of virtual environments: Design, implementation, and applications* (pp. 999-1026). Mahwah, New Jersey: Lawrence Erlbaum Associates, Inc.

Kahan, M., Tanzer, J., Darvin, D., & Borer, F. (2000). Virtual reality-assisted cognitive-bahavioral treatment for fear of flying: Acute treatment and follow-up. *Cyberpsychology and Behavior*, *3*, 387-392.

Kamphuis, J.H., Emmelkamp, P.M.G., & Krijn, M. (2002). Specific phobia. In Hersen, M. (Ed.), *Clinical behavior therapy, adults and children* (pp. 75-89). New York: John Wiley & Sons.

Klein, R. A. (2000). Virtual reality exposure therapy in the treatment of fear of flying. *Journal of Contemporary Psychotherapy*, *30*, 195-207.

Krijn, M., Emmelkamp, P.M.G., Biemond, R., de Wilde de Ligny, C., Shuemie, M. J., & van der Mast, C.A.P.G. (2004). Treatment of acrophobia in virtual reality: The role of immersion and presence. *Behaviour Research and Therapy*, *42*, 229-239.

Loomis, J.M. (1992) Distal attribution and presence. *PRESENCE, Teleoperators and Virtual Environments*, 1(1), 113-119.

Loomis, J.M. (1993). Understanding synthetic experience must begin with the analysis of ordinary perceptual experience. *IEEE Symposium on Research Frontiers in Virtual Reality* (pp. 54-57). San Jose, California.

Maltby, N., Kirsch, I., Mayers, M., & Allen, G.J. (2002). Virtual reality exposure therapy for the treatment of fear of flying: A controlled investigation. *Journal of Consulting and Clinical Psychology*, *70*, 1112-1118.

Merians, A.S, Jack, D., Boian, R., Tremaine, M., Burdea, G.C., Adamovich, S.V., Reece, M., Poizner, H. (2002). Virtual reality-augmented rehabilitation for patients following stroke. *Physical Therapy*, *82*, 898-915.

Mühlberger, A., Herrmann, M. J., Widemann, G., Ellgring, H., & Pauli, P. (2001). Repeated exposure of flight phobics to flights in virtual reality. *Behaviour Research and Therapy*, *39*, 1033-1050.

Mühlberger, A., Widemann, G. & Pauli, P. (2003). Efficacy of a one-session virtual reality exposure treatment for fear of flying. *Psychotherapy Research*, *13*, 323-336.

Naiman, A. (1992). Presence, and other gifts. *PRESENCE, Teleoperators and Virtual Environments*, 1(1), 145-148.

North, M.M., and North, S.M. (1994). Virtual environments and psychological disorders. *Electronic Journal of Virtual Culture, 2*(4), 37-42(ep.).

North, M.M., North, S.M., and Coble, J.R. (1995a). An effective treatment for psychological disorders: Treating agoraphobia with virtual environment desensitization. *CyberEdge Journal, 5*(3), 12-13.

North, M.M., North, S.M., and Coble, J.R. (1995b). Effectiveness of virtual environment desensitization in the treatment of agoraphobia. *International Journal of Virtual Reality, 1*(2), 25-34.

North, M.M, North, S.M., and Coble, J.R. (1996a). *Virtual Reality Therapy, An innovative paradigm*. CO: IPI Press.

North, M.M., North, S.M., and Coble, J.R. (1996b). Effectiveness of virtual environment desensitization in the treatment of agoraphobia. *PRESENCE, Teleoperators and Virtual Environments. 5*(4).

North, M.M., North, S.M., and Coble, J.R. (1996c). Application: Psychotherapy, Flight Fear Flees, *CyberEdge Journal, 6*(1), 8-10.

North, M.M., and North, S.M. (1996d). Virtual psychotherapy. *Journal of Medicine and Virtual Reality, 1*(2), 28-32.

North, M.M., North, S.M., and Coble, J.R. (1997a). Virtual environment psychotherapy: A case study of fear of flying disorder. *PRESENCE, Teleoperators and Virtual Environments. 6*(1).

North, M.M., North, S.M., and Coble, J.R. (1997b). Virtual Reality Therapy Combating Fear of Public Speaking. Medicine Meets Virtual Reality.

North, M.N., North, S.M., Virtual reality combats obsessive-compulsive disorders (OCD), (2000). Medicine Meets Virtual Reality 2000 Conference.

Riva, G., (1997a). The virtual environment for body image modification (VEBIM): development and preliminary evaluation. *PRESENCE, Teleoperators and Virtual Environments. 6*(1).

Riva, G., (1997b). Virtual Reality in Neuro-Psycho-Physiology, IOS Press.

Rizzo, A.A.; Buckwalter, J.G.; Bowerly, T.; Van Der Zaag, C.; Humphrey, L.; Neumann, U.; Chua, C.; Kyriakakis, C.; Van Rooyen, A.; Sisemore, D. (2000). The virtual classroom: A virtual reality environment for the assessment and rehabilitation of attention deficits. *Cyberpsychology and Behavior*, *3*, 483-499.

Rizzo, A.A., Buckwalter, J.G., & van der Zaag, C. (2002). Virtual environment applications in clinical neuropsychology. In Stanney, K.M. (Ed.), *Handbook of virtual environments: Design, implementation, and applications* (pp. 1027-1064). Mahwah, New Jersey: Lawrence Erlbaum Associates, Inc.

Rothbaum, B.O., Hodges, L.F., Anderson, P.L., Price, L., & Smith, S. (2002). Twelve-month follow-up of virtual reality and standard exposure therapies for the fear of flying. *Journal of Consulting and Clinical Psychology*, *70*, 428-432.

Rothbaum, B., Hodges, L.F., Kooper, R., Opdykes, D., Williford, J., and North, M. (1995a). Effectiveness of computer-generated (virtual reality) graded exposure in the treatment of acrophobia. *American Journal of Psychiatry, 152(4)*, 626-628.

Rothbaum, B.O., Hodges, L.F., Opdyke, D., Kooper, R., Williford, J.S., and North, M.M. (1995b). Virtual reality graded exposure in the treatment of acrophobia: A case study. *Journal of Behavior Therapy, 26(3)*, 547-554.

Rothbaum, B.O., Hodges, L.F., Smith, S., Lee, J.H., & Price, L. (2000). A controlled study of virtual reality exposure therapy for the fear of flying. *Journal of Consulting and Clinical Psychology*, *68*, 1020-1026.

Sheridan, T.B. (1992). Musing on telepresence and virtual presence. *PRESENCE, Teleoperators and Virtual Environments. 1*(1), 120-126.

Schare, M. L., Scardapane, J.R., Berger, A.L., Rose, N., & Berger, S. (1999). A virtual reality based anxiety induction procedure with driving phobic patients. Presented at Association for Advancement of Behavior Therapy, November, 1999, Toronto.

Shapiro, F. (1995). *Eye movement desensitization and reporocessing*. New York: The Guilford Press.

Stanney, K. (1995). Realizing the full potential of virtual reality: Human factors issues that could stand in the way. *IEEE Proceedings of Virtual Reality Annual International Symposium '95*. Research Triangle Park, North Carolina, 28-34.

Strickland, D., Marcus, L., Hogan, K., Mesibov, G., and McAllister, D. (1995). Using virtual reality as a learning aid for autistic children. *Proceedings of the Autism France 3rd International Conference on Computers and Autism* (pp. 119-132). Nice, France.

Tate, D., L., Sibert, L., & King T. (1997). Virtual environments for shipboard firefighting training. *Proceedings of the 1997 Virtual Reality Annual International Symposium.*

Valente, Shardon M. (2002). Obsessive-Compulsive Disorder. *Perspectives in Psychiatric Care*, *38*, 1.

Varner, D. (1993). Olfaction and VR. *Proceedings of the Conference on Intelligent Computer-Aided Training and Virtual Environment Technology*, Houston, TX.

Wald, J., & Taylor, S. (2000). Efficacy of virtual reality exposure therapy to treat driving phobia: A case report. *Journal of Behaviour Therapy and Experimental Psychiatry*, *31*, 249-257.

Wiederhold, B.K. & Wiederhold, M.D. 1998. A review of virtual reality as a psychotherapeutic tool, CyberPsychology & Behavior 1(1), 45-52.

Wiederhold, B.K., Gevirtz, R., & Wiederhold, M.D., (1998). Fear of flying: a case report using Virtual Reality Therapy with physiological monitoring, CyberPsychology & Behavior.

In: Toward a Science of Clinical Psychology
Editor: Luciano L'Abate, pp. 321-336
ISBN: 978-1-60456-062-6


*Chapter XVII*

# METHODOLOGICAL PSYCHOTHERAPY

***Piero De Giacomo, Andrea De Giacomo, Francesco Margari, Rita Masellis and Wanda Santamato***

## ABSTRACT

This chapter is based on the view that in the future the field of psychotherapy may resort to different cognitive tools from the traditional ones, thanks to contributions from other disciplines like artificial intelligence, algebra, and logic. Starting from these premises, in this chapter we report data on our research that could mark the start, or first step along a new line of reflection and application in the field of psychological and psychotherapeutic interventions.

The formal basis underlying this research is the Elementary Pragmatic Model, a model of the mind, interactions and changes that is not considered in detail herein because it has already been presented in many publications and reviews (Silvestri 1980, De Giacomo, 1992, De Giacomo 1993, L'Abate et al., 2000, L'Abate & De Giacomo 2003, De Giacomo et al, 1997, 2000, 2007).

This chapter, therefore, deals only with experimentation based on the use and development of a specific test of the Elementary Pragmatic Model (EPM), the SISCI test (acronym of Synthesis and Scission) evaluated in the 1970s and fully defined in the 1980s (L'Abate & De Giacomo, 2003). It is based on Holtzman's Inkblot figures but adopted in our research in a different way from the usual procedure, as described below (Holtzman, 1961). The possible application of the method to families has also been described (Pierri, 1992).

In current research, we adopted a SISCI procedure in which sentences with a strong psychological impact replaced the 90 figures of the Holtzman test. We define this procedure as SISCI-Sentences to differentiate it from the previous SISCI-Figures procedure. These sentences were generated from the interpretation of dreams according to the EPM (De Giacomo et al., 2004). Briefly, each dream was recorded in a computer program and processed, freely in a first step and then on a grid based on the EPM classification. At the end of processing each dream, a sentence will emerge describing the participant's knowledge of him/herself and/or of the world. This method generated an extremely large number of sentences that were adopted to create reflections on the self and the world (De Giacomo and Iadicicco, 2001).

From among the 500 sentences that emerged from this procedure, a group of expert psychologists and psychiatrists, including also the authors of this work, selected 90 sentences. The 90 sentences are presented one at a time to participants, who are asked to write down on a specific chart which sentences they liked best, or which had the strongest impact on them. Subsequently, participants are shown, one at a time, forty sentences (randomly selected) defined as other possible choices by most viewers. Finally, participants are asked to make the same choice as in the first step, again on the complete set of 90 sentences. In short, the test involves a choice of sentences with a strong psychological impact in Stage 1, followed by a set "perturbation" phase in Stage 2 (definable as presenting the "world of others" through random selection), and then in Stage 3 making another choice among the same set of 90 sentences. This three-step procedure yielded an algebraic process that can quantify the percentage of times a given subject chose, in the second stage, a sentence they had not chosen in the first and that was not present in the randomized choices ( U1 Antifunction ); the percentage of times the subject chose, in the second stage, a sentence they had not chosen in the first but that was present in randomized choices (U2 Acceptance ); the percentage of times the subject choose, in the second stage, a sentence that he had chosen in the first but that was not present in the randomized choices ( U3 Maintenance ), the percentage of the times the subject had chosen the same sentence, present among the randomized choices, in both stages ( U4 Sharing ).

Thus, the calculation of the coordinates (based on the three steps of the test: first choice, randomized selection choice, second choice) is as follows:

1. Two alternatives, according to whether, in Stage 3, participants choose (n001) or do not choose (n000) a sentence that was not chosen in Stage 1 and was not presented in Stage 2.
2. Two other alternatives according to whether, in Stage 3, participants choose (n011) or do not choose (n010) a sentence not chosen in Stage 1 but which was shown in Stage 2.
3. Another two alternatives, according to whether, in stage 3, participants choose (n101) or do not choose (n100) a sentence that was chosen in stage 1 but was not shown in stage 2.
4. Finally, two other alternatives according to whether, in stage 3, participants choose (n111) or do not choose (n110) a sentence that was chosen in Stage 1 and was shown in Stage 2.

These 8 alternatives represent the four main Coordinates in the EPM. According to the relative frequencies in which those four possibilities occur in the same participant, four Coordinates are developed:

a. Antifunction: $U1 = n(001)/(n(001)+n(000))$;
b. Maintenance: $U2 = n(101)/(n(101)+n(100))$;
c. Acceptance: $U3 = n(011)/(n(011)+n(010))$;
d. Sharing: $U4 = n(111)/(n(111)+n(110))$.

Results were calculated in terms of these Coordinates and of sixteen functions obtained following the mathematical computation described in De Giacomo, 2007. Scoring is based on the changes occurring in the overall responses of participants from the first to the second presentation. It is measured on the basis of repeated interactions, described by the patterns of sixteen functions (F0 to F15): a standard calculated as the mean of patterns obtained from normal participants. At each interaction a change occurred in the participants' pattern according to the EPM Table of Paradoxes (L'Abate & De Giacomo, 2003, pp. 122-123). In this way, after a certain number of interactions, the participant's state is always found to be crystallized in only three, simpler final states F0, F3, F15. Previously published experiments (L'Abate & De Giacomo, 2003, De Giacomo et al. 2007) show that normal participants have different results from pathological participants and also that the patterns of the coordinates, functions and final states derived, change after psychological intervention based on the sentences.

One question we needed to answer at the start of this study pertained to whether it is more efficacious to use questions or sentences; this question underlies the issue of whether the use of questions or sentences is more efficacious in psychotherapy in general. To answer

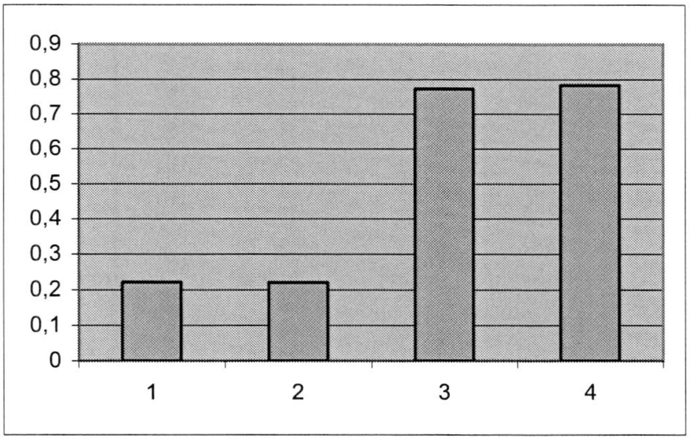


Figure 1: Mean values of the Coordinates in 98 students of Medicine using the SISCI-Questions

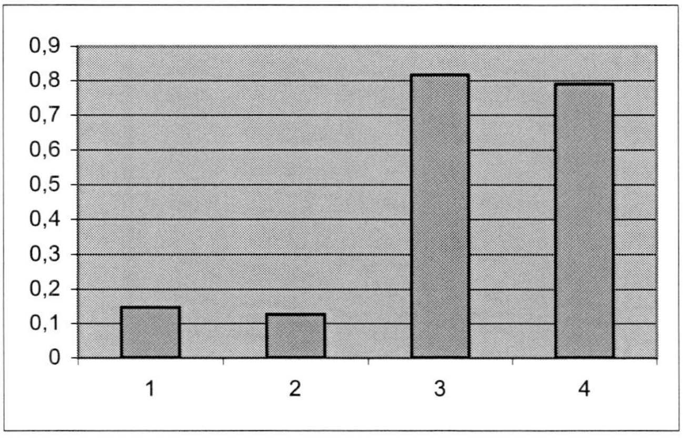


Figure 2: Mean values of the Coordinates in 98 students of Medicine using the SISCI-Sentences

this question and so choose between the two options, we carried out an experiment with 98 medical students using the same three-stage organization characteristic of SISCI: a) the subject's first choice among 90 elements, b) the choice among 40 of the 90 elements selected by the experiment operator, generally chosen by randomization , c) the subject's second choice, again among the 90 elements.

The list of 90 sentences and 90 questions used in this experiment is reported rispectively in table 1 and in table 2.

The results are described in Figures 1 and 2 and table 3.

Table 3 shows the statistical differences found when comparing the SISCI-Sentences to the SISCI-Questions. There was a significant difference for three of the four coordinates (U1 antifunction that appears lower, U2 acceptance that appears lower, U3 maintenance that appears increased, while U4 shows no significant difference.). Following this outcome, we decided to use the sentences not the questions, because with the sentences the pattern of coordinates was more strongly differentiated, better characterized in the sense of less chaos (coordinate U1 antifunction) and there was greater acceptance of the participant's own world (coordinate U3 maintenance). This choice supports the idea that psychotherapeutic interventions may be more efficacious when based on statements than on questions .

After choosing the SISCI-Sentences, we administered a further series of studies with normal and pathological participants. Their results have been already been published or are in press (De Giacomo et al. 2007; De Giacomo et al. in press).

An original as yet unpublished work examined whether the results were the same or different when participants with a pathological pattern of functions were set to interact with "themselves" or with the group of junior residents in the psychiatry training group, and if the latter case was true whether the results were nearer or further from the overall results in the pathological group.

This research showed a reduction of chaos (impossibility of choosing) and an increase in nullification or a "mental vacuum" when interacting with the pattern of Junior residents in comparison with interacting with their own pattern. The results are shown in Figure 3, figure 4 and Table 4.

Our interest in the use of sentences in the field of psychotherapy is owed to an experience common to many psychotherapists (De Giacomo et al., in press) when patients treated several years earlier return for a visit or accompany another patient. Sometimes, they refer that a certain sentence used with them many years earlier was very important, and acted as a kind of compass for their lives, an element around which they organized their minds. The issue of using sentences with a strong psychological impact in psychotherapy is linked to the problem of how to make sentences more effective. (De Giacomo et coll., 2004, 2006) There are various possibilities: a) creating expectations about the sentence that will be said to them, b) referring the previously described experience with patients seen years before who describe the importance in their lives of a certain sentence said to them; c) asking the subject to repeat the chosen sentence at each session or visit ; d) asking the subject to work on the sentence, by considering the reason why they chose it, for instance, how it fits into their convictions, what associations it arouses in them, what episodes in their life it evokes, how they would extend the sentence from their own point of view, what story they would build on it; e) creating a metaphorical structure that encourages acceptance of the sentence; f) asking the person who should accept the sentence to create a mental vacuum or another mental state (see mental states of the EPM, Wikipedia 2006) and then tell them the sentence; g) using the sentence in

**Table 1.**

| LIST OF THE 90 QUESTIONS ADOPTED FOR THE SISCI-QUESTIONS |
|---|
| 1) Which event or experience taught me most? |
| 2) What is the thing you wish for most? |
| 3) What do you like about yourself and what would you change? |
| 4) What excites you? |
| 5) Which bad experience would you cancel from your mind? |
| 6) What is the worst thing that ever happened to you? How did you get over it? |
| 7) What is my strength? |
| 8) Who is the dearest person to you, among the ones you know? |
| 9) What question would center the core of my mind? |
| 10) Do you think that your life experiences helped you to improve your knowledge of the world or of yourself? |
| 11) What element, event or situation of the past has an influence upon my present choices and my way of being? |
| 12) What is the thing I shun most and in what way? |
| 13) What is the gift you would like to receive most? |
| 14) Speak of the most recurring thought that comes to light when you are alone. |
| 15) What or who do I think is indispensable in my life, almost necessary to life? |
| 16) What situation causes you embarrassment? |
| 17) What is for you necessary and fundamental? |
| 18) What relation can you define between living and dreaming? |
| 19) Have you ever been completely happy and satisfied in your life? |
| 20) What would you change in your life? |
| 21) Describe the most important decision you had to take. |
| 22) What is the greatest satisfaction you had in life? |
| 23) What is your main purpose in life? |
| 24) What among your dreams did you make come true? |
| 25) If you could change yourself, what would you change? |
| 26) Am I always myself, or do I hide behind a mask? |
| 27) Think about something that made you suffer but changed your life positively. |
| 28) When I am with others am I myself or do I play a part? |
| 29) What would you do if you had no limits and prohibitions? |
| 30) If you could change your identity for a day, who would you like to be? |
| 31) Am I disposed to open my mind to another person? |
| 32) What would you not change in your life for any reason? |
| 33) Which situations had I to face in my life that made me grow and mature? |
| 34) How do I try to overcome obstacles? |
| 35) Is it important what people think of me? |
| 36) If you had to make a list of the values in which you believe, which would be the first ones? |
| 37) When was the last moment you lived when you felt happy? |
| 38) Which activities among the ones you practice are satisfying for you? |
| 39) What metaphor would you choose to describe yourself in relation to other people? |
| 40) What would make you happy at this moment? |
| 41) If you could change the world as you like, how would you rebuild it? |
| 42) What was the most important step in your life? |
| 43) If you could be a VIP for a day, who would you like to be? |
| 44) Who are you? If you had to define yourself with an adjective, which one would you choose? |
| 45) What is the worst accusation that people can make against you? And the best compliment? |
| 46) If I was on a solitary isle, who would I take with me? |
| 47) What is my greatest hope? |

48) Am I happy because of other people's happiness?
49) Can you sum up in a metaphor the way you feel at this moment?
50) What is the most beautiful dream you had?
51) Think about the last time you laugh.
52) How could we be aware of present happiness?
53) What is the most beautiful memory for me?
54) Do you think you are more like a sphere, a square or a triangle?
55) Have you ever desired with eagerness anything, struggling to obtain it at any cost, and fearing it when you were almost able to grasp it?
56) Have you ever loved anybody?
57) Who is the first person to whom you would address a letter?
58) Does it happen to you more frequently to talk or to argue with yourself?
59) What is the most precious thing I possess?
60) what would make me happy?
61) What does strike you in a person that you meet for the first time?
62) What do people who know me see of positive in me?
63) What do I see of positive around me?
64) In which occasions I feel the need to hide my real I? And why?
65) Let imagine yourself in some years time: what would you see?
66) Have you ever pretend to be someone that you are not?
67) Which characteristics must possess someone to become one of your friends?
68) To which extent the desire to be accepted to other people conditions your way of being?
69) Do you think it is worth engaging yourself in something that perhaps you will never obtain?
70) In your opinion our future depends on destiny?
71) Certainties in my life.
72) What do I see when I look in the mirror?
73) What in your opinion is the sense of life?
74) What do you like most and what would you change?
75) Am I able to be myself with other people?
76) What is my dream in the drawer?
77) In what way could I improve myself?
78) Where and with whom would you like to be in this moment?
79) Do I really believe in what I am doing?
80) If you had to thank anybody making a balance of your life, who would you thank and why?
81) If you were an animal what animal would you be?
82) Is it easier for you to think before acting or acting without thinking?
83) If you would practice a sport, it would be a team sport, or a sport to be practiced alone?
84) To whom would you give life?
85) Have you ever realized something you really wanted?
86) Close your eyes, estranging from everything: what is the first thing that comes to your mind?
87) Have you ever had a high opinion of yourself and in what circumstances?
88) Am I able to teach anything to anyone?
89) To define what I expect from life and from the world.
90) To say what in this moment could make you happy.

**Table 2.**

**List of the 90 sentences adopted for the SISCI-Sentences**

1. It is one thing to creatively pursue a goal and another thing to creatively pursue the goal of pursuing a goal.
2. Sometimes telling yourself I'm nobody can help you.
3. If you're surprised that some event has led to some other event this means that a new door is opening for you.
4. Can you afford to abandon yourself to self-abandon?
5. Think about the succession and instantaneousness of events.
6. To sail away, after hoisting the sails you need to wait for the wind.
7. Compare your dream with the dream of your dream.
8. Find something that completely fulfils you.
9. Your mindset means that the way you see is the way you see yourself.
10. Be what you are.
11. Jealousy is like a dictatorship that grows out of uncertainty.
12. Wear glasses that allow you to see what you can't see.
13. When there's confusion all around you look for a meaning.
14. A sexual rapport doesn't last for ever.
15. To get back to creatively pursuing a goal you need to take account of a universe where all choices are possible.
16. It is one thing to find a way and another thing to find the way to find a way.
17. Dictatorship grows out of the fulfillment of a dream.
18. If you generate uncertainty in your conversational partner he or she will go away.
19. Sometimes you launch into delirium or a daydream so as not to tell yourself "I'm nobody".
20. There's constancy in constancy, constancy in change and constancy in non-existence.
21. The fear of making a mistake makes you make worse mistakes.
22. You can only explain life and death in terms of pairs.
23. Your fear that they will chase you and kill you grows out of uncertainty and abstraction.
24. Doubt persists until the world gives you some answers.
25. If you fight against confusion it can destroy your mind.
26. Sometimes your mind is forced to keep repeating things because it is a prey to doubt (that arises because of creatively pursuing goals and getting back negative answers).
27. When doubt interacts with doubt it destroys your mind.
28. There are sentences and formulas that can program your mind.
29. In order for things that show they have a meaning to have that meaning, you need to accept some postulates.
30. Abstraction is the launching-pad of dreams.
31. It is one thing to accept and another thing to accept that you accept.
32. If the outside world is a metaphor and you keep to your own world the outside world will become too accepting a world.
33. There are sixteen ways of betraying.
34. If you have to go into the world of madness go in as a pseudo-altruist.
35. Mary, Mary, quite contrary is what one turns into if one is creatively pursuing a goal and starts to doubt oneself.
36. You can't have some things without some other things.
37. There are words and sentences that can untie knots in your mind.
38. You're anxious because you want to give birth to yourself.
39. If I doubt about doubt I blot out doubt.
40. Anger coupled with confusion blots out everything.
41. The image of a ship can let you sail away.
42. You can answer an insult in sixteen different styles.
43. Suspicious people have something to hide.
44. One of the ways to creatively pursue a goal is by making order out of chaos.
45. Between death and chaos my world and my path unfold.
46. When someone or something hurts you, ask yourself if your hurt wasn't also due to your attitude of acceptance of the principles according to which it was what hurt you that hurt you.
47. My path through life as an individual is based on nice things, things that I like and that tend towards my world.

48. Have the courage to see yourself as you are.
49. Creatively pursuing a goal is inextricably linked to doubt about achieving it.
50. Sometimes in dreams you fulfill your dreams.
51. Even dreams can make you stronger.
52. Sometimes the world goes your way but too much and so unexpectedly that it is more bad than good. Catching a giant octopus can also be dangerous.
53. It's possible to pursue a goal even if there is no goal: I creatively pursue a goal without there being a goal, I pursue a process without there being anything in that process.
54. Some sentences can open up worlds.
55. On the subject of the wolf in sheep's clothing, remember that when the wolf eats you he is true to his nature as a wolf.
56. When you think of the difficulties are you in difficulty?
57. Attacking back when you're attacked means conforming to the other person's behavior towards you.
58. Sometimes you can react and change, but other times you end up in a final state of either absolute rigidity or total confusion or else you're completely blotted out.
59. If you accept the world and the world accepts you, you will go on accepting the world.
60. Put things in order.
61. You need to turn to the abstract in order to get new answers.
62. Once you have found a path that gratifies you, you need to be able to find that path again in the future.
63. Putting things in order means aiming for a certain type of organization that fulfils an inner need, it's a way of making oneself feel better, perhaps of making oneself stronger.
64. Sometimes when you're creatively pursuing a goal you get lost on the outskirts.
65. "Arrange the world so that it gives you the answer you want".
66. If you're always in operative mode learn to be metaphorical, learn to dream. Mediation may even cause fading of the imagination.
68. Your uncertainty can paralyze those who depend on you.
69. Paranoia is when doubt is coupled with dictatorship.
70. Be careful! Pseudo-altruism can generate dislike.
71. Taking the path to delirium means going towards the abstract rather than towards doubt and oblivion.
72. Sometimes we compensate for uncertainty by gratifying ourselves in various ways.
73. The fear of feeling bad makes me feel bad.
74. Madness is a mixture of creatively pursuing a goal, of abstraction and of being blotted out.
75. There is uncertainty and there is the need to escape from uncertainty.
76. Sometimes reality is like a dream fulfilled.
77. If you creatively pursue the goal of dreaming you will end up in an abstract world.
78. Make sure you can distinguish between sharing and accepting.
79. You're looking for something that can completely fulfill you.
80. If you're in a bad situation and you passively accept it you're setting the stage for dictatorship.
81. Negative-uncertain-anguished answers to the world go hand in hand.
82. The meeting of two dictatorships leads to confusion.
83. If the world is uncertain set yourself up as a dictator.
84. Pursuing a goal and having doubts go hand in hand.
85. Some sentences are passwords that open up the heart of our mind.
86. Something can't change.
87. If you try be successful then creatively pursuing a goal will take you towards the world's world.
88. It often happens that external dictatorship turn into internal dictatorship.
89. In each situation you should identify and distinguish the various goals you're pursuing and the various keys to each of them.
90. Many paths lead to doubt.

**Table 3: statistically significant difference for three of the four coordinates between the use of the SISCI- Sentences and SISCI-Questions for 98 medical students**

| | Sisci sentences N = 98 | | Sisci questions N = 98 | | |
|---|---|---|---|---|---|
| | Mean | SD | Mean | SD | p value |
| U1 (Antifunction) | 0.1474 | 0.1095 | 0.2210 | 0.1822 | p ≤ 0.0001 extremely significant |
| U2 (Acceptance) | 0.1268 | 0.1041 | 0.2207 | 0.1876 | p ≤ 0.0001 extremely significant |
| U3 (Maintenance) | 0.8169 | 0.1375 | 0.7737 | 0.1585 | p ≤ 0.0114 significant |
| U4 (Sharing) | 0.7904 | 0.1628 | 0.7838 | 0.1628 | p ≤ 0.7414 not significant |

**Table 4: statistically significant differences between the means for the final states in patients whose functions interacted with "themselves" and with the junior residents in the psychiatry training group.**

| | Patients - themselves N = 20 | | Patients – Junior residents N = 20 | | |
|---|---|---|---|---|---|
| | Mean | SD | Mean | SD | p value |
| F0 | 0.09712 | 0.05348 | 0.1658 | 0.0004892 | p ≤ 0.0001 extremely significant |
| F3 | 0.4411 | 0.01275 | 0.4685 | 0.003826 | p ≤ 0.3494 not significant |
| F15 | 0.1687 | 0.07008 | 0.07608 | 0.0001735 | p ≤ 0.0001 extremely significant |

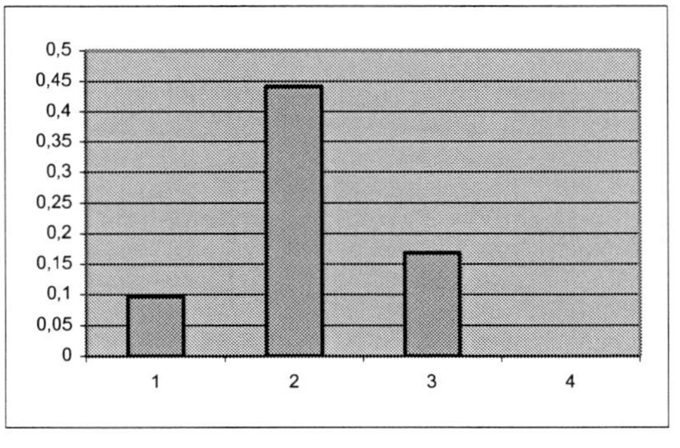


Figure 3: Mean final states in patients whose functions interacted with "themselves".

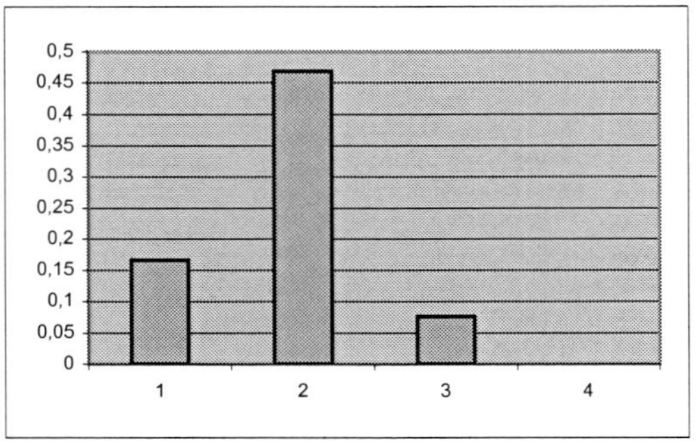


Figure 4: mean final states in patients whose functions interacted with those of the junior residents in a psychiatry training group

those moments when the patients asks the therapist to "say something, i.e. to provide an input, perhaps by asking whether it would be particularly important for them; h) resorting to a mnemonic technique.

Another possibility is to use the structure of the EPM in participants who are working with the Sisci sentences as described above. We conducted a preliminary experiment in 48 students of psychology, and after doing the test, they were asked to work on the sentences freely, by writing for half an hour every day for a week, on the 100 (chosen the first time, not chosen in the randomized choices and not chosen the second time) and 110 sentences (chosen the first time, chosen in the randomized choices but not chosen the second time) and then, after this work period they repeated the Sisci sentences test. A statistically significant difference was found for the coordinate U2-acceptance, that appeared increased (Table 5).

The expected result predicted an increase for both coordinates U2 (acceptance) and U3 (maintenance). Instead, we found only one increase, of the coordinate U2 (acceptance) but not of U3 (maintenance). In any case a response was obtained and this led us to judge our approach to be efficacious. The aim of our work is to make our intervention ever more incisive, by increasing the length of time for work on the sentences, for example, or using the types of intervention mentioned above.

## A Method of Counseling Online based on the Elementary Pragmatic Model

This section aims at describing a new method to counsel online derived from the EPM.

### The structure of our Counseling On Line service

Another study, this time not based on the SISCI-Figures but based instead on sentences deriving from the Elementary Pragmatic Model and on a test based on this same model (L'Abate & De Giacomo, 2003) was done online in the context of creating Counseling Online service.

The "Counseling Online" service with the EPM starts with an enquiry made by the managers of the service for whichever goal the user hopes to achieve, in other words a "contract".

The first time the user enters the "virtual room", she or he must enroll, supplying personal details, an email address and giving informed consent to the treatment of sensitive personal data.

After registering, the user is communicated her/his Nickname via e-mail, and her/his password for accessing the Counseling; these data are subsequently digitized in the appropriate text area at each access. The program continues with a brief text message which reminds the user of the Counseling aims, followed by a welcoming message.

A scheme of the sequence of sessions is reported below:

## First Session

- Joining ( initial contact )
- Individuation of the goal to be pursued: a greater self-awareness.

A list of 31 sentences is presented, from which the user chooses the sentence that has the greatest psychological impact on her/him: Table 6

The user is given the prescription to work on the sentence by elaborating freely during the course of the session. This prescription expects the user to work on the sentence also taking into account the following points:

a. the reason for the choice
b. how the sentence fits into her/his system of convictions
c. what associations it evokes in her/him
d. how s/he would rewrite the sentence according to her/his point of view so as to make it correspond most closely to her/his world
e. what story s/he would build around the sentence

**Table 5: comparison of mean coordinates of Sisci sentences in 48 students of psychology before and after free work on the sentences.**

| | SISCI-Sentences 13 November 2006 N = 48 | | SISCI-Sentences 4 December 2006 N = 48 | | |
|---|---|---|---|---|---|
| | Mean | SD | Mean | SD | p value |
| U1 (Antifunction) | 0.1193 | 0.09191 | 0.092 | 0.1011 | $p \leq 0.0671$ not quite significant |
| U2 (Acceptance) | 0.1346 | 0.09547 | 0.08770 | 0.08087 | $p \leq 0.0011$ very significant |
| U3 (Maintenance) | 0.8196 | 0.1720 | 0.8357 | 0.1905 | $p \leq 0.6132$ not significant |
| U4 (Sharing) | 0.7782 | 0.2097 | 0.8434 | 0.1842 | $p \leq 0.0830$ not quite significant |

After this "homework" phase, the user is given a grid with sixteen spaces (corresponding to the sixteen styles of response to the sentences generated with the Elementary Pragmatic Model) and is asked to mark on this grid the impact the sentence has had on her/him. The impacts considered in the program, based on the sixteen relational styles of the EPM are as follows:

1) It nullifies you;
2) It seems to you strange;
3) It just makes you read the text;
4) It makes you understand and think about other possibilities;
5) It makes you shut yourself away;
6) It leads you to oppose it;
7) It confirms your way of seeing things;
8) It seems to you an imposition;
9) It leads you to a passive acceptance;
10) It leads you to acceptance in your own interests;
11) It leads you to complete acceptance;
12) It leads you to a surprised, enthusiastic acceptance;
13) It leads you to doubt;
14) It makes you think in metaphorical terms;
15) It leads you to mediate different ways of seeing things;
16) It leads you to confusion.

The next step is to present the user with the test "Self-View Questionnaire" (L'Abate & De Giacomo, 2003, pp. 395-396). The purpose of this test is to provide a guide to reflection on how s/he sees her/his relationship with others according to the sixteen relational styles proposed by the EPM, as regards the present, past and future.

At this stage the session can proceed in two different ways:

a. if the user feels like it and the therapist is willing, s/he can ask for feedback, so as to discuss together the previous work on the sentence, otherwise
b. the user is referred to the next session. ( There must be an interval of at least 24 hours between sessions).

## The First Statistical Data Collected in our Counseling Online Service

We have collected preliminary statistical data on a sample of users who concluded the entire program completing the 10 sessions, performing all the tests, and answering all the questions proposed. The sample consisted on 139 users, 113 females and 26 males. The period of observation and the data collection on the sessions lasted from 2005 to 2007.

The first 5 sentences most commonly chosen by the men in the sample are the following: "Having a goal is already achieving a goal" ( 9,23%), "Project yourself towards the other person's world" (7,69%), "Being a perpetual poet is not compatible with life" (6,54%), "Much unhappiness derives from the fact that you want to do one thing and the other whereas in fact you can do one thing or the other"( 6,15%), "Enter the world of doubt" (5.77%). The first 5 sentences most commonly chosen by the women are the following: "Project yourself towards the other person's world" (9.03%), "Wear dream-tintd glasses" ( 7.08%), "Having a goal is already achieving a goal" (6.99.%), "The way you see my relationship with you is not necessarily the way I see my relationship with you" (6.90%). "Much unhappiness derives from the fact that you want to do one thing and the other whereas in fact you can do one thing or the other" ( 6.73%).

By completing the test "Self-view questionnaire" proposed at the end of each session, after working on the chosen sentence with "a strong emotional impact" was found to be a very effective tool for helping the user to become more self-aware and to understand her/his interactive characteristics, as referred to the present, past and future.

The large quantity of data that can be obtained from users who have completed the test, repeated at each of the ten sessions of the program, can be analyzed in great depth and seem to be important. They are not yet sufficient for definitive statistical analysis but they are indicative of a possible assessment methodology.

Herein we have analyzed the available population sample, as said before consisting of 139 users, 113 women and 26 men, who completed the program and carefully and fully answered the test. Of the *sixteen functions*, we have selected three, corresponding to the *3 final states* that constitute the 5th level of the MPE, representing a kind of essence, or "skeleton" of the human mind : Nullification (F0), Maintenance of one's own world (F3) and Chaos – the impossibility of making a choice (F15).

For each of these states we have created a "weighted" scale, ranging from the best situation with a maximum score of 12, to the worst, with a score of 1. We then processed the data related to these three states and compared those obtained at the first and at the last sessions. We found that:

The mean values for the user population, as regards the state F0 – Empty/Absent (nullification), changed from 16.78205 at the first session to 15.74359 at the last, demonstrating a decrease in F0 corresponding, according to the hypothesis suggested by these data, to a user perception of an improvement.

The mean values for the user population as regards the state F3–Tenacious/Egocentric changed from 10.17949 at the first to 10.98718 at the last session, corresponding again to the participants' perception of an improvement.

Finally, for the state F15 - Confused/Chaotic, we can see a decline from the mean value of 12.67949 at the first session to 11.35897 at the last. This change can also be hypothesized to indicate a perceived improvement.

At present, these data can only indicate a possible methodology for assessing any changes in self-perception occurring during the experience, as well as offering a grid that can help users to understand and assess themselves.

**Table 6.**

**31 sentences of the Conseling Online based on the Elementary Pragmatic Model**

1. Much unhappiness derives from the fact that you want to do one thing and the other whereas in fact you can do one thing or the other.
2. If you meet a deliberately contrary person and you adopt a creative, sharing attitude they will be able to feel doubt.
3. Being a perpetual poet is not compatible with life.
4. If you are hostile to yourself any attempt to solve a problem creatively will be transformed into doubt and uncertainty.
5. Wear dream-tinted glasses.
6. Project yourself towards the other person's world.
7. Enter the world of doubt.
8. The way you see my relationship with you is not necessarily the way I see my relationship with you.
9. Having a goal is already achieving a goal.
10. Hurting someone hurts yourself.
11. If you are a doubter and you want to become an upholder of your world, give yourself gifts you really like, do things that lead towards your world.
12. Uncertainty, doubt, ambivalence, doubtfulness, being swayed by the waves, if this is a state that repeats, repeats, repeats itself, in the end it nullifies you, it kills your mind.
13. In every situation there is one way that is already ready and organized, and an uncertain way that has to be organized, but sometimes it is difficult to find that first way.
14. There are negative things that fascinate you.
15. When a situation is against you, you will have to go through a phase of doubt before finding the road in the direction of the search for the solution.
16. Wear worry-tinted glasses.
17. Give me a hand by not giving me a hand.
18. If the starting point is not clear all the next steps will be unclear.
19. If you pursue a goal creatively, if the outcome is positive, in other words it leads towards your world, this will make you stronger.
20. If you say they are better it will make them worse, if you say they are well it will make them ill.
21. When you think you're a great person, the almighty or a genius, or your work seems to you very important and headed for great results and great success, tell yourself: <<I'm in a dream-attack>>.
22. What seems definite is not in fact definite if it is seen only as a content and not as a container, that is, if it is put in brackets, let's say in a certain frame.
23. True luck is when you get something unexpected that you like.
24. To wear or not to wear suspicion-tinted glasses: you are wearing suspicion-tinted glasses.
25. If you want to keep your creativity feed off chaos.
26. Teasing is a way of attacking softened by a component of pseudoaltruism that hides a way of using teasing to strengthen one's own position.
27. Losing control of yourself is sometimes like becoming your own enemy, or forgetting something (emptying your mind completely) is sometimes the same as becoming your own enemy.
28. Hang some abstract pictures on the walls of your home, add some abstract constructions to the constructions of your mind.
29. If you are a contrary person, con-fusion kills you.
30. If you want to make a contrary person uphold their world show yourself to be a pseudoaltruist.
31. Sequences are interrupted either by nullification or by absolute inflexibility or by total confusion.

IV ) *Users' opinion*

At the end of the therapy, the users were asked to assign a score to the Counseling Online experience, on a scale ranging from 1 ( the minimum) to 5 (the maximum). We found that all the men voted the program to be easy, 34.62% giving it a score of 4/5 and 61.54% of 5/5. Among the women, 27.43% assigned the maximum score and 55.75% gave it 4/5. As regards usefulness, 19.23% of the men gave it the maximum score of 5/5 and 46.15% gave it 4/5, while 11.5% of the women assigned a score of 5/5 and 43.36% gave it 4/5. Finally, 61.54% of the men found the experience with the counseling project satisfying; 42.31% assigning a maximum score of 4/5 and 19.23% of 5/5. Among the women, 47.79% found it satisfying; 37.17% assigning a score of 4/5 and 10.62 % a score of 5/5.

The Counseling Online service seems to be effective. It helps to increase self-awareness and the understanding of the outside world by presenting an unusual way of seeing things, being based on an original theory of mind organization that is not confined to good sense or the traditional psychological lines of thought.

The next step could be that of creating a completely automated pathway, an "intelligent" program that could capture the essential aspects of the organization of human thoughts and hence affections, and thus make it possible to help users to achieve a higher level of well-being.

## Conclusion

The foregoing methodological approach needs to be refined and re-evaluated. However, it demonstrates how it is possible to link theory with practice and practice with research.

## References

Bateson, G. (1980). *Mind and nature.* Glasgow UK: Fontana/Collins.

De Giacomo, P. (1992). The elementary pragmatic model: from theory to therapeutic practice. *Annuali Istituto Superiore di Sanità.* 28, 169-76.

De Giacomo, P. (1993). *Finite systems and infinite interactions. The logic of human interaction and its application to Psychotherapy.* Norfolk, CT: Bramble Books.

De Giacomo, P., De Giacomo, A., Sgobio, A. (2004). Applicazione clinica di un metodo di elaborazione dei sogni basato sul Modello Pragmatico Elementare per migliorare la conoscenza di se stessi e della propria vita psichica in rapporto col mondo. *Ricerche in Psichiatria.* Vol. I – n.1 Gen/Apr. CIC Ed. Intern.

De Giacomo, P. & Iadicicco, R. (2001). *Manuale di Zen Occidentale: La logica della saggezza.* Rome, IT: Edizioni Hermes.

De Giacomo, P., L'Abate, L., Santamato, W. et al. (2007). "Compass" sentences with strong psychological impact in family therapy: Preliminary investigations. *Journal of Family Psychotherapy, 18*, 45-69.

De Giacomo, P., Margari, F., Pupino, M.E., Storelli, M., De Giacomo, A., Giovannelli, M., & Masellis, R. (2006). Counseling online basato sul Modello Pragmatico Elementare: Descrizione e primi dati statistici. http://www.polit.org/ital/piero2006.htm

De Giacomo, P., Mich, L., Storelli, M., De Nigris, S., et al., (2004). A method of counseling online using the Elementary Pragmatic Model. In D. Macer Ed., *Challanges for bioethics from Asia* (pp 102-108). Bangkok Japan: Eubios Ethics Institute.

De Giacomo, P., Pierri, G., Santoni Rugiu, A., Buonsante, M., Vadruccio, F., Zavoianni, L. (1997). Schizophrenia: a study comparing a family therapy group following a paradoxical model plus psychodrugs and a group treated by the conventional clinical approach. *Acta Psychiatrica Scandinavia, 95*, 183-188.

De Giacomo, P. & Santoni Rugiu, A. (2000). The Elementary Pragmatic Model. In K. J.

Miller & J. S. Mizes (Eds.), *Comparative treatments for eating disorders* (pp. 236-257). New York: Springer.

Holtzman, W. H. (1961). *Holtzman Inkblot Technique (Forms A and B).* New York: Psychological Corporation

L'Abate, L., De Giacomo, P., McCarty, F., De Giacomo, A. & Verrastro, G. (2000). Testing three models of intimate relationships. *Contemporary Family Therapy: An International Journal, 22*, 103-122.

L'Abate, L. & De Giacomo, P. (2003). *Intimate relationships and how to improve them. Integrating theoretical models with preventive and psychotherapeutic applications.* Westport, CT: Praeger.

Pierri, G. (1992). Methods for evaluating normal and pathological couples and families according to the Elementary Pragmatic Model. *Annuali Istituto Superiore di Sanità, 28*, 177-184

Silvestri, A., De Giacomo, P., Pierri, G., Lefons, E., Pazienza, M.T., Tangorra, F. (1980). A Basic Model of Interacting Participants, *Cybernetics and Systems: An International Journal. 11*, 113-127. http://it.wikipedia.org/wiki/Modello Pragmatico Elementare

In: Toward a Science of Clinical Psychology
Editor: Luciano L'Abate, pp. 337-352
ISBN: 978-1-60456-062-6


*Chapter XVIII*

# Validation of the Continuum of Likeness in Intimate Relationships

***Mario Cusinato and Walter Colesso***

## Abstract

The construct of similarity is central in the identity-differentiation process to understand individual differences and distinguish among different degrees of functionality over the life cycle (L'Abate & Cusinato, 2007) and it is still current and popular in relationship science (Acitelli, Kenny, & Hall, 2001; Cole & Teboul, 2004; Cupach & Metts, 1995). Theoretical research studies on the similarity construct in intimate relationships, developed in the second part of the last century, flourished within a myriad of analogous terms, such as identification, attraction, imitation, etc., mainly according to a dichotomous perspective (Griffitt, 1974; Heider, 1958; Schneider, Hastof & Ellsworth, 1979). Nevertheless, several authors have proposed analogous concepts or terms according to three or more degrees (Harvey, 1966; Johnson, 1982; Kelly, 1955; Kohlberg, 1962; Levinger, 1964; Mahler, 1968; Rotter, 1966; Witkin, 1965).

L'Abate (1976) illustrated and discussed a continuum of likeness with six degrees of differentiation at three different levels in differences and similarities. This formal model proposes that people make choices (consciously and/or unconsciously) moving from one pole to the other but at different levels according to their stage of life, their functional level of relational competence, their individual history, their sex, socio-cultural status, etc. The model may be outlined as a bell-shaped distribution, where functionality is placed toward the center and dysfunctionality toward the extremes. Therefore, the choices of a functional individual will be according to the same bell distribution with few items at the two extreme degrees and many more items in the central degrees. The shift from the formal model to its empirical verification is a chapter only just sketched and still waiting to be written. A recent work (Cusinato & L'Abate, in press) tries to give satisfactory answers by proposing a paper-and-pencil self-report - subsequently translated into a computerized form (Likeness Continuum Profile, LCP) - later replaced by a laboratory experiment of clinical psychology (Likeness Continuum Task, LCT).

This chapter documents three successive studies carried out to validate this likeness continuum. In the first, the LCP was administered to high-school and undergraduate students, followed by a comparison between LCP and LCT data. In the second study, the LCT was administered to non-clinical participants, data were first analyzed together, and then sub-groups according to sex, age, and status were selected. In the third study, two different types of clinical subjects were considered with LCT data.

The construct of similarity considered here concerns personal and interpersonal contexts. It is "perceived similarity because it exists in the eyes of subjective beholders (including researchers) rather than in objectively observable behavior" (L'Abate, 1999, p. 192). It is particularly connected with the construction of the personal self - that is the birth and development of personal identity - while individuals live intimate relationships first with their parents and siblings and, then, with their kin, peers, and other meaningful people of their life context.

# PART 1: FROM SIMILARITY TO LIKENESS CONTINUUM

## Clarifying the course of the similarity construct

As already mentioned, psychologists began to take an interest in the concept of similarity only in the second part of the last century with few exceptions. The literature highlights complexity and little clarity both at theoretical and methodological level. First of all, we need to distinguish and link different concepts: similarity, identification, attraction, imitation. Then, the relations between similarity and differentiation have to be defined, evaluated and justified. The major theoretical framework in the area of likeness is the Social Comparison Theory (Festinger, 1954), later revised in Temporal Comparison Theory (Albert, 1970), an umbrella term under which many empirical researches were implemented.

Particularly meaningful works were realized by some researchers and/or research teams who were able to highlight some reference points: (a) Byrne (1971): comparison runs among similar people who seem attractive and satisfied; (b) Lynn (1969): different similarity degrees must be distinguished; (c) Lickona (1974): at developmental level, bonds change while individual likeness is progressively interpreted on the differentness background; (d) Duck (1975): attitude motivation has to emerge because different motivations can underlie similar attitudes. In a nutshell, we can say that likeness promotes affiliation but at certain conditions because first a need for uniqueness emerges and then for differentiation.

Along this research line, relevant and serious methodological problems are underlined over and over again: (a) a controlled laboratory setting offers results that are different from a real life setting; (b) research studies based on brief meetings differ from longitudinal studies able to focus at best on lasting relationships and to distinguish different stages; (c) some research studies are difficult to replicate because non-standardized techniques and tools were originally applied; (d) individuals or groups studied are frequently unrepresentative of the population and subgroups are often distinguished by rough criteria; (e) lastly, studies are concentrated mainly on white middle class people.

Specific application areas concern mate selection, marital relationships, and parent-child relationships. About the first, the question at the beginning of the research is: 'Is attraction/choice made based on similarity or complementarity?' As regards the second ambit, 'Does marital satisfaction derive from similarity or complementarity?' And for the third: 'In which way does conformity combine with autonomy?' Answers are neither linear nor simple, because the developmental and functionality degrees of relationships have to be taken into account. As a rule, we can say that children assert themselves in comparison with their parents and, even when they protest, their parents are their referents. Similarity exists as an important variable in adult relationships, i.e., it exists to a degree and various gradations should be detected and determined along a continuum. "Formation of personal self-categories is not a matter of differences, but a matter of relative similarities and differences. Personal identity is made possible because of self-other differentiation in terms of some shared higher-order identity that provides a context for social comparison. This implies quite clearly that similarity and difference go hand in hand in defining the personal self. Thus, even at the personal level, self-definition is inherently social, contextual, and relational. This emphasis represents an important point of departure from dominant social-cognitive models of the personal self, which treat self-schemata as absolute rather than as relative properties of the perceiver" (Onorato & Turner, 2002, p. 151). The crucial aspect is really the continuum: "Similarity in classification is fundamental and functionally many faceted... Once identity is abandoned, similarity changes its nature from being a binary-valued characteristic to a multi-valued one, and in some sense continuous." (Bergman, Magnusson, & El-Khouri, 2003, p. 54)

This similarity continuum underlies the development of important relationships and concerns the sense of identity acquired developmentally in relations with intimate people, first of all with the mother. L'Abate (1976, 1985, 1997, 2005) formally describes it with six ranges (three of similarity and three of differentiation) that produce a bell-shaped continuum, in line with the Gaussian curve with the two aspects of dysfunctionality placed at each extreme. L'Abate notes that, so far, this model has been expanded and applied to a variety of areas: most functional individuals behave in the middle in most ranges of this distribution; a few functional individuals may behave in either the same-opposite ranges in one or two areas; a smaller number of semi-functional individuals are unable to function in the middle of most areas.

## Identity Differentiation Over the Life Cycle

The continuum results from the elaborating process of self-identity, that is, the image of ourselves, which is largely refined as we grow. An early autistic stage in the first months of life is apparently followed by a symbiotic stage until the end of the third year, a projective-omnipotent stage between 4 and 6 years of age, and an autonomous-homonymous stage thereafter. Especially in heterosexual development, there may be stages initially defined by sexual awakening (13-15), practicing-dating (14-17), acceptance/rejection of sexual roles (16-19), and eventually, permanence of sexual choices (18-25). The latter is the stage when the teenager begins to separate emotionally, if not physically or financially, from his/her parents, sometimes with conflict, sometimes without. When the adolescent reaches the age of 16, he/she begins to reorganize self-identity boundaries in terms of sexual and interpersonal choices and the similarity continuum can be run on every range in a more or less functional way, when the process outcome may be defined as identity elaboration, considering the answer to the question "Who am I?". This process does not take place in a vacuum. It occurs within a continuous interplay of transactions with caregivers, siblings, peers, teachers, co-workers, bosses, friends, lovers, and even enemies. This interplay shapes how one sees oneself and how one chooses to integrate the various identities that are continuously considered over the course of the lifetime. Thereafter, how one sees oneself is the outcome of a process of comparison with intimates and non-intimates, "a comparison of similarities and differences along a continuum, and not just solely in terms of a binary similar-different process that still dominates the relevant literature" (L'Abate, 2005, p. 215). Through this process of modeling and identification, the individual learns how to relate to him/herself and to others. Differentiation can be described according to three levels. At the highest, individuals learn to define themselves and develop a positive sense of identity according to their modality of identity/differentiation with intimate others. At the intermediate level, they learn to differentiate and develop a borderline sense of self from intimate others through a process of sameness-oppositeness. At the lowest level, individuals learn to differentiate themselves and develop a defective sense of identity according to a symbiotic and alienated sense with intimate others.

## The Continuum of Likeness Builds Relational Competence

The continuum is needed to account for how we become differentiated developmentally and build a sense of identity as individuals having relationships with others. Thereafter, identity derives from the ability of loving, negotiating, and sharing exchange modalities between and among intimate others (being, doing, and having; cf. L'Abate, 1995). The most functional is the ability to love and to negotiate, balancing how being is considered appropriately in relation to doing and having along the life cycle, the more differentiated one will become and vice versa. No single range by itself, isolated from other ranges, can conceivably describe identity in intimate relationships. Each range needs a counterpart to define itself according to a combination of two ranges dialectically related to each other. In concrete, individuals vary, into a dialectical logic, along the different ranges of the Gaussian curve. The dimension of psychopathology appears as an accentuation of the two extremes of the distribution, assimilation and alienation. At the intermediate level, emotional and mental health is expressed as sameness and opposition, whereas creativity lies in the center, in the ranges of similarity and differentness, where the likelihood of functionality in most relationships is high and differences are reconciled with a minimum of conflict. By the same token, the two intermediated ranges predict a semi-functionality and at the two extremes dysfunctionality is at the highest. Hence, a sense of identity based on integration of similarity and differentness will be more functional and "healthier" than a sense of identity developed from sameness and oppositeness. Similarly, a sense of identity based on assimilation and alienation can be most incomplete and dysfunctional.

As mentioned before, the crossing from the formal model to its empirical verification is a chapter only just sketched and still waiting to be written: "Evidence to support the existence and influence of an underlying continuum of likeness in intimate relationships is fraught with many theoretical and empirical issues. Such a continuum may indeed exist; however, how influential is this continuum? How does the continuum of likeness stack up against criteria of validity and reliability? How can it be tested in the future? And how is it related to other relevant personality propensities, relationship styles, functionalities, and dysfunctionalities? The answers to these questions remain open." (L'Abate, 1997, p. 174)

## Operationalization of the Continuum of Likeness in View of Empirical Enterprises

The three studies reported in this chapter represent a contribution to the filling of this gap. Initially a paper-and-pencil self-report was created, followed by a laboratory test of clinical psychology.

The "Likeness Continuum Profile" (LCP) self-report starts from two taxonomies concerning important personal qualities and important people, and has already been validated (Cusinato & Pastore, 2001). A first version uses the taxonomy of important intimate people (9 items: from a partner to a teacher/coach/counselor) evaluated by the subject on the six levels of the likeness continuum: (a) accepting or refusing each level (with the choice: Yes/No); (b) if Yes, with which intensity (three options: sometimes, often, always), concerning the present, the past, and the future. The questionnaire asks for 27 comparisons for every item, in total 324 items. Some preliminary research showed the procedures as too complicated, if not even too long.

In the next version (Cusinato, 2003), a new taxonomy was introduced (9 personal qualities) to produce questions closer to individual experiences: "With this person... (one at a time, from the first to the ninth) and comparing him/her with this quality (one at a time, from the first to the ninth), do you choose this level of similarity (among six levels, one at a time)? Answer: Yes/No. The subjects were invited to make a total of 486 choices. However, as a little uncertainty had transpired in some empirical trials about whether respondents would effectively and adequately distinguish the six likeness ranges, a brief introduction on the meaning of the six ranges was included in the administration. The new application appeared in any case too long, soon tiring respondents who might end up producing random choices. The second part of the administration was also changed into: "With this person... and comparing him/her with this aspect... to which level (among six) of identity-differentiation do you act?" This last version asks for 81 comparisons with an additional answer opportunity, NA (not applicable). Besides, it was decided to transform the paper-and-pencil test into software that should facilitate introduction to the test and choice comparison, and also offer the respondent an immediate feedback at the end of the test. Some data analyses - presented below - found interesting aspects even if, as concerns the evaluation of the continuum, the respondents appear to prefer one range (i.e., the emerged pole) and put the others on the opposite pole (i.e., the submersed one), also showing restrictive and little distinguished evaluation of the continuum (Scilletta, 2001).

The discussion on the obtained results led to the translation of the LCP into a four-step laboratory task of clinical psychology "Likeness Continuum Task" (LCT, Cusinato & L'Abate, in press). In the first step ("personalization") the subject is invited to consider the nine items of the taxonomy "people of your life context" and to identify a real person for each item describing in his/her own words quality of relationship. In the second step ("test training") the six ranges are introduced with their definitions and comprehension is tested with examples proposed by the researcher/clinician and/or the subject. In the third step ("coin placement") the subject is provided with ten 5-cent coins and invited to place them (one at a time) on an A3 sheet of paper with six cells corresponding to the ranges of the continuum; this step addresses relationships with each of the 9 individuals (one at a time).

Instructions are: "Compared to this person... do you recognize yourself in 'a' (i.e., "I completely assimilate to")? Yes/No. If *Yes*, please place a coin on that cell; if *No*, please go on to 'b' and consider that statement". After reviewing the six modalities, the subject still has at least four coins and then he/she is invited to continue the level comparison: "Which degree do you think to strengthen? Please place a coin, one at a time, on the proper statement". And so on up to the last coin. All evaluations concerning the first person are registered in an *ad hoc* answer sheet. After this, the relationship with the second person is considered, then with the third, and so on up to the ninth. In the fourth phase ("inquiry") the subject is asked to explain his/her coin distribution and produce some real examples to check the right use of the continuum (in particular, concentration on the extremes). The subject may modify the distribution or distinguish the present from the past (everything is obviously registered).

# PART 2: LIKENESS CONTINUUM TASK

Three successive studies are presented in order to verify: (a) if the subjects are able to distinguish among the ranges along the continuum in two evaluation modalities (LCP and LCT); (b) if the continuum of a large group, comparable to a non-clinical population sample, has a bell-shaped distribution to verify the formal model; (c) how and to what extent sub-groups follow the bell-shaped distribution, based on specific independent variables (for example, sex or particular family context) or on specific stages of the life cycle, or levels of dysfunctionality; (d) which relationships with important persons of their life context induce subjects to activate which modalities along the likeness continuum. Log-linear analyses - applied to all interaction tables - offer the basic issues of the three studies; dichotomous scores, both as regards identity and differentiation, are than deducted from the sum of the three ranges. Mentioned standard $z$ scores are those exceeding $z$ for $p = .05$* or $p = .01$ **, or $p = .001$***.

## STUDY 1: The continuum of likeness in high-school students and undergraduates

Likeness is named a "hidden ingredient" because it may range from being consciously spoken to unconsciously unspoken at each end of an awareness dimension, and from clear to confused, mixed, and unclear along a clarity dimension (Cusinato & L'Abate, in press). For this reason, the paper-and-pencil self-report profile created for monitoring the six dialectical conditions has to be tested. Its refinement will be positively verified if data obtained from its administration to non-clinical participants appear distributed according a bell-shaped continuum; secondary, a contribution for its validity could come from different distribution of the continuum, for example, of two sub-groups divided for age or sex.

## Participants

High-school students attending an Institute of the Milan hinterland and undergraduate students from Padua University attending a course in Family Psychology were asked to fill in the Likeness Continuum Profile. The high-school students were 117: 18 males and 99 females, $M$ = 17.3 with a range of 16-19 years; the undergraduate students were 117 too: 18 males and 99 females, $M$ = 23.5 with a range of 22-26 years.

## Method

The last version of the Likeness Continuum Profile (LCP), a paper-and-pencil self-report translated into a computerized form, was administered in a computer laboratory to 20 participants at a time. The application time was 23 minutes on average with a range of 15-35 minutes and data were immediately available for log-linear analyses.

## Results

The results are summarized in Figure 1. The likeness continua of the two groups are traced out in the shape of histogram with the bell-shaped distribution as comparison background according the formal model. The table below the histograms shows the standard z scores of the two groups exceeding $z$ for $p$ = .05, .01, .001.

## Discussion

In both groups, the obtained variance of the continuum shows different levels of similarity with intimates, but not too much according to the bell-shaped distribution proposed by the formal model. After investigating the process used by the subjects in choosing the different levels, a dichotomized decision may be supposed: after identifying one level as acceptable (according to their relational experience and/or by self-presentation), the subjects treat this as the emerged pole; all other levels are compressed in the submersed pole. So, subjects do not offer an accurate representation of all the relational choices.

The high-school students stress the levels of *assimilation*, *similarity*, and *alienation*; the undergraduates those of *sameness*, *oppositeness*, and *differentness*. The two groups show also dissimilar development degrees on likeness. In addition, high-school students stress identity, undergraduates the differentiation in dichotomous derived scores. Reviewing the distribution of the six likeness degrees for the 9 intimate items, undergraduates emphasize the *differentness* modality with children, school-fellows, and intimate others, the young students with partner, mother, and father. In addition, these underline *assimilation* vs. *oppositeness* with their younger siblings.

In conclusion, results offer some stimulating suggestions concerning developmental evolution but reveal some limitations, i.e. poor elicitation of the continuum. Probably a self-report test may be an unsuitable tool for catching the variability of identity-differentiation felt with important people; probably the awareness is not rightly helped and supported.

Therefore, an alternative modality (LCT) was created and tentatively applied to a group of 27 undergraduates selected with independent variables - sex: females; age: $M$ = 24.1, and personal status: single - similar to those of the 27 subjects chosen from the previous LCP application. The results are summarized in Figure 2.

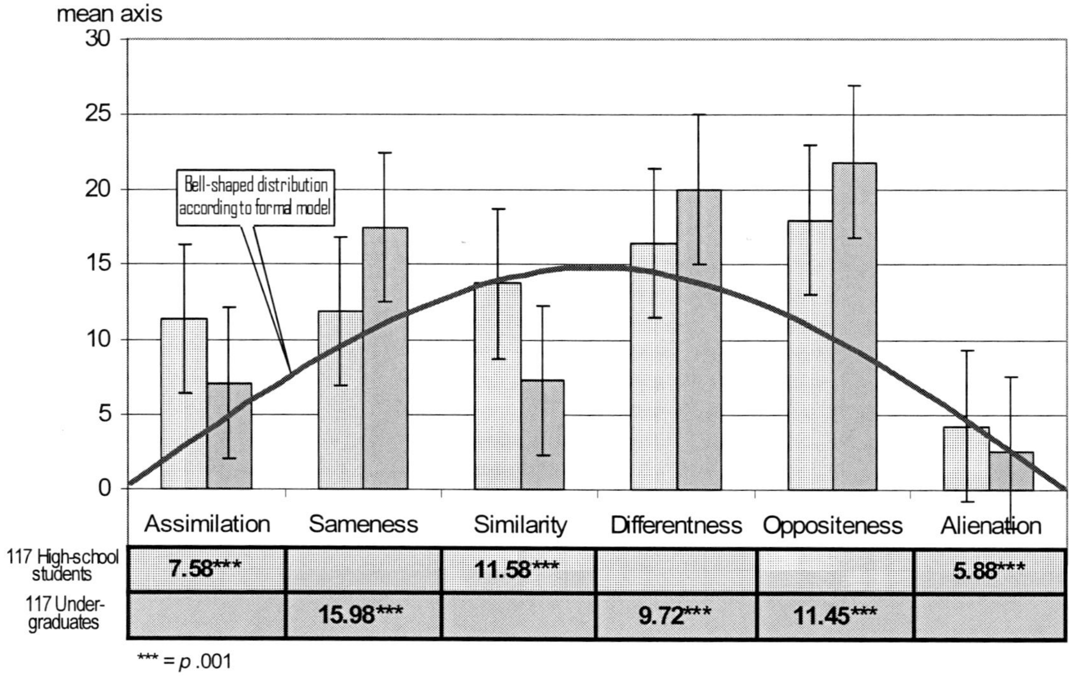


Figure 1. LCP Data Analyses of High-school Students *vs.* Undergraduates

Keeping the bell-shaped distribution as comparison background, LCT continuum levels appear to follow the distribution much more than LCP levels; only *differentness* exceeds the distribution. In addition, while the dichotomous LCP differentiation conditions are higher than identity conditions, in the LCT it is vice versa: a larger band of recognized identity is monitored when the likeness continuum appears more carefully elicited.

## STUDY 2: The continuum of likeness in LCT with non-clinical individuals

The results of the tentative first LCT applications needed to be confirmed by a more pondered study that adequately monitored the main independent variables: sex, age, and personal status. It should ascertain the consistency of the adopted instructions and monitor variations along the developmental stages and across different conditions, too. In particular, the additional charge of the three identity conditions and the sliding of the three differentiation conditions toward the centre of the continuum might be evaluated as spurious or, in some way, structural.

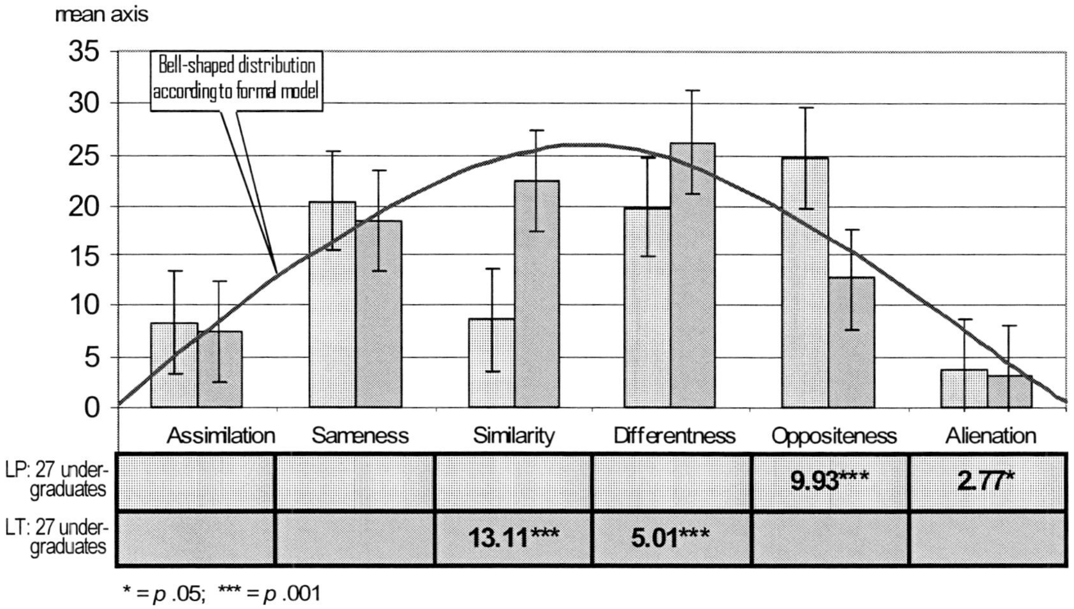


Figure 2. Likeness Continuum in LCP *vs.* LCT

## Participants

The participants were 222 non-clinical subjects, 91 males and 131 females, ($M$ = 27.29; age range = 14-62 years) who had volunteered to take part in a laboratory task in order to verify the extent to which each participant saw him/herself like the significant individuals of his/her setting, that is to say the degree of similarity or differentiation. The data obtained were strictly confidential and were supplied only to those participants that requested them.

From the participants, two groups were selected. They were chosen individually in order to compare data by sex: 69 males and 69 females ($M$ = 26.84; age range = 14-46 years) (First analysis). For a subsequent comparison, 40 participants per four age ranges (50% males and 50% females) were selected: sub-group 14-19 y. o.; sub-group 20-28 y. o.; sub-group 29-36 y. o.; sub-group 37-46 y. o. (Second analysis). Finally, a third selection considered four sub-groups comparable by status (42 participants each sub-group, 50% males and 50% females): singles ($M$ = 24.19, range = 15-44 years), fiancés/fiancées ($M$ = 24.90, range = 20-37 years), married ($M$ = 36.43, range =20-58 years) (Third analysis).

## Method

LCT was applied individually (Cusinato & L'Abate, in press) upon filling in the Informed Consent Form. The task time averaged 37 minutes, with a range of 25-55 minutes. Obtained data were first analyzed together, then per sub-groups.

## Results

Figure 3 shows the derived likeness continuum histogram with the bell-shaped distribution as comparison background according to the formal model and standard *z* scores.

## Discussion

Empirical data seem to confirm the formal model even if differentiation degrees slip a little to the center and identity degrees are somewhat blown. Thus, the analyses repeat the first obtained performances; nevertheless, different reasons may be proposed: i.e. inaccurate instructions, mainly female participants, self-presentation biases and other, but the "hidden ingredient" quality of likeness may not be excepted so that people are more aware of identity modalities and are inclined to recognize the more central grades of differentiation as reported standard *z* scores attest.

Analyses of "six dialectical conditions x intimate relationships" (Table 19.3) show the participants' orientations along the continuum. *Assimilation* is significantly selected for "partner" (i.e., boy-friend/girl-friend, fiancé/fiancée, or spouse: 14.97***), "mother" (3.83***), "children" (i.e., natural or acquired children, young siblings, or babies: 6.19***), and "educator" (3.01*); very little selected for "school-fellows" (– 7.58***) and "co-workers" (– 9.00***). *Sameness* is selected particularly for "children" (4.09***) and very little for "siblings" (– 3.74*) and "school-fellows" (– 3.08*); *Similarity* for "educator" (7.57***) and little for "co-workers" (– 3.51*). On the differentiation slope, *Differentness* is significantly selected for "co-workers" (3.48**) and little for "mother" (– 3.88***) and "father" (– 4.09***); *Oppositeness* selected for "father" (3.78**), "siblings" (7.99***), and "co-workers" (4.07***), little for "partner" (– 7.45***), "children" (7.99***), and "others" (-3.86***); *Alienation* is selected particularly for "partner" (– 3.11*) and "others" (– 3.82***). Summarizing the results, *Assimilation* excels in relationships with "partner", "mother", and "children"; *Oppositeness* with "father" and "siblings"; *Alienation* with "school-fellows" and "co-workers". Relationships with "friends" and "others" are expanded on the continuum.

Subsequent analyses compared the various sub-groups mentioned before.

*Analysis 1: LCT likeness continuum of male vs. female sub-groups.* Male participants stress *Assimilation* (4.09***) and *Opposition* (2.69**); female participants *Sameness*" (2.56**), *Similarity* (6.68***) and *Differentness* (4.12***), so that the two sexes live relationships differently: more centralized conditions for females, more extreme ones for males.

*Analysis 2: LCT likeness continuum of four age sub-groups.* Their histograms follow roughly the bell-shaped distribution with some variations. Teenagers and thirty-year-olds give distributions without significant *z*: therefore, they stress a little, probably for different reasons, the external conditions and drop a little the central ones. The twenty-year-olds' subgroup stresses *Assimilation* (4.93***); the forty-year-olds' subgroup *Sameness* (4.77***) and *Differentness* (2.80*). Analyses of "six dialectical conditions x intimate relationships" show people connected with the six conditions: in *Assimilation*, "partner" is chosen by all four sub-groups (respectively 3.77**, 4.40***, 5.07*** and 6.04***; in *Opposition*, "siblings" by the first three sub-groups (respectively 4.38***, 3.56**, and 3.95***); in *Assimilation*, "children" by the third and fourth group (respectively 4.65*** and 7.35***); in *Alienation*, "school-fellows" by the first (3.49**), the third (4.58***), and the fourth group (5.76***); "co-workers" by the fourth (3.97***).

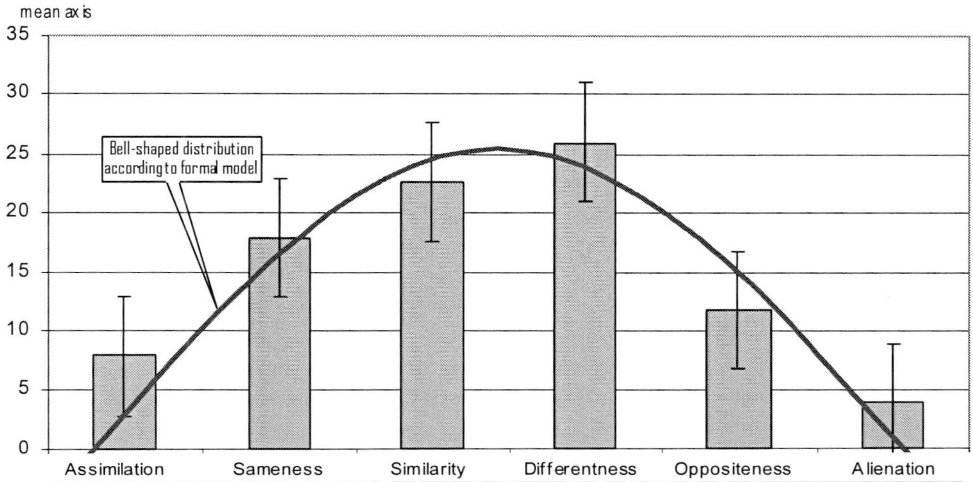


| | Assimilation | Sameness | Similarity | Differentness | Oppositeness | Alienation |
|---|---|---|---|---|---|---|
| 222 Non-clinical | **– 22.24*** ** | **24.11*** ** | **41.85*** ** | **53.64*** ** | **– 3.33*** | **– 38.63*** ** |

* = *p* .05; *** = *p* .001

Figure 3. LCT Likeness Continuum of Non-clinical Participants

*Analysis 3: LT likeness continuum of three status sub-groups.* Their histograms follow roughly the bell-shaped distribution with variations. The Singles' group stresses *Assimilation* (4.46***) and drops *Sameness* (– 2.91*) and *Similarity* (– 3.23**); engaged people show a distribution without significant *z:* a little stressed external conditions and a little dropped central ones, they are balanced between identity and differentiation; the married people group stresses *Sameness* (3.97***) and *Similarity* (3.16**), and drops *Alienation* (– 2.80**). Analyses of "six dialectical conditions x intimate relationships" show people connected with the six conditions: in *Assimilation*, "partner" and "children" are dropped by the singles (respectively – 6.24*** and – 6.44***) and stressed by married people (respectively 5.58*** and 8.32***); in *Differentness*, fiancés/fiancées choose "mother" (3.68**) and "children" (3.82***); in *Similarity* "co-workers" (3.16*); in *Sameness*, married people stress "partner" (4.07***) and "children" (5.98***).

## STUDY 3: The continuum of likeness in LCT with clinical individuals

The previous study attested the likeness continuum of non-clinical individuals traced according to a bell-curve. Clinical people should trace a different continuum in accordance with the specificity of their clinical condition: more marked shifting aside in serious pathologies, less marked in semi-functional conditions. This study verified the likeness continuum of anorexics and psychotics: the former should strength the sameness condition, the latter the assimilation condition without neglecting dialectical shifts (L'Abate & Cusinato, in press).

## Participants

Two different types of clinical subjects were considered: female anorexics (Cozzi, 2004) and male and female psychotics (Longhin, 2003). In both groups, a control sub-group of non-clinical people was identified one by one and co-opted in the study. Both clinical groups were also sub-divided into two sub-groups according to their clinical conditions.

The first group included 20 female anorexics (*M* = 18.90 years; range 14-24) subdivided in (a) in-patient group: 10 anorexics (mean age 18.70; range 14-24; symptoms for an average of 4 years) in-patients at a private clinic, and (b) out-patient group: 10 anorexics (mean age 19.10; range 15-24; symptoms for an average of 5 years) being treated at a public medical service. Both institutions are in North-East Italy.

The second group included 20 psychotics (*M* = 35.81 years; range 26-44) followed at the public health services of the Padua district: 10 males (*M* = 34.40) and 10 females (*M* = 37.80). It was divided according to type of care: 10 subjects (*M* = 33.50; range 27-40) were followed in a day-hospital service; 10 subjects (M = 36.13 y. o.; range 26-43) lived in sheltered structures. The individuals from the first sub-group had a longer psychiatric history, but their situation was defined as low crisis risk; the individuals from the second sub-group had only recently started their psychiatric history and were at high crisis risk.

## Method

Clinical participants were asked to perform LCT as part of the routine evaluation program. Control group participants were identified inside the involved clinical institutions and were asked to take part in the study illustrated in the preliminary Informed Consent Form application. Administration to clinical participants lasted much longer than administration to the control group. In particular, psychotics often asked for more sessions to complete the application and were more inclined to co-operate with a person they were familiar with. The elicitation of some examples of specific choices (Step 4: Inquiry) started some sort of awareness that the examiner had to be prepared to manage.

## Results

Figure 4 summarizes the results obtained by $z$ analyses of the two clinical groups and their correspondent control groups. As in previous figures, the respective histograms appear with the bell-shaped distribution as comparison background according to the formal model and standard $z$ scores.

## Discussion

As shown in the histograms and the *z* tables, the two control groups follow the bell-curve trend with the two specificities already known; this trend is not evident in the two clinical groups: anorexics strengthen the choice of *Assimilation* (11.52***), psychotics simultaneously "Assimilation" (6.36***) and *Alienation* (6.70***) - supported by *Opposition* (3.64***). For the first time, a test of dialectical shifts between the two extreme conditions is performed.

As already said, analyses of six dialectical conditions x intimate relationships show the participants' orientations along the continuum toward their important relations. Anorexics live their relational ambivalence strengthening, on the identity slope, *Assimilation* (5.31***) and similarity (3.51**) with the doctor in attendance and, on the differentiation slope, *Oppositeness* with "mother" (3.01*) and *Alienation*" (6.58***) with "school-fellows". Psychotics strengthen *Differentness* with "friends" (3.96***), *Alienation* with "father" (4.40***) and "co-workers" (3.93***). *Anorexic sub-groups*: a comparison between in-patient and out-patient anorexics gives similar histograms even if *Differentness* is more greatly strengthened in the first sub-group (3.86***) and *Alienation* in the second (2.39*) according to the stage of their illness.

*Psychotic sub-groups*. The two Likeness Continua are different: the day hospital sub-group moves toward differentiation, the protected accommodation sub-group toward identity. Analyses of continuum x intimates underline *Alienation* for "father" in both sub-groups - as already mentioned -, *Assimilation* for "partner" (3.22*) in the first sub-group, and for "friends" (3.30*) and "doctor in attendance" (3.22*) in the second.

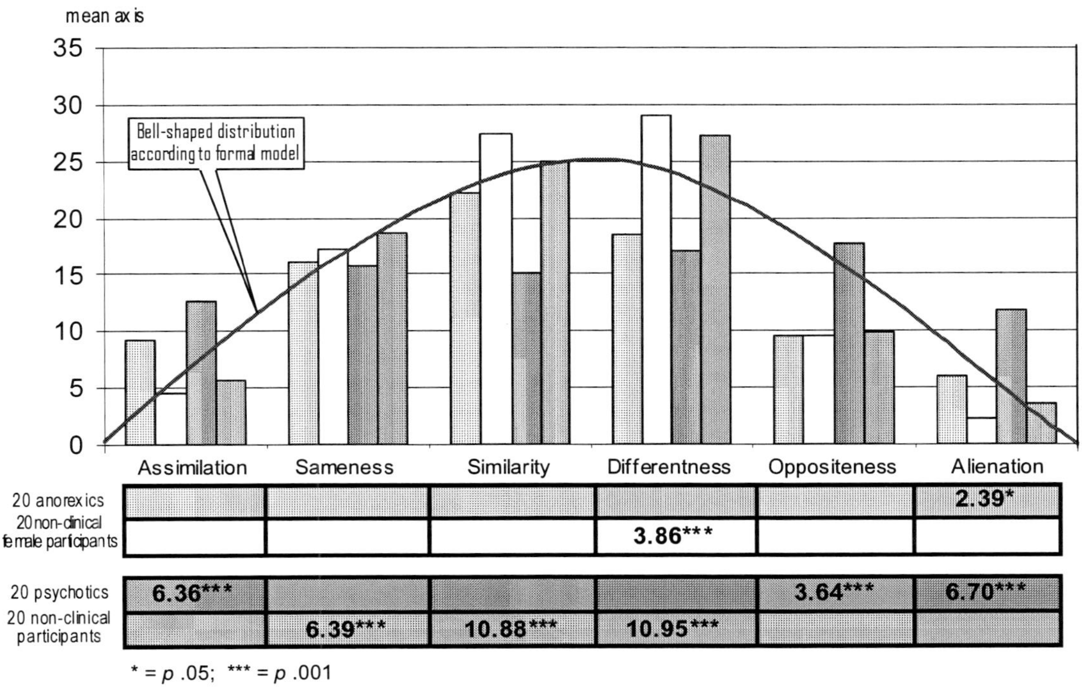


Figure 4. LCT Likeness Continuum of Clinical Groups *vs.* Non-clinical Participants

## Conclusions

The studies illustrated in this chapter highlight that the continuum of likeness can be operationable even if the test process shows some complexity. The obtained results attest again likeness as a "hidden ingredient" in intimate relationships. LCT is confirmed to offer more strength in eliciting the six continuum conditions than LCP. In fact, analyses of data obtained by LCT application to various non-clinical groups give continuously a bell-shaped distribution according to the formal model and they testify in favor of validity of both the task and the conceptualization. Clinical group data of the third study trace different continua and give evidence of the elicitation process activated by the subjects.

Several aspects still remain to be explained, first of all the overestimation of identity conditions and the slipping of identity differentiations to the center of the continuum. Different reasons may be proposed: erroneous instructions, mainly female participants, self-presentation biases, participants' possible task awareness. However, quality of likeness may not be excluded as the "hidden ingredient" by which people are more aware of identity modalities and inclined to better recognize the central grades of differentiation. In the second place, another reason for this complexity involves examiners' training, especially what is needed to understand the precise meaning of similarity-difference in the second step of the task, and the elicitation of examples explaining the choices made in the fourth step. If task adequacy can be guaranteed by the typical training for dealing with non-clinical participants, the administration of the task to clinical individuals requires specific competencies to cope with their difficulties. The acquisition of these competencies allows matching at best evaluation and intervention; actually, LCT offers numerous indications to gain clarity on and awareness of likeness experiences.

In the third place, the studies illustrated suggest the replacement of the supplied taxonomy of important others with an elicited one when working on a case study or as regards treatment, because participants are not always able to interpret the taxonomy roles ideographically and therefore find it difficult to appropriately appraise their relationships.

Lastly, useful stimuli can certainly come from further research. The above studies have confirmed that elicitation of the likeness continuum is a complex process that requires a certain degree of awareness and that can be realized through suitable strategies. Functional individuals will let their relational experiences surface thus producing a positive pattern of likeness continuum; less functional or dysfunctional individuals will show more or less dysfunctional aspects. On that account, a pre- and post-test LCT - with the use of suitable measures of identity-differentiation - would highlight improvement in functional people and decline in less functional or dysfunctional ones. The application of this hypothesis to suitable research designs and its subsequent implementations can be useful for the likeness construct to become a little less hidden relational ingredient.

## References

Acitelli, L. K., Kenny, D. A., & Hall, P. (2001). The importance of similarity and understanding of partners' marital ideals to relationship satisfaction. *Personal Relationships, 8*,

167-185.

Albert, M. (1970). Temporal comparison theory. *Psychological Review, 84*, 485-503.

Bergman, L. R., Magnusson, D., & El-Khouri, B. M. (2003). *Studying individual development in an inter-individual context*. Mahvah, NJ: Earbaum.

Byrne, D. (1971). *The attraction paradigm*. New York: Academic Press.

Cole, T., & Teboul, J. C. B. (2004). Non-zero sum collaboration, reciprocity, and the preference for similarity: Developing an adaptive model of close relational functioning. *Personal Relationships, 11*, 135-160.

Cozzi, F. (2004). *Competenza relazionale e anoressia nervosa [Relational competence and anorexia nervosa]*. Unpublished dissertation in psychology. Padua: University of Padua.

Cupach, W. C., & Metts, S. (1995). The role of sexual attitude similarity in romantic heterosexual relationships. *Personal Relationships, 2*, 287-300.

Cusinato, M. (2003). *A task of relational competence. Instruction manual*. Treviso, Italy: Centro della Famiglia.

Cusinato, M., & L'Abate, L. (in press). Likeness: A hidden ingredient in family therapy. *American Journal of Family Therapy*.

Cusinato, M., & Pastore, M. (2001). Uno strumento di valutazione dell'importanza di sé in rapporto all'altro. Analisi delle strutture tassonomiche in prospettiva evolutiva [An evaluation tool of self-importance in relationships to others. Analyses of taxonomic structures from a developmental perspective]. *Età Evolutiva, 69*, 5-18.

Duck, S. (1975). Attitude similarity and interpersonal attraction: Right answers and wrong reasons. *British Journal of Social and Clinical Psychology, 14*, 311-312.

Festinger, L. (1954). A theory of social comparison processes. *Human Relations, 7*, 117-140.

Griffitt, W. (1974). Attitude similarity and attraction. In T. L. Huston (Ed.), *Foundations of interpersonal attraction* (pp. 285-308). New York: Academic Press.

Heider, F. (1958). *The psychology of interpersonal relations*. New York: Wiley.

Harvey, O. J. (1966). System structure, flexibility, and creativity. In O. J. Harvey (Ed.), *Experience, structure, and adaptability* (pp. 39-65). New York: Springer.

Johnson, J. R. W. (1982). *The logical typing of the symmetrical complementary, and parallel relationship typology: A follow-up study*. Unpublished doctoral dissertation, Georgia State University, Atlanta.

L'Abate, L. (1976). *Understanding and helping the individual in the family*. New York: Grüne and Stratton.

L'Abate, L. (1994). *A theory of personality development*. New York: Wiley.

L'Abate, L. (1997). *The self in the family. A classification of personality, psychopathology, and criminality*. New York: Wiley.

L'Abate, L. (1999). Being human: Loving and hurting. In A. C. Richard, & T. Schumrum (Eds.), *Invitation to dialogue. The legacy of Sidney Jourard* (pp. 81-90). Dubuque, IO: Kent/Kendall.

L'Abate, L. (2005). *Personality in intimate relationships. Socialization and psychopathology*. New York: Springer.

L'Abate, L, & Cusinato, M. (2007). Linking theory with practice: Theory-derived interventions in prevention and family therapy. *The Family Journal. Counseling and Therapy for Couples and Families, 15*, 318-327.

Levinger, G. (1964). Note on need complementarity in marriage. *Psychological Bulletin, 61*, 153-157.

Lickona, T. (1974). A cognitive-developmental approach to interpersonal attraction. In T. L. Huston (Ed.), *Foundations of interpersonal attrac*tion (pp. 31-59). New York: Academic Press.

Longhin, L. (2003). Competenza relazionale di psicotici [Psychotics' relational competence]. Unpublished dissertation in psychology. Padua: University of Padua.

Lynn, D. B. (1969). *Parental and sex role identification: A theoretical formulation.* Berkeley, CA: McCurchan.

Kelly, G. (1955). *The psychology of personal construct.* New York: W. W. Norton.

Kohlberg, L. (1969). Stage and sequence: The cognitive-developmental approach to socialization. In D. A. Goslin (Ed.). *Handbook of socialization theory and research* (pp. 347-480). Chicago, IL: Rand McNally.

Mahler, M. S. (1968). *On human symbiosis and the vicissitudes of individuation.* New York: International University Press.

Onorato, R. S., & Turner, J. C. (2002). Challenging the primacy of the personal self: The case for depersonalized self-conception. In Y. Kashima, M. Foddy, & M. Platow (Eds.), *Self and identity: Personal, social, and symbolic* (pp. 145-178). Mahvah, NJ: Earbaum.

Rotter, J. B. (1966). Generalized expectancies for internal versus external control of reinforcement. *Psychological Monograph, 80* (Whole No. 609).

Schneider, D., Hastof, A., & Ellsworth, P. (1979). *Person perception.* Reading, MA: Addison-Wesley.

Scilletta, C. (2001). *Versione computerizzata della Prova di Competenza Relazionale. Esplorazione delle opportunità teoriche ed applicative [Computerized version of the Task of Relational Competence. Explorations of theoretical and applicative opportunities].* Unpublished dissertation in psychology. Padua: University of Padua.

Witkin, H. A. (1965). Psychological differentiation and forms of pathology. *Journal of Abnormal Psychology, 70*, 317-336.

# SECTION V. CONCLUSION

In: Toward a Science of Clinical Psychology
Editor: Luciano L'Abate, pp. 355-383

ISBN: 978-1-60456-062-6


*Chapter XIX*

# WORKING AT A DISTANCE FROM PARTICIPANTS: WRITING AND NONVERBAL MEDIA

*Luciano L'Abate*

## ABSTRACT

To become truly a science clinical psychological evaluations and interventions should be as much as possible free from biases and opinions based on personal whims and wills of professionals. Both evaluations and interventions should be based on reproducibly inter-subjective methods. This statement means that evaluations and many interventions should take place with participants at a distance from professional clinical psychologists and instead in the hands and minds of middle-level and bachelor-level semi-professionals using mechanical devices and standard instruments. Why? Because only at a distance from participants can professionals make decisions based on objective evidence rather then on personal or professional biases. To maintain distance from participants, increase objectivity, and therefore avoid personal biases, it is crucial for doctorate level clinical psychologists and even psychotherapists to work through intermediaries, be they human or mechanical.

## TOWARD A HIERARCHY OF PERSONNEL AND EQUIPMENT: INCREASED USE OF MIDDLE-PROFESSIONAL AND TECHNICAL LEVEL PERSONNEL

In reviewing the present status of mental health professions, Robiner (2006) in his section on the use of least expensive providers concluded:

> "...as concerns about costs and quality are balanced, the roles of relatively more intensively trained professionals (i. e, psychologists) are likely to change. Increasingly, their roles may focus on their knowledge and skills in supervision, management,

research, and program development, and less on the direct provision of clinical services."(Robiner, 2006, p. 615).

The laboratory method, therefore, is one way to hasten this prediction, especially in relationship to a hierarchical organization of personnel and equipment. This hierarchy (Table 20.1) implies the use of middle-and technical-level personnel akin to paralegals in law and physician assistants in medicine. The use of middle-level psychological sub-para- and middle level personnel and technicians has existed since the establishment of laboratory evaluation (L'Abate, 1968) and of neuropsychology.

DeLuca (1989) reviewed the historical, professional, and legal precedents for using technicians. He delineated a rationale for their deployment and examined deployment patterns current at the time. He also argued that: "The utilization of technicians affords the neuropsychologist with optimal standardization, reliability, and validity of the assessment process. Moreover, the practice is highly cost-effective and efficient (p. 3)." He also discussed how many state psychological associations and boards as well as third-party health providers have attempted to "supplant or eliminate this practice (p. 3)."

DeLuca and Putman (1993) argued that "The use of the professional/technician model or, more specifically, the laboratory method in clinical psychology and clinical neuropsychology has many advantages: (1) objective data collection; (2) more efficient use of the psychologist's time; and (3) cost-effectiveness (p. 100). They analyzed differential practices in the utilization of psychological technicians and investigated the "widespread" use of technicians among neuropsychologists, supporting the increase in efficiency and cost-effectiveness. They cited this writer's applications of the laboratory method to psychodiagnostic assessment, monitored play therapy, and the evaluation and enrichment of couples and families. They also cited Durlack's (1979) findings about the comparative effectiveness of para-professional versus professional helpers in psychotherapy.

The arguments by DeLuca and Putman are buttressed by advances in the increased use of homework assignments (Kazantzis & L'Abate, 2007) and of low-cost approaches to promote physical and mental health (L'Abate, 2007c) as discussed in Chapter 1 of this volume and expanded below. Rather than a professional/ technician dichotomous distinction, it is preferable to envisage a hierarchical ladder of personnel according to different levels of education, interest, and skill (Table 19.1).

In spite of De Luca and Putman's arguments about the advantages of the laboratory method in neuro-psychology, this method has not been adopted in many clinical psychology specialties. One reason for this neglect is the glut of professionals and semi-professionals in the field of mental health who are not concerned with seemingly academic research but who are concerned instead with the every day very real and legitimate issue of making a living, according to a private practice rather than to a public health model. As long as that is the case, the laboratory method may be used in academic, medical, and institutional settings but not in private or independent practice. To increase possible applications of the laboratory method, we need to explore how to combine talk, the traditional medium of communication and healing in both evaluation and psychotherapy, with two other thus far neglected media: writing and non-verbal approaches. The combination of all three media should lead to synergistic outcomes and possibly increase efficacy and cost-effectiveness in clinical psychology endeavors. Furthermore, with the inclusion of all three media in clinical practices, we should be able to see which participants can communicate and perhaps heal more effectively using one medium over the other two. Using exclusively one medium, such as talk, we never allow professionals as well as participants to find which medium works best for which participants.

**Table 19.1: Toward a Hierarchy of Clinical Psychology Personnel**

| Educational Level | Skills and Responsibilities |
|---|---|
| Board Displomate | Supervision and support of doctorate level professionals |
| | Leadership in research and in conceptualization of laboratory procedures, evaluations and interventions, and results. |
| Doctorate | Crisis intervention |
| | Development of treatment plans based on conclusions from evaluation based on reason for referral, history, interview, objective tests, and final diagnosis |
| | Decision making and delegation of specific evaluative and therapeutic responsibilities, matching problem with solution, matching treatment plans with specific therapists. |
| | Supervision and support of master- and bachelor- level personnel Quality control, maintenance of ethical, professional, and scientific standards. |
| | Interpretation and report writing from laboratory evaluations |
| Master or equivalent | Carrying out most verbally talk-based and non-verbal therapeutic, para-therapeutic and pre-therapeutic responsibilities, including protracted f2f and online contacts with participants including self-help protocols. |
| Bachelor or equivalent | Administration and scoring of standard psychological tests either by hand or by computer. |
| | Administration and follow-through of structured low-cost interventions to promote physical and mental health, preventive psycho-educational skill-training programs. |
| High school or equivalent | Clerical responsibilities, filing, answering phone calls, routine tasks. |

*Adapted from L'Abate, 2003, p. 230.

## In Search of Cost-effective Methods in Psychotherapy

The grand visionary of psychotherapy, Nicholas A. Cummings (Thomas & Cummings, 2000) predicted that psychotherapy practices would change from the one-to-one model of traditional psychoanalysis to more cost-effective group psychotherapies, which, of course, would include also the most natural group there is, the family. He also predicted that managed care would lead to the industrialization of psychotherapy, and an increase in psycho-educational programs, such as those found in this volume. To make psychotherapy even more cost-effective, he recommended also the principle of "Give homework in the first session and every therapy session thereafter." (p. 272). This principle has been followed to the letter by the recent publication of a complete handbook on the subject (Kazantzis & L'Abate, 2007).

Kazantzis and L'Abate (2007) included most schools of psychotherapy and most clinical conditions to demonstrate that homework assignments, in addition to being cost effective, produce positive outcomes. Hence, there is no longer a rationale to justify passivity, non-active participation, and non-directiveness in psychotherapy. Perhaps the three major Rogerian requirements of unconditional regard, warmth, and empathy may have been useful in working with functional or semi-functional participants. However, these requirements, in my humble opinion, may fail in producing improvements in acting-out personality disorders, participants with chronic psychiatric disorders, as well as couples and families. Hence, there is a need to include the two other media of communication in our evaluative and healing practices to deal with conditions that may be refractory to words.

What Cummings did not predict, and perhaps there was no way at predicting at that time (1994), that writing would become a major vehicle of service delivery as the very next advance in the meta-morphosis from talk-based (tb) psychotherapy practiced face-to-face (f2f) to the practice of online psychotherapy at a distance.

## The Internet and its Implications for the Laboratory Method

Clinics, hospitals, colleges, universities, and public libraries where computers are available can and will be increasingly used for delivery of selected mental health protocols, especially to help people who are reluctant, unwilling, or unable to seek medical, psychiatric, or mental health services requiring f2f tb contacts. Potential participants, be they individuals, couples, or families, who may not need f2f tb treatment, could use such programs on an enrichment or preventive basis. For those who have already consulted established mental health professionals, computers can become an additional or alternative, cost-effective source of help for many mental health concerns, as already is the case (Strecher, 2007).

Implications for the use of computer-Internet approaches are relevant to the delivery of both preventive and therapeutic treatment approaches. If it can be demonstrated that properly programmed computers allow easy access to participants (individuals, couples, and families) who: (1) would not otherwise access existing mental health facilities or; (2) may not need f2f tb treatment; but (3) can use self-administered programs, a new, cost-effective delivery system could be opened up. This delivery system would reach more participants per unit of professional time than it was possible heretofore. This approach would in no way decrease or diminish the function of existing mental health personnel. It would enhance this function by empowering existing mental health professionals to reach more people per unit of professional time through this approach than was possible heretofore through f2f talk. This is why a granduate program in structured online approaches is included in Appendix A.

The Internet has changed the way psychological evaluations and interventions are and will be delivered in the not too distant future (Fogg, 2003; Hsiung, 2002; Maheu, Pulier, Wilhelm, & McMenamie, 2005; Maheu, Whitten, & Allen, 2001). As Strecher (2007) commented on the use of the Internet for evaluation:

"A prerequisite for interactivity is the ability to understand the needs of the user, and now more than a decade of studies have demonstrated that well-designed computer-based assessments can at least rival the validity of assessments using paper-and-pencil methods, trained interviewers, or clinicians."(pp. 56-57).

The chaotic nature of evaluations and interventions in f2f tb practices will become even more chaotic when practiced online. It is important, therefore, to rely more and more on standardized uniform practices, SOPs of the LM that will assure that those practices go hand in hand with research. Rather than research versus practice going along two separate and independent tracks, as it has happened in the past and it is still happening in the present, the LM would allow for *both* practice *and* research to move along two sides of the same track tied together rather then separately, as in a monorail. Unfortunately, the open nature of the Internet will allow a great many unqualified charlatans to abuse of this medium to reach and scam a great many people in need of help. How can clinical psychologists avoid being compared to the charlatans and scammers who are already crowding the Internet? Here is where the importance of proper evaluation is crucial to let uninformed potential participants avoid falling in the hands of unqualified charlatans. Professionals will be differentiated from non-professionals on the basis of their following scientifically replicable objective procedures that will allow to evaluate participants in ways that are not usually followed by non-professionals.

Qualified professionals, of course, will need to be knowledgeable of the fundamentals and vast opportunities of the Internet (Crumlish, 1996; Goldman, 1994; Maloy, 1996; Marusich & Blackthorn, 1998; McGuire, Stillborne, McAdams, & Hyatt, 2001; Sadowski, Campbell-Koella, & Keene, 2001)

### *Laboratory Evaluation Online*

Evaluating potential participants online poses quite a few ethical and professional problems (L'Abate, 2001, 2002). How do we know the person we are evaluating is the person we think we are evaluating? How about issues of confidentiality? Who will know what results will be found? Who will receive these results, the one we evaluated or someone else? These are professional and ethical issues that clinical psychologists who want to join the 21st century will need to grapple with and resolve. Encryptions and passwords might be one way to solve problems of direct communication with intended participants including issues of privacy and confidentiality. This is why a considerable amount of information needs to be included in training clinical psychologists to operate online, especially in relation to ethical and professional issues (Fogg, 2003; Gackenbach. 1998; Hsiung, 2002; Jones, 1995; Maheu, Pulier, Wilhelm, & McMenamin, 2005; Maheu, Whitten, & Allen, 2001; Pulier, Mount, McMenamin, & Maheu, 2007; Schwartz, 1984).

If psychological interventions are occurring online, why should there not be also evaluations online? A suggested theory-derived, partially validated battery of paper-and-pencil , self-report instruments for adults is included in Appendix A within a proposal for a graduate training program of online structured interventions. However, one important aspect of online evaluation lies in achieving more reliable diagnoses at a distance, without ever seeing participants f2f or talking with them. As aberrant such a possibility may be to many psychotherapists, one must keep in mind that many life-death decisions are made every day online in medicine. Provided there are sufficient technical and professional guidelines and restrictions, there is no reason why reliable diagnoses may not be obtained online (Morrison & Stamps, 1998). What would be the use of this much information available online if it cannot be applied to real live participants? For instance, a semi-structured interview (L'Abate, 1992), that includes weights to distinguish between functional and dysfunctional answers, could be administered as part of an online test battery suggested in Appendix A.

### *Laboratory Interventions Online*

The methodology to evaluate and intervene online is found in the pioneering work of Seligman et al., 2005). That research should be considered as the harbinger of things to come in prevention and psychotherapy in this century. Along the same lines, I have proposed using the dictionary as a first step in helping people understand themselves by acquiring terms that are more relevant and specific to their conditions than a catch-all diagnosis. For instance, instead of attributing a non-specific and often times threatening diagnosis of "depression", why not ask participants to define (in writing) and give two examples of depression-related terms from any list of terms related to that condition, as found in many objective tests and questionnaires (L'Abate, 2007a)? By asking participants to rank-order which items apply to them more than other items, instead of a catch-all term, depression may become much more specific and real to the individual by relying on a restricted number of items than all of those contained in the test. This approach can become grist for the therapeutic mill by administering homework assignments specifically designed to elaborate on the origin, intensity, duration, and rate of a specific behavior pattern. This approach has been adopted in a great many workbooks or protocols (L'Abate, 2008) and in proposing written interventions with couples (L'Abate, 2007b).

By the same token, rather than trying to use psychological tests to determine psychopathology, why not ask participants to rate themselves on positive activities above and beyond whatever conflicts may be the reason for referral, as suggested in Chapter 1 of this volume? After looking at the positive individual and multi-relational aspects of their relationships, participants are asked to define and give two examples of terms related to dysfunctional patterns in their relationship. The rank-order of these patterns allows therapists to work on one pattern at a time f2f or to administer each pattern as homework assignments that are specific to the partners' conflicts (L'Abate, 2007b).This approach, of course, implies a more directive stance than some psychotherapists may be willing to assume.

## DIRECTIVENESS IN PSYCHOTHERAPY: ARGUMENTS AND EVIDENCE FOR A RADICAL PROPOSAL

Directiveness in psychotherapy is related to how much homework is assigned above and beyond f2f tbcontacts. Directiveness ranges from no homework and just talk at one extreme of a continuum to the radical extreme of this proposal, psychotherapy consisting mainly of gradually assigned homework with less and less reliance on f2f talk and progressively greater reliance on homework. This proposal is based on three recent advances that heighten the importance of directiveness in psychotherapy: (1) increase in the use of in-between session homework; (2) introduction of prescriptive low-cost approaches to promote physical and mental health, and (3) greater reliance on distance writing as an alternative or adjunct to talk.

The purpose of this section is to argue for and to give supporting conceptual, empirical, and practical evidence for a seemingly radical and possibly extreme position along a continuum of directiveness in psychotherapy. This continuum is defined by two extremes of minimum directiveness or even non-directiveness at one extreme and a maximum of directiveness at the other extreme. The term "directiveness " is defined here as the assumption or appropriation of a directive role in psychotherapy. That role consists of giving (or not-giving), administering (or not administering) to participants (clients, consumers, patients) instructions, recommendations, suggestions, for in-between- or extra-session activities, practice exercises, prescribed tasks, handouts, worksheets, or homework assignments. How much homework, if any is assigned, therefore, becomes a criterion of directiveness not considered in major, representative psychotherapy texts that did not include also the role of extra- or in-between sessions homework (Bongar & Beutler, 1995; Norcross, 1986; Roth & Fonagy, 1996; Sperry, Brill, Howard, & Grisson, 1996; Zeig, 1997). What is proposed here means *empirically based directiveness*.

The major predictor of therapeutic outcome, agreed upon by a great deal of research, is without a doubt, the therapist's empathic understanding, unconditional positive regard, warmth, spontaneity, congruence, and genuiness (Luborsky, Crits-Christoph, Mintz, & Auerbach, 1988, pp. 138-140). These characteristics fall within the expressive *communal* therapeutic style relevant, if not crucial, to the establishment of a therapeutic alliance. That alliance is responsible for producing a great part of the variance in the positive outcome of psychotherapy (Bongar & Beutler, 1995; Fonagy, Target, Cottrell, Phillips & Kurtz, 2002; Hubble, Duncan, & Miller, 1999; Safran & Muran, 1995; Snyder & Ingram, 2000). Since so much has been written about this style in psychotherapy texts, this style is of paramount importance to the therapeutic process and outcome, but it will not be the focus of this section.

That communal style, no matter how important, is secondary to the purpose of this section that is focused on a second predictor of therapeutic outcome, and that is: therapist directiveness (Luborsky et al., 1988). This quality refers to the therapist *agentic*, instrumental methods that constitute how directive (or non-directive) a therapist is in practice. Beutler, Machado, and Neufeldt (1994, pp. 255-256) in reviewing the evidence for therapist "action-oriented" directiveness reported "contradictory findings" perhaps due to how directive therapists may have been, suggesting that: "Perhaps moderate levels of directiveness facilitate outcomes while high levels do not. *The absence of standard and comparable measures of therapist directiveness prevent an analysis of this possibility* (underline mine, p. 256)."

This possibility has been explored and exploded by the historical meta-analysis of Kazantzis, Deane, and Ronan (2001). They provided the first-hand evidence for the direct connection between assignment of homework and increased, positive therapy outcome. This evidence has been substantiated in a variety of studies in cognitive-behavioral therapy (Kazantzis, Deane, Ronan, & L'Abate, 2005) and more recently in Kazantzis and L'Abate's treatise (2007) that includes major schools of psychotherapy and major clinical populations and modalities of treatment.

Consequently, on the basis of that evidence, directiveness can be evaluated by the extent to which psychotherapists or a particular school of psychotherapy use and administer in-between sessions or extra-session activities, tasks, or "practice exercises" as homework assignments to participants (children, youth, single adults, couples, and families). In the past I have used the term "assignment" for lack of a better word, but, on the basis of the many critical comments about this term (Kazantzis & L'Abate, 2007), I have opted for a more neutral and hopefully more acceptable, less scholastic term like "practice exercises." Whether that is an appropriate choice remains to be seen.

## Three Recent Advances in the Therapeutic Repertoire

Three recent advances are bound to influence and impact the practice of psychotherapy as we know it by expanding the range and options of preventive, para-therapeutic, and pre-therapeutic practices available to psychotherapists: (1) greater reliance on writing as an alternative or as an adjunct to face-to-face (f2f) talk; (2) increased attention to extra- or in-between session homework; and (3) introduction of prescriptive low-cost approaches to promote physical and mental health. Older or already established para-therapeutic practices, consisting of structured psycho-educational social training programs have existed for more than a generation, even though they has not been used by most psychotherapists, constituting a tier of preventive approaches unfortunately separate from traditional therapeutic practices (De Maria, 2003; Fonagy et al., 2002; L'Abate, 1990; Mrazek & Haggerty, 1994). These approaches, although relevant, cannot be covered here as well approaches included in the empirically supported therapies movement (Dobson & Craig, 1998; Nathan & Gorman, 2002). Nonetheless, eventually both approaches will be reconsidered as part of this proposal.

## Distance Writing in Psychotherapy

More and more psychological practice will include working at a distance from participants, in some cases without ever seeing them f2f (L'Abate, 1992). This conclusion may seem aberrant to those psychologists and psychotherapists who place sole value in their personal presence and in the power of the spoken word. Yet, a variety of sources and even evidence suggest that this trend, distance writing, will increase and become the norm in the future. The major source for this trend is the Internet which, as already noted, is revolutionizing the way mental health services are already and will be increasingly delivered in this century.

F2f talk has been traditionally the major if not the sole mode of communication (and healing) in most schools of psychotherapy (Norcross, 1986; Norcross & Goldfried, 1992; Snyder & Ingram, 2000), whether they use or not use homework assignments, or whether they conceive of psychotherapy as an art or a science, including the empirically-based psychotherapy movement (Dobson & Craig, 1998; Nathan & Gorham, 2002). These schools have one major quality in common and that is: they are all based on f2f contacts and on talk as the major if not the sole medium of communication and healing between participants and psychotherapists. To decrease the inevitable therapist's variability, some schools use therapy manuals to assure protocol replicability. What most homework assignments, on the other hand, have in common is an increasing reliance on writing rather than talking (Kazantzis & L'Abate, 2007), as in prescriptions, instructions, written handouts, worksheets, or workbooks, as discussed below.

## Working at a Distance from Participants

Working at a distance from participants through writing is not a new position. Scientific, medical, legal, governamental, educational, and industrial fields rely on the written medium to accumulate a body of knowledge that is basic for the advancement of that particular field. Science progresses on the basis of reproducible operations described through written records, not just words. Most medical practices rely on medications administered and recorded through written prescriptions to participants at home, only rarely in the physician's office. Skyscrapters are built on the basis of printed blue-prints, not words. Governmental organizations rely on written records to establish past experiences and evidence. Educational fields may rely initially on the spoken words of teachers, but ultimately, knowledge by students is stored in their class-notes and in their assigned readings and assessed by written examinations. Even preaching, where words may be the main medium of communication, is based on the written word of a Bible, Koran, Torah, or other written documents.

Psychotherapy (and preaching?), therefore, remains the last bastion of human activity that rests mainly or solely on talk rather than on written documentation. Psychotherapy notes may represent a written record, but we still do not know how accurate and self-serving those notes may be. Furthermore, we do not know how those notes are related to the process and progress in psychotherapy. No mention of therapy notes was made in the psychotherapy treatises cited in this section and in other sources not included here. DeVries (2006) for instance, suggested that senior citizens take notes in therapy sessions. Consequently, if progress is to be achieved in helping troubled people it is already occurring and it will increasingly occur through distance writing rather than f2f talk, as on the Internet (Maheu, Pulier, Wilhelm, McMenamin, & Brown-Connolly, 2004), where helpful relationships are established every day without f2f contact.

## TYPES OF WRITTEN HOMEWORK

There are at least six different types of writing that can be used as homework assignments or practice exercises: (1) open-ended, (2) autobiographical, (3) expressive, (4) guided, (5) programmed, and (6) automatic.

### *Open-ended*

This type of writing includes diaries, journals, and gathering of personal information. Most of the literature and research on this type of writing can be found in Levine and Calvanio (2007)

### *Autobiographical*

The results of "The Nun Study" (Snowden, 2001) brought to real life the importance of reliving one's life in writing rather than through talk. Literature and research on autobiography is found in Demetrio and Borgonovi's review (2007)

### *Expressive*

This type includes what is now called the "Pennebaker's Paradigm," writing for 15-20 minutes a day for four consecutive days about one's secret traumas and hurts heretofore not shared with anyone else (Esterling, L'Abate, Murray, & Pennebaker, 1999; Esterling & Pennebaker, 2001; Lepore & Smyth, 2002; Pennebaker, 2001). Most of the recent literature and research on this paradigm is reviewed by Kasewiwic, Slatcher, and Pennebaker (2007).

### *Guided*

Rather than a categorical type of writing, guided writing represents a continuum ranging from written comments or questions to written homework practice exercises using diaries, journals, autobiographies, expressed writing (Gambesca & Weeks, 2007, p. 355; L'Abate, 2002, pp. 55-58) It could consists of letters written but never mailed to completing questionnaires or structured interviews (De Vries, 2007; Twohig, Pierson, & Hayes, 2007; Niemeyer & Winter, 2007).

### *Programmed*

This type of writing involves written handouts, worksheets, or practice exercises assigned in-between sessions. When these practice exercises focus on a specific topic over an extended period of time, they are called workbooks. There is an increasing plethora of workbooks produced by John Wiley and Sons, Guildford, New Harbiger Publications, Haworth Press, and Springer. Many other publishers are rushing to produce workbooks for clinical and non-clinical conditions (Jordan & L'Abate, 1995; L'Abate, 1986, 1992, 1996, 2004a, 2004b, 2007b; L'Abate & De Giacomo, 2003).

As Twohig, Pierson, and Hayes (2006) concluded about the function of workbooks in psychotherapy: "...workbook-based therapy might be more effective than therapy without the workbook (2006, p. 128)." A meta-analysis of workbooks administered with minimal or without personal contact between trainers and participants produced a medium effect size of .44 (Smyth & L'Abate, 2001), suggesting that even without a therapist, workbooks can produce significant effects. Workbooks in out-patient psychotherapy with individuals, couples, and families, in comparison to participants who did not receive workbooks, contrary to a prediction cost-effectiveness, did not shorten the number of therapy sessions. Instead, workbooks produced a statistically significant increase in the number of sessions (L'Abate, L'Abate, & Maino, 2005). Whether this increase was due to greater involvement in the process of change by participants is a possibility that needs to be evaluated (Bohart & Tallman, 1999). On the other hand, Goldstein's use of a problem-solving workbook reduced by half the number of hospital days in decompensating women with personality disorders in Buenos Aires (L'Abate & Goldstein, 2007).

Workbooks can be classified along a variety of dimensions that include type of population (children, youth, single adults, couples, and families), level of functionality (high, medium, low), type of dysfunctionality (internalization versus externalization), fixed versus flexible format, paradoxical versus straightforward style, and reason for referral versus test-derivation (L'Abate, 1996; 2004a, 2004b, 2997b). Workbooks vary also along a dimension of theory-derived versus theory-independent. For instance, a workbook about arguing and fighting in couples, among others, was derived from clinical practice. Workbooks about depression, negotiation, parenting, and self-differentiation were derived completely from models in a relational theory of personality socialization in intimate relationships (L'Abate, 2005). Consequently, their theoretical derivation makes workbooks a more dynamic and interactive way of evaluating theoretical models than static self-report, paper-and-pencil tests.

#### *Automatic*

There is no sufficient and reliable evidence to support this type of writing except to fulfill an amateurish and entertainment function.

The types of writing included in this section can become a tier of their own in a proposed graduate-degree program for online administration of structured interventions (Appendix A).

## Increased Attention to Homework: Toward a Continuum of Directiveness in Psychotherapy

Given a continuum of directiveness defined by two extremes of giving or not giving in-between-sessions homework, the extreme in non-directiveness is represented by the Rogerian position derived from humanistic and existential schools of thought and of psychotherapy (Rogers, 1980). This school does not give suggestions, directions, or homework assignments, unless suggested by participants themselves (Witty, 2007). *Being* emotionally available or the *Presence* and intimacy of the therapist, his or her continuous Awareness of what is said to express empathy, unconditional regard, intimacy, and respect for participants are more important factors than actual behavioral *Performance* (information and services) or *Production* (money and possessions). Essentially, this school bases its approach on a purely *communal* style with a minimum of agency on the part of the therapist. The Performance of the therapist, except for what has been said in-session, and Production of results are either irrelevant or unimportant. Stress lies on Awareness and on the emotional availability by therapists for participants. This Awareness is much more important than Performance or

Production. Greater Awareness may or may not accidentally or incidentally lead toward greater effectiveness in Performance and Production of participants, but it is not guaranteed.

Another aspect of the non-directive, existential and humanistic schools relates to how much evaluation and validation enter into assessing the outcome of these approaches. If psychotherapy is perceived essentially as an art, whatever a therapist does or says is justified on grounds that the personal and subjective experience of the therapist supercedes any external, objective measure of therapist's effectiveness: Performance or Production. The personal Presence and moment-to-moment experience of the therapist is the end-all of the process. No external criteria are necessary to validate that experience. Consequently, even though Rogers was the first to introduce tape-recordings of therapy sessions, the results from this process remain pretty much in the air, given the seemingly anti-empirical stance taken by followers of this school (Witty, 2007). These considerations, therefore, would locate this school in the supportive, communal extreme in a continuum of directiveness.

A position close to the extreme of non-directiveness is represented by the psychoanalytic school that, in some cases relies on homework assignments of dream analysis. Here "Insight" seems synonymous with Awareness. Stricker (2007), for instance, comments that "...there is little specific role for homework in traditional psychoanalytic psychotherapy (p. 102)". A middle point in this continuum is represented by emotion-focused experiential therapy (Ellison & Greenberg, 2007), where feelings and "empowerment" are the major thrust of this approach and homework is assigned ad hoc, seemingly without a specific general rationale or systematic plan. Perhaps, another school in the middle of this continuum could be interpersonal psychotherapy (Young & Mufson, 2007).

The extreme of directiveness is represented by the cognitive-behavioral schools, where homework assignments constitute the bulk or core of the psychotherapeutic process (Beck & Tompkins, 2007; Kazantzis, Deane, Ronan, & L'Abate, 2005; Ledley & Huppert, 2007). Stress on Performance and Production may or may not lead toward greater Awareness. If and when Awareness occurs, it is accidental or incidental to the outcome. Awareness is not guaranteed because the major goal of therapy is to learn skills in Performance and in Production rather than in Being Present and Awareness. Hence, this school fits within the agentic, instrumental method of therapy and tends to see psychotherapy as a scientific enterprise, not as an art or as a religion. For this school, psychotherapy is essentially a science and thus it can be evaluated and validated objectively just like any other scientific pursuit.

Consequently, a major aspect of this school is reliance on empirical evaluation of psychotherapy outcome and a systematic analysis, i.e., dismantling, of what factors enter in producing that outcome (therapeutic alliance, personality of the therapist, level and type of dysfunctionality in participants, etc.), including replicable manuals to increase uniformity and reduce variability in psychotherapy to assure empirical validation of treatment outcomes (LeCroy, 1994; Van Hasselt & Hersen, 1998).

## Dimensions of Directiveness in Homework Assignment

Even though these obviously overlapping dimensions are phrased with an either-or dichotomy, it is understood that each dimension could represent a continuum in its own rights (Lambert, Harmon, & Slade, 2007).

### As hoc versus Systematic Homework

Homework can range all the way from tasks or practice exercises given at the spurt of the moment to thought-out homework based on previously conceived and planned treatment strategies. Examples of the former can be found in psychoanalytic psychotherapy (Stricker, 2007), interpersonal psychotherapy (Young & Mufson, 2007). Examples of the latter can be found in cognitive-behavioral contributions (Beck & Tompkins, 2007) and in the treatment of borderline personality disorders (Lindenboim, Chapman, & Linehan, 2007).

### Specificity versus Generality

Homework can vary along a dimension of specificity at one end and generality at the other end. Examples of the former are found in the work of Lindenboim, Chapman, and Linehan (2007). Examples of the latter can be found in the work of emotion-focused experiential therapy (Ellison & Greenberg, 2007), among others (Nelson, Castonguay, & Barwick, 2007).

### Theory-derived versus Theory-independent

Dream-analysis, for instance, would be a theory-derived type of homework. Except for assignments in the behavioral-cognitive school, most assignments seem to be theory-independent. This dimension will be reviewed below in relationship to programmed writing.

## Low-cost Prescriptive Approaches to Promote Physical and Mental Health

Recently a whole compendium (L'Abate, 2007c) of research-based, low-cost approaches to promote physical and mental health introduced and added a completely new tier within the traditional distinction among primary, secondary, and tertiary prevention approaches (L'Abate, 1990; Mrazek & Haggerty, 1994). This compendium includes a classification of research supporting the use and prescription of inexpensive approaches, self-initiated or administered by others, to promote physical and mental health. Whether these approaches enter within the tier of universal primary prevention or whether they constitute a separate tier of their own remains to be seen. Nonetheless, these approaches can be added synergistically to preventive and psycho-therapeutic practices to lower their costs and perhaps increase their efficacy and effectiveness.

## Primary Approaches

Each approach constitutes a chapter in the list given below. Including authors's names and full references would take more space than necessary. The interested reader will see the evidence supporting each topic in the original compendium. Therefore, each chapter is listed by topical title only. These approaches, supported by evidence, possess important policy and public health implications that, for reasons of space, cannot be discussed in detail here (L'Abate, 2006a, 2007).

### Nutrition

Primary approaches are basic to survival, including nutrition, diets, Omega-3 fatty acids, vitamins, supplements, and herbs.

### Non-verbal

These approaches include pleasant activities, like meditation, relaxation, exercise, dancing, gardening, or playing cards, among others.

## Secondary Approaches

Secondary approaches devoted exclusively to writing will be considered in grater detail in the next section.

*Secondary Relational Approaches* include close physical contact between parent and infant, massage and prolonged non-erotic touch, affection like hugging, holding, huddling, and cuddling (3HC), love-making, emotional intimacy, as in the sharing of hurts and fears of being hurt, forgiveness for errors and transgressions, and spirituality.

## Tertiary Multi-relational Approaches

Among others, these approaches include friends, support groups, animal companions, emotional intelligence, the Good Behavior Game for aggression in classrooms, and peer-wise tutoring. The latter two topics are not contained in the original compendium but are enclosed in a position paper (L'Abate, 2006b).

What does this new tier of inexpensive, prescriptive approaches mean for the practice of psychotherapy and especially for the practice of directiveness in psychotherapy? It means that, at least from a public health viewpoint, the maximum good for the most people at the least possible cost, less expensive approaches can be used before, during, or after f2f talk therapy. They can also be used to evaluate the motivation of participants to change. Instead of psychological tests that find it difficult if not impossible to evaluate this motivation, this new tier, as well as a second tier of structured, psycho-educational, social training programs, administered in groups, like assertiveness training, couple enrichment, parenting, etc. (De Maria, 2003; L'Abete, 1990), can be prescribed in a successive sieves or stepped treatment approach, as suggested in this proposal below.

## A Radical Proposal

Even though the cognitive-behavioral school may seemingly represent the most extreme of directiveness, by relying mainly on using homework assignments or practice exercises more or less systematically, I would assume, argue, and support an even more extreme, radical, if not drastic position, that is: *psychotherapy should consist of a maximum of homework assignments and a minimum of f2f contacts and talk.* Instead of talk being the major if not the sole medium of communication and healing between participants and professionals, the major medium of communication between participants and professionals should be administration of in-between sessions tasks through written instructions or prescriptions, handouts, worksheets, and workbooks or protocols.

The process of psychotherapy, therefore, should take place at distance from therapists, in the home where behavior needs to be changed rather than in the therapist's office, where behavior is changed in the presence and activity of the therapist. Whether that behavior generalizes outside of the therapist's office depends on participants practicing it in their own homes. The behavior to be changed should occur at home, not in the therapist's office. Psychotherapy, therefore, would consist of a process with a minimum of reliance on f2f contacts and on talk and maximum reliance on homework practice exercises (Jordan & L'Abate, 1995; L'Abate, 1986, 1990, 1991, 1992, 1997a, 1997b, 1999, 2001, 2002, 2003a, 2003b, 2004a, 2004b, 2005, 2997a, 2007b; L'Abate & De Giacomo, 2003). This progression in assignment of more complex homework as therapy progresses is especially evident in the work of sex therapists (Gambiscia & Weeks, 2007) and others (Kazantzis & L'Abate, 2007).

Given this thesis, the process of therapy, as routinely performed in medical practices, for instance, would start with participants desirous of professional help completing the least expensive sieve, that is: completing a simple task at a distance from the therapist, progressing then though various, more complex and expensive, intervening sieves, and finally progressing to the most expensive sieve and that is: seeing and talking with the therapist f2f. Incidentally, this approach has been implemented for years by Gould (2001) with thousands of participants. That pioneering work planted the original seed, among other seeds, for this proposal (L'Abate, 2004b).

## The Practice of Successive Stages in Psychotherapy

The introduction of "successive sieves" (L'Abate, 1990), which are now called "stepped treatments" or "successive stages," as an example, could be one way to address the problem of discriminating among different levels and types of functionalities and dysfunctionalities, ranging from the serious to the superficial and the trivial from the troublesome (Davison, 200l; Haaga, 2000; Newman, 2000; Otto, Pollack, & Maki, 2000; Sobell & Sobell, 2000; Wilson, Vitousek, & Loeb, 2000). This approach does stress the importance of differentiating among degrees and types of dysfunctionalities and at least three preventive approaches to deal with them: primary, secondary, and tertiary prevention. This conceptual and rather practical solution would distinguish among different levels of prevention. This distinction would reflect on the fact that most therapists are not interested or even knowledgeable about using primary and secondary methods to deal with many problematic but not severe issues that make up the majority of present day private practice, except for crisis intervention for really serious problems (De Maria, 2003; L'Abate, 2006a, 2006c, 2006d).

To use an analogy from medicine, successive stages mean taking first a home-measure of severity, that is, body temperature through a thermometer. Second, if an aspirin does not reduce the fever level overnight and no other home-remedy is successful, then an office-visit is scheduled. There blood pressure measurement and blood analyses will help determine whether more extensive and expensive evaluations should be taken, CT-scan, EKG, etc. By the same token, a screening check-list of positive activities, as suggested above, as well as an initial screening battery of short self-report tests to measure levels of functioning, such as an objective questionnaire to evaluate level of functioning from historical family and developmental background can be administered online and scored by computer (L'Abate, 1992, 1996, 2007d), plus brief, self-report paper-and-pencil inventories to evaluate levels of depression and anxiety and a list of personal concerns, may be sufficient to reach some conclusion on whether (1) a self-help group for a specific addiction may be more efficient and sufficient than f2f tb psychotherapy with a professional, or (2) whether a specific, psycho-educational or psycho-social skill training program administered by a middle-level professional may be sufficient, and less expensive, for immediate purposes, or (3) administration of specific written protocols for homework assignments.

An inverse successive stages approach was used years ago, when families who terminated family therapy, were administered enrichment programs to decrease the chances of a relapse (Kochalka, Buzas, L'Abate, McHenry, & Gibson, 1987). By the same token, to avoid and prevent lapses and relapses, additional psychoeducational social skills programs could be administered after termination of treatment. However, as DeMaria (2003) commented on this issue, private practitioners do not refer their patients to anybody else unless a primary care physician is needed for medication but never to other practitioners for preventive skills training or similar programs. This proprietary trend is dangerous to our participants and to our profession.

These stages can be simplified and summarized into:

Stage 1. Administration of simple paper-and-pencil self-report rating scales followed by recommendations for assignment to either low-cost approaches to promote physical and mental health (L'Abate, 2007c) or (homework assignments of specific self-help protocols through mail, fax, or Internet (Kazantzis & L'Abate, 2007) to evaluate motivation to change rather than relying only on words. Stage 2. Admission to a therapy groupwith added homework assignments, or Stage 3. Admission to f2f tb individual, couple, or family therapy with a professional helper.For couples or families the reader is referred to L'Abate (2007d)

Even though this proposal uses only three stages, they are used for illustrative purposes. Each stage can be broken down into more specific sub-steps according to the nature of the problem and the ideological and experiential proclivities of the psychotherapist. A summary of these stages is illustrated in Table 19.2.

**Table 19.2 Progressive Stages in Psychotherapy**

Stage 1. To be performed and completed as homework, with minimum help from professional (Kazantzis & L'Abate, 2007).

a. Internet support groups, and/or mantras suggested by Seligman et al., (20005)
b. When Internet is not available let participants try one of the low-cost approaches of their choice that is more consistent with their likes, needs, and wants (L'Abate, 2007b)
c. Indiividual, couple, or families activities (Table 2).
d. Non-targeted protocols or workbooks for life-long learning for individuals, couples, and families (L'Abate, 2007a).
e. Autobiographies (Demetrio & Borgonovi, 2007), dairies, journals and personal information (Levine & Calvanio, 2007)

Stage 2. Structured online interventions for targeted populations at risk for breakdown and deterioration (co-dependents, adult children of alcoholics, victims of sexual abuse, etc.).

a. Completion of tasks in Stage 1: Successful versus unsuccessful?
b. Expressive writing ("The Pennebaker Paradigm"; Kasewics, Slatcher, & Pennebaker, 2007)
c. Targeted self-help protocols for specific conditions such as externalization and internalization personality disorders (Clusters B and C of DSM-IV; L'Abate, 2007a).
d. Specific task assignments for specific conditions or concerns (Kazantzis & L'Abate, 2007).

Stage 3. Face-to-face talk with professional, crisis interventions, psychotherapy.

a. Completion of Stages 1 and 2: Successful versus unsuccessful?
b. Face-to-face intervention with medication
c. Medication with hospitalization or incarceration.

## Stage 1

For instance, a low-cost approach from the list of approaches given above could be presented to potential participants, asking whether they are following any of those approaches listed above and found in a rating sheet provided in Chapter 1 of this volume. A depressed participant could use physical exercise to bolster medication and/or f2f psychotherapy. A conflictual couple could choose to go dancing once a week before seeing the therapist the next day. A family with small children may be asked to hug, hold, huddle, and cuddle two or three times a week to see what happens afterwards. Not all the low-cost approaches listed above might be included in this sieve. Forgiveness, for instance, may have to be practiced after an hurt or transgression is shared over the phone or online with the therapist. Joining a specific support group online may be another task to be accomplished before seeing the therapist.

## Stage 2

A second task, among many possible ones, could be joining a psycho-educational, social skills training program, either in groups or on the internet. The issue here, as in the previous sieve, lies in participants successfully completing homework on their own to demonstrate their interest and involvement in change for the better.

## Stage 3

This stage, seeing and talking with a therapist f2f, would take place once homework assignments are completed. Seeing and talking with a therapist, therefore, should be contingent on completing some kind of assignment or practice exercise, no matter how trivial the assignment may seem. Perhaps the hours-long pre-op process necessary before a patient is wheeled in to a surgeon might illustrate this analogous process. Essentially, this proposal follows a successive sieves approach suggested years ago (L'Abate, 1990) and now called stepped treatment, starting with the least expensive approach, not involving professional contacts and moving on, when necessary, to the most expensive sieve, talking with a professional f2f.

Of course, this proposal is cognizant of individual differences in participants, as suggested by Harwood, Sulzner, and Beutler (2007). Assignments for internalized disorders, for instance, would be quit different from those for externalizing disorders. The latter were unfortunately left out from the recent review (Kazantzis & L'Abate, 2007), but are included in the work of McMahan (McMahan & Arias, 2004; Reed, McMahan, & L'Abate, 2001). This topic, tailoring assignments to individual personalities, is too important to be dealt with in few sentences. Therefore, it cannot be included here, but the interested reader is referred to the paradigm suggested by Harwood, Sulzner, and Beutler (2007).

This proposal is in line with a view of psychotherapy as a science versus a view of psychotherapy as an art. Consequently, a science is composed of replicable methods rather than variable and non-replicable individual whims or wills of psychotherapists. Homework assignments can be quantified and assessed in their frequency, rate, quality, and replicability. Words are difficult and expensive to quantify and replicate unless manuals are used or tape-recorded for research purposes. However, the use of manuals and tape-recordings is limited to research-orientated academicians rather than to most psychotherapists on Main Street.

If psychotherapists and mental health professionals were to follow a hierarchical organization (Table 20.1), as done in most fields of endeavor, according to levels of education and training and technical specialization, with semi- and para-professional personnel, many of these stages could be administered by this personnel before reaching the full-fledged professional. Instead of accepting directly potential participants for expensive and chancy f2f tb psychotherapy, given the easy availability of a promotional (L'Abate, 2007), a preventive tier (Kazantzis et al., 2005; Kazantzis & L'Abate, 2007) and a psycho-educational tier (De Maria, 2003; Roth & Fonagy, 1996), it is now possible to prescribe the least expensive approach. This approach could be chosen, for instance, by participants themselves from the list given in Chapter 1 of this volume, to see whether they can learn from them on their own.

If participants fail to learn from any promotional approach available to them, or are already involved in one of those approaches but need more help, then perhaps a structured psycho-educational approach may be tried, as in assertiveness training, couples enrichment, parenting groups, or the like. Only after failing to profit by any of these approaches can a participant be admitted to f2f psychotherapy. Even then, seeing a professional should be contingent on participants or intimates completing questionnaires or objective self-information forms or structured interviews in the waiting room (L'Abate, 1986; 1992). Only on completion of these tasks either as homework or in some tasks in the therapist's office, can one be accepted into f2f, talk-based psychotherapy. Even then, participants need to agree to complete in-between sessions practice exercises through signing a written contract (L'Abate, 1986). Under these conditions, if participants are seen f2f without previous task completion, a reversed sieves approach could be implemented to see whether participants can use more than words to work for change in their lives.

Eventually, administration of practice exercises could be based on a gradual increase in spacing between f2f sessions and homework. For instance, one could begin with one hour of homework for one hour of f2f talk-based psychotherapy. Depending on costs, this spacing could increase to two hours of homework for one hour of psychotherapy, going all the way to 3 to 4 hours of homework for one hour of psychotherapy. Ultimately, this homework could occur online without ever seeing or talking with a therapist f2f.

This radical position is justified and supported by the following conceptual arguments and by some empirical evidence. F2f talk is too (1) variable, (2) difficult to control, and (3) even though effective in some ways, inefficient to deal with the mass of mental health problems besetting our nation (L'Abate, 1997b, 1999; New Freedom Foundation, 2003; United States Public Health Service, 1999); (4) expensive and available mainly to participants who can afford it, using just language to solve problems, or have time and energy to spend with professionals.

## Ethical and Professional Issues

This proposal is not free from ethical and professional issues, including among many, requiring the signature of participants after reading and keeping a copy of an informed consent form (L'Abate, 1986, 2001, 2002, 2004a), with caveats to assure that who signs the informed consent form is indeed the person who is receiving the treatment. A thorough developmental/historical background, acquired through a structured interview that also measures levels of psychopathology (L'Abate, 1992) must be a second requirement of all participants, either through the mail, online, or in the therapist's waiting room. Intimates should be included in the treatment or should be fully cognizant of how the process of treatment is taking place. If and when possible, at a minimum, a battery of self-administered, paper-and-pencil tests, such as the Beck Depression Inventory and a screening rating scale (Sajatovic & Ramirez, 2001), would be highly desirable to assess the level of functioning and establish a baseline to evaluate progress and outcome of treatment.

## The Importance of Nonverbal and Psychomotor Activities

The purpose of this section is to provide a rationale for adding and including nonverbal and psychomotor activities to augment positive outcomes in psychotherapy practices (Foulds & Harrington, 1974; De Winter & Drozdek, 2004; Fallon-Cyr & Fallon-Cyr, 2002; Fortini & Tissot, 1997; Hays, 1999; Martinsen, 2005; Penedo & Dahn, 2005; Torres, Mendez, Merino, & Moran, 2002). Interestingly enough, supporting Rosenbaum's (2005) thesis about the neglect of psychomotor activities in psychology, no references about this topic could be found in leading personality psychology treatises. References about non-verbal behavior were found in communication and relationship science (Burgoon, & Bacue, 2003; Wilson, Shi, Tirmestein, Norris, & Rack, 2006). Among the many possible psychomotor therapy programs, Pesso's System/Psychomotor approach seems to have attracted greater attention in the USA and abroad (Howe, 1991; Pesso, 1969, 1973), with some empirical albeit indirect support (Knapen Van der Vliet, Van Coppenolle, David, et al. 2005). Two main issues with these techniques lie in their cost: (1) for how long do they require professional training, and (2) can they occur without professional training after they have been learned to criterion. If professional training is extensive and continuously required for an extended period of time, their advantage of being group-administered and, therefore, relatively cost-effective, may be offset by the length of professional training requited. For instance, I practiced Thai Chi for four years. However, I needed the continuous example and demonstration from a trainer to follow the practice, since the movements required seemed too complicated for me to learn on my own. Apparently the same process took place in other members of the group, since no one left to practice on their own.

The addition of the psychomotor medium should produce synergistically positive effects in the outcome of tb f2f psychotherapy. Some nonverbal activities do not require movement or psychomotor activities, even though instructions and training may be conducted verbally on in writing online, such as relaxation and meditations (McGrady, 2007; Smith, 1985). Nonverbal and psychomotor activities, on the other hand, in addition to those mentioned above, require movement and include pleasant, pleasurable, and positive activities (Anderson, 2007), expressive movement, such as dancing (Dulicai & Schelly Hill, 2007), as well as physical exercise and sports (Calogero & Pedrotty, 2007). These latter are easy to learn, to the point of being self-initiated, last for a life-time, and do not show any negative side-effects.

As Rosenbaum's (2005) argued, human motor behavior has been neglected by psychology and, as L'Abate (1997b, pp. 315-322) maintained, also by psychotherapy. Possibly, the reasons for this neglect are historical, after all psychotherapy started by being based on talk rather than on non-verbal behavior. Consequently, non-verbal and psychomotor behaviors have not been validated as much as talk-based psychotherapy. Furthermore, unless they are administered in groups, nonverbal activities may not be as cost-effective or as age-or gender-appropriate as talk. Non-verbal behavior, supposedly, is reserved for children and not for adults.Yet, there is ample evidence that nonverbal activities do produce lastingly positive effects, as reviewed by the chapters listed above and by the meager evidence also cited above. These activities can be self-taught or are easy to administer and to learn. Therefore, they are inexpensive and cost-effective (L'Abate, 2007c). They can be administered by middle-level professionals or by professionals as homework assignments.

Psychomotor does not mean only one approach, which may have been validated, but it includes also to other activities implicit in play and games (Cartacci, 2006; L'Abate, 2007d). There is plenty of evidence included in a recent volume to indicate that there is a plethora of positive (psychomotor) activities that can be either self administered or administered by others to almost everyone, regardless of age, gender, eduction, and socio-economic status. These approaches have been validated repeatedly, are self-initiated, last for a life-time, and have no negative side-effects (L'Abate, 2007c). They are so inexpensive and so easy to administer and to learn that mental health professionals cannot longer claim ignorance or inability to administer them. Very likely, professionals themselves use them in their own lives, yet they may be loath to require the same of their participants.

## Resistance to Change in the Psychotherapy Profession

As long as f2f talk remains the major or sole medium of communication, the *status quo* in psychotherapy will prevail. It will take an extreme, even iconoclastic position like the one proposed here, to produce controversy, conflict, and possible change in a profession that claims and proclaims to produce change in others but that cannot or will not change its own practices. These changes could allow psychotherapists to help a wider range of populations that need help than would be possible solely through f2f talk.

Given the possibility of synergistic outcomes and possible cost-effectiveness, one needs to ask why additional media, such as distance writing and non-verbal approaches are not included in most psycho-therapeutic practices? A ready answer to this question would focus on training. We rely on our past training and experience and, if both approaches work for us, why change? Is past training sufficient to explain this resistance? It is ironic that a profession dedicated to produce changes in others cannot produce changes in its own practices (L'Abate, 1997a, 1999). The psychotherapy profession is still stuck at the personal f2f tb contact and the personal presence and words of the psychotherapist as the two *sine-qua-non* conditions to produce change in its participants. As a result, no other, possibly even more therapeutic and cost-effective approaches and media, are considered.

As already noted, another issue that has been brought out by De Maria (2003) relates to the fact that more psycho-therapists do not refer their clients to receive different and cheaper alternatives, such as psycho-educational skill training, enrichment programs, or other structured interventions that could benefit participants. This proprietary inclusive control and exclusion of other possibly even more advantageous approaches speaks to the need to educate participants to learn about the availability of less expensive, more specific, and perhaps even more useful alternatives than the presence of a professional and over-reliance on the f2f spoken word.

## Conclusion

The inclusion of writing and non-verbal interventions is an inevitable addition and change in the further differentiation of any discipline, specifically f2f tb psychotherapy, into more and more specific functions. The need to rely on cost-effective methods and approaches will inevitably lead toward professionals working at a distance from participants and to rely more and more on middle-professional and technical-level personnel with greater use of mechanical devises to get the job done. Only in this fashion the profession of clinical psychology will be able to fulfill its mission of the greatest good for most people at the least possible cost.

In an ideal clinical psychology laboratory there would be specialists with various levels of education, interest, and skill. There may be middle-level professions specializing in online interventions (see Appendix A). There may be middle-level professionals specializing in non-verbal approaches. There could be middle-level professionals specializing in group techniques. There may be middle-level professionals specializing with children and their families. Over all these specialties there would be a doctorate level professional to make sure that there is accountability and verifiability in the evaluation of all these interventions on a before-after interventions basis.

## References

Anderson, J. S. (2007). Pleasant, pleasurable, and positive activities. In L. L'Abate (Ed.), *Low-cost approaches to promote physical and mental health: Theory, research, and practice* (pp. 201-217). New York: Springer.

Beck, J. S., & Tompkins, M. A. (2006). Cogniitive therapy. In N. Kazantzis & L. L'Abate (Eds.), *Handbook of homework assignments in psychotherapy: Research, practice, and prevention* (pp. 51-63). New York: Springer Science

Beutler, L. E., Machado, P. P. P., & Allstetter Neufeldt, S. (1994). Therapist variables. In A. E. Begin & S. L. Garfield (Eds.), *Handbook of psychotherapy and behavior change* (pp. 229-269). New York: Wiley.

Bohart, A. C., & Tallman, K. (1999). *How clients make therapy work: The process of active self-healing*. Washington, DC: American Psychological Associaton.

Bongar, B., & Beutler, L. E. (Eds.).(1995). *Comprehensive textbook of psychotherapy: Theory and practice*. New York: Oxford University Press.

Burgoon, J. K. (1994). Nonverbal signals. In M. L. Knapp & G. R. Miller (Eds.), *Handbook of interpersonal communication* (pp. 229-284). Thousand Oaks, CA: Sage

Burgoon, J. K., & Bacue, A. E. (2003). Nonverbal communication skills. In J. O. Greene, & B. R. Burleson (Eds.), *Handbook of communication and social interaction skills* (179-219). Mahwah, NJ: Erlbaum.

Calogero, R., & Pedrotty, K. (2007). Daily practices for mindful exercise. In L. L'Abate (Ed.), *Low-cost approaches to promote physical and mental health: Theory, research, and practice* (pp. 142-160). New York: Springer.

Cartacci, E. (2006). Per una terapia dell'esperienza: Principi e metodi in psicomotricita' (For a therapy of experience: Principles and methods in psychomotricity). *Saggi: Child development & disabilities, 32*, 15-23.

Crumlish, C. (1996). *The Internet for busy people*. Berkeley, CA: Osborne/McGraw -Hill.

Davison, G. C. (2000). Stepped care: Doing more with less? *Journal of Consulting and Clinical Psychology, 68*, 580-585.

DeLuca, J. W. (1988). Neuropsychology technicians in clinical practice: Precedents, rationale, nad current deployment. *The Clinical Neuropsychologist, 3*, 3-21.

DeLuca, J. W., & Putman, S. H. (1993). The professional technician model in clinical neuro-psychology: Deployment characteristics and practice issues. *Professional Psychology: Research and Practice, 24*,100-106.

De Maria, R. (2003). Psychoeducation and enrichment: Clinical considerations for couple and family therapy. In T. L. Sexton, G. R. Weeks, & M. S. Robbins (Eds.). *Handbook of family therapy* (pp.411-430). New York: Brunner/Rutledge.

Demetrio, D., & Borgonovi, C. (2007). Teaching to remember ourselves: The autobiographical methodology. In L. L'Abate (Ed.), *Low-cost approaches to promote psysical and mental health: Theory, research, and practice* (pp. 251-270). New York: Springer Science.

DeVries, H. M. (2006). Older adults. In N. Kazantzis & L. L'Abate (Eds.), *Handbook of homework assignments in psychotherapy: Research, practice, and prevention* (pp. 175-185). New York: Springer Science

DeWinter, B., & Drozdek, B. (2004). Psychomotor therapy: Healing from action. In J. P. Wilson & B. Drozdek (Eds.), *Broken spirits: The treatment of traumatized asylum seekers, refugees, war and torture victims* (pp. 386-402). New York: Brunner/Rutledge.

Dobson, K. S., & Craig, K. D. (Eds.).(1998). *Empirically supported therapies: Best practice in professiona l psychology*. Thosand Oaks, CA: Sage.

Dulicai, D., & Schelly Hill, E. (2007). Expressive movement. In L. L'Abate (Ed.), *Low-cost approaches to promote physical and mental health: Theory, research, and practice* (pp. 177-200). New York: Springer.

Durlack, J. A. (1979). Comparative effectiveness of paraprofessional and professional helpers. *Psychological Bulletin, 86*, 80-92.

Ellison, J. A., & Greenberg, L. S. (2006). Emotion-focused experiental therapy. In N. Kazantzis & L. L'Abate (Eds.), *Handbook of homework assignments in psychotherapy: Research, practice, and prevention* (pp. 65-82). New York: Springer Science

Esterling, B. A., L'Abate, L., Murray, E., & Pennebaker, J. M. (1999). Empirical foundations for writing in prevention and psychotherapy: Mental and physical outcomes. *Clinical Psychology Review, 19*, 79-96.

Esterling, B. A., & Pennebaker, J. M. (2001). Focused expressive writing, immune functions, and physical illness. In L. L'Abate (Ed.), *Distance writing and computer-assisted interventions in psychiatry and mental health* (pp. 47-60). Westport, CT: Ablex.

Fallon-Cyr, M., & Fallon-Cyr, M. (2002). The Halomi method and body-centered

psychotherapies. In S. Shannon (Ed.), *Handbook of complementary and alternative therapies in mental health* (pp. 331-354). San Diego, CA: Academic Press.
Fogg, B. J. (2003). *Persuasive technology: Using computers to change the way we think and do*. San Francisco, CA: Morgan Kaufmann.
Fonagy, P., Target, M., Cottrell, D., Phillips, J., & Kurtz, Z. (2002). *What works for whom? A critical review of treatments for children and adolescents*. New York: Guilford.
Fortini, K., & Tissot, S. (1997). For a typologyof body-mediated therapies. In J. Guimon (Ed.), *The body in psychotherapy* (pp. 94-106). Basel, Switzerland: Karger.
Foulds, M. L., & Harrington, P. B. (1974). Effects of psychomotor group therapy on ratings of self and others. *Psychotherapy: Theory, Research, and Practice, 11*, 351-354.
Gackenbach, J. (Ed.). (1998). *Psychology and the Internet: Intrapersonal, interpersonal, and transpersonal implications*. San Diego, CA: Academic Press.
Gambescia, N., & Weeks, G. (2006). Sexual dysfunction. In N. Kazantzis & L. L'Abate (Eds.), *Handbook of homework assignments in psychotherapy: Research, practice, and prevention* (pp. 351-366). New York: Springer Science
Goldman, N. (1994). *The complete idiot's pocket reference to the Internet*. Indianapolis, IN: Alpha Books.
Gould, R. L. (2001). A feedback-driven computer program for outpatient training. In L. L'Abate (Ed.), *Distance writing and computer-assisted interventions in psychiatry and mental health* (pp. 93-111). Westport, CT: Ablex.
Haaga, D. A (2000). Introduction to the special section on stepped models of psychotherapy. *Journal of Consulting and Clinical Psychology, 68*, 547-548.
Harwood, T. M., Sulzner, J. M., & Beutler, L. E. (2007). Directions of homework in psychotherapy prevention. In N. Kazantzis & L. L'Abate (Eds.), *Handbook of homework assignments in psychotherapy: Research, practice , and prevention* (pp. 445-454). New York: Springer Science
Hays, K. (1999). *Working it out: Using exercise in psychotherapy*. Washington, DC: American Psychological Association.
Howe, L. P. (1991). Origins and history of Pesso System/Psychomotor therapy. In A. Pesso & J. S. Crandell (Eds.), *Moving psychotherapy: Theory and application of Pesso System/Psychomotor therapy* (pp. 3-31). Cambridge, MA: Brookline Books.
Hsiung, R. C. (Ed.). (2002). *E-therapy: Case studies, guiding principles, and the clinical potential of the Internet*. New York: W. W. Norton.
Hubble, M. A., Duncan, B. L., & Miller, S. D. (1999). *The heart & soul of change: What works in therapy*. Washington, DC: American Psychological Association.
Jones, S. G. (Ed.). (1995). *CyberSociety: Computer mediated communication and community*. Thousand Oaks, CA: Sage.
Jordan, K,, & L'Abate, L. (1995). Programmed writing and therapy with symbiotically enmeshed patients. *American Journal of Psychotherapy, 49*, 225-236.
Kacewicz, E., Slatcher, R. B., & Pennebaker, J. W. (2007). Expressive writing: An alternative to traditional methods. In L. L'Abate (Ed.), *Low-cost approaches to promote psysical and mental health: Theory, research, and practice* (pp. 271-284).New York: Springer Science.
Kaufman, G. B. Jr. (1991). Childhood loss and postural insecurity: A thererical and empirical

validation of Pesso system/psychomotor. In A. Pesso & J. S. Crandell (Eds.), *Moving psychotherapy: Theory and application of Pesso System/Psychomotor therapy* (pp. 59-65). Cambridge, MA: Brookline Books.

Kazantzis, N., Deane, F. P., Ronan, K. R. (2000). Homework assignments in cognitive and behavioral therapy: A meta-analysis. *Clinical Psychology: Science & Practice*, *7*, 189-202.

Kazantzis, N., Deane, F. P., Ronan, K. R., & L'Abate, L. (Eds.).(2005). *Using homework assignments in cognitive-behavioral therapy*. New York: Routledge.

Kazantzis, N., & L'Abate L (Eds.).(2007). *Handbook of homework assignments in psychotherapy; Theory, research, and prevention*. New York: Springer Science.

Knapen, J., Van der Vliet, P., Van Coppenolle, H., David, H., el al. (2005). Comparison of changes in physical self-concept, global self-esteem, depression and anxiety following two different psycho-motor therapy programs in nonpsychotic psychiatric patients. *Psychotherapy and Psychosomatics*, *74*, 353-361.

L'Abate, L. (1968). The laboratory method in clinical psychology: An attempt at innovation. *The Clinical Psychologist*, *21*, 182-183,

L'Abate, L. (1977). *Enrichment: Structured interventions with couples, families, and groups*. Washington, DC: University Press of America.

L'Abate, L. (1986). *Systematic family therapy*. New York: Brunner/Mazel.

L'Abate, L. (1990). *Building family competence: Primary and secondary prevention strategies*. Newbury Park, CA: Sage.

L'Abate, L. (1991). The use of writing in psychotherapy. *American Journal of Psychotherapy*, *45*, 87-98.

L'Abate, L. (1992). *Programmed writing: A self-administered approach for interventions with individuals, couples, and families*. Pacific Grove, CA: Brooks/Cole.

L'Abate, L. (1997a). The paradox of change: Better them than us! In R. S. Sauber (Ed.), *Managed mental health care: Major diagnostic and treatment approaches* (pp. 40-66). Bristol, PA: Brunner/ Mazel.

L'Abate L (1996). Workbooks for better living *<www.mentalhealth-help.com>*

L'Abate, L. (1997a). Distance writing and computer-assisted training. In R. S. Sauber (Ed.), *Managed mental health care: Major diagnostic and treatment approaches* (pp. 133-163). Bristol, PA: Brunner/ Mazel.

L'Abate, L. (1997b). *The self in the family: Toward a classification of personality, criminality, and psychopathology*. New York: Wiley.

L'Abate, L, (1999). Taking the bull by the horns: Beyond talk in psychological interventions. *The Family Journal: Therapy and Counseling for Couples and Families*, *7*, 206-220.

L'Abate L (Ed.).(2001). *Distance writing and computer-assisted interventions in psychiatry and mental heath*. Westport, CT: Ablex.

L'Abate, L (2002). *Beyond psychotherapy: Programmed writing and structured computer-assisted interventions*. Westport, CT: Ablex.

L'Abate, L. (2003a). *Family psychology III: Theory building, theory testing, and psychological interventions*. Lanham, MD: University Press of America.

L'Abate, L.. (2003b). Treatment through writing: A unique new direction. In L. Sexton, G. Weeks, & M. Robbins (Eds.), *Handbook of family therapy* (pp. 397-409). New York:

Brunner-Rutledge.

L'Abate L (2004a). *A guide to self-help workbooks for clinicians and researchers.* Binghamton, NY: Haworth.

L'Abate L (Ed.).(2004b).*Using workbooks in mental health; Resources in prevention, psychotherapy, and rehabilitation for clinicians and researchers.* Binghamton, NY: Haworth.

L'Abate, L. (2005). *Personality in intimate relationships: Socialization and psychopathology.* New York: Springer-Science.

L'Abate, L. (2007a). A completely preposterous proposal: The dictionary as vehicle of behavior change in the family. *The Family Psychologist, 23,* 39-42.

L'Abate, L. (2007b). A proposal for including distance writing in couple therapy. *Journal of Relationship and Couple Therapy , vol.* pages..

L'Abate, L. (2007c). (Ed.). *Low-cost approaches to promote physical and mental health: Theory, research, and practice* . New York: Springer.

L'Abate, L. (2007d). *Sourcebook of self-help protocols in mental health.* New York: Springer Science.

L'Abate, L. (2007e). What I really believe about family therapy. *Journal of Family Psychotherapy, 18,* 33-44.

L'Abate, L. (in press). *Handbook of play and playful behavior throughout the life cycle.* Westport, CT: Greenwood.

L'Abate L., & De Giacomo, P. (2003). *Intimate relationships and how to improve them: Integrating theoretical model in prevention and psychotherapy applications.* Westport, CT: Praeger.

L'Abate, L., & Golstein, D. (2007).Workbooks for the promotion of mental health and life-long learning. In L. L'Abate (Ed.), *Low-cost approaches to promote physical and mental health: Theory, research, and practice* (pp.285-302). New York: Springer Science.

L'Abate, L., L'Abate, B. L., & Maino, E. (2005). A review of 25 years of part-time professional practice: Written homework assignments and length of psychotherapy. *American Journal of Family Therapy, 33,* 19-31.

Lambert, M. J., Harmon, S. C., & Slade, K. (2007). Directions for research on homework. In N. Kazantzis & L. L'Abate (Eds.), *Handbook of homework assignments in psychotherapy: Research, practice, and prevention* (pp. 407-422). New York: Springer Science

LeCroy, G. W. (1994). *Handbook of child and adolescent treatment manuals.* New York; Lexington Books.

Ledley, D. R., & Huppert, J. D. (2006). Behavior therapy. In N. Kazantzis & L. L'Abate (Eds.), *Handbook of homework assignments in psychotherapy: Research, practice, and prevention* (pp. 19-32). New York: Springer Science

Lepore, S. J., & Smyth, J. M. (Eds.).(2003). *The writing cure: How expressive writing promotes health and well-being.* Washington, D.C.: American Psychological Association.

Levine, M., & Calvanio, R.(2007). The recording of personal information as an intervention and as an electronic health support. In L. L'Abate, (Ed.), *Low-cost approaches to promote physical and mental health: Theory, research, and practice* (pp. 227-250). New

York: Springer-Verlag.

Lindenboim, N., Chapman, A. L., & Linehan, M. M. (2007). Borderline personality disorder. In N. Kazantzis & L. L'Abate (Eds.), *Handbook of homework assignments in psychotherapy: Research, practice, and prevention* (pp. 227-245). New York: Springer Science

Luborsky, L., Critss-Christoph, P., Mintz, J., & Auerbach, A. (1988). *Who will benefit by psychotherapy? Predicting therapeutic outcomes*. New York: Basic Books.

Maheu, M. M., Pulier, M. L., Wilhelm, F. H., McMenamin, J. P., & Brown-Connolly, N. E. (2004).*The mental health professional and the new technologies: A handbook for practice today*. Mahwah, NJ: Erlbaum.

Maheu, M. M., Whitten, P., & Allen, A. (2001). *E-health, telehealth, and telemedicine: A guide to start-up and success*. San Francisco, CA: Jossey-Bass.

Maloy, T. K. (1996). *The Internet research guide*. New York: Allworth Press.

Martinsen, E. W. (2005). Exercise and depression. *International Journal of Sport and Exercise Psychology,* 3, 469-483.

Marusich, C., & Blackthorn, S. (1998). *Internet commerce for dummies*. Foster City, CA: IDG Books.

McGrady, A. (2007). Relaxation and meditation. In L. L'Abate (Ed.), *Low-cost approaches to promote physical and mental health: Theory, research, and practice* (pp. 161-176). New York: Springer.

McGuire, M., Stillborne, L., McAdams, M., & Hyatt, L. (2001). *The Internet handbook for writers, researchers, and journalists*. New York: Guilford.

Meier, M. J. (1992). Modern clinical neuropsychology in historical perspective. *American Psychologist*, 47, 550-558.

Morrison, M. R., & Stamps, R. F. (1998). *DSM-IV Internet companion: A complete guide to over 1500 web sites offering information on mental health, keyed to DSM-IV*. New York: W. W. Norton.

Nathan, P. E., & Gorman, J. M. (Eds.).(2002). *A guide to treatments that work*. New York: Oxford University Press.

Neimeyer, R. A., & Winter, D. A. (2006). Personal construct therapy. In N. Kazantzis & L. L'Abate (Eds.), *Handbook of homework assignments in psychotherapy: Research, practice, and prevention* (pp. 151-170). New York: Springer Science

Nelson, D. L., Castonguay, L. G., & Barwick, F. (2007). In N. Kazantzis & L. L'Abate (Eds.), *Handbook of homework assignments in psychotherapy: Research, practice, and prevention* (pp. 425-441). New York: Springer Science

New Freedom Commission on Mental Health (2003). *Achieving the promise: Transforming mental healthcare in America: Executive summary*. Rockville, MD: DHHS Publication No. SMA-03-3831.

Newman, M. G. (2000). Recommendations for a cost-effective model of psychotherapy allocation using generalized anxiety disorder as an example. *Journal of Consulting and Clinical Psychology, 68*, 549-555.

Norcross, J. C. (Ed.).(1986). *Handbook of eclectic psychotherapy*. New York: Brunner/Mazel.

Norcross, J. C., & Goldfried, M. R. (Eds.).(1992). *Handbook of psychotherapy integration.*

New York: Basic Books.
Otto, M. W., Pollack, M. H., & Maki, K. M. (2000). Empirically supported treatments for panic disorder: Costs, benefits, and stepped care. *Journal of Consulting and Clinical Psychology, 68*, 556-563.
Penedo, E. J., & Dahn, J. R. (2005). Exercise and well-being: A review of mental and physical activity. *Current Opinion in Psychiatry, 18*, 189-193.
Pennebaker, J. M. (2001). Explorations into the health benefits of disclosure: Inhibitory, cognitive, and social processes. In L. L'Abate (Ed.), *Distance writing and computer assisted interventions in psychiatry and mental health* (pp. 34-44). Westport, CT: Ablex.
Pesso, A. (1969). *Movement in psychotherapy*. New York: New York University Press.
Pesso, A. (1973). *Experience in action: A psychomotor psychology*. New York: New York University Press.
Pulier, M., Mount, T., McMenamin, J., & Maheu, M. (2007). Computers and the Internet. In L. L'Abate (Ed.), *Low-cost approaches to promote physical and mental health: Theory, research, and practice* (pp. 303-319). New York: Springer.
Robiner, W. N. (2006). The mental health professions: Workforce supply and demand issues and challenges. *Clinical Psychology Review, 26*, 600-625.
Rogers, C. R. (1980). *A way of being*. Boston, MA: Houghton Mifflin.
Rosenbaum, D. A. (2005). The Cinderella of psychology: The neglect of motor control in the science of mental life and behavior. *American Psychologist, 60*, 308-317.
Roth, A., & Fonagy, P. (1996). *What works for whom? A critical review of psychotherapy research*. New York: Guildford.
Sadowski, A., Campbell Koella, J., & Keene, M. (2001). *The Mayfield quick view guide to the internet for students of psychology and the research in progress*. Mountain View, CA: Mayfield.
Safran, J. D., & Muran, J. C. (Eds.).(1995). *The therapeutic alliance*. New York: Wiley.
Sajatovic, M., & Ramirez, L. F. (2001). *Rating scales in mental health*. Hudson, OH: Lexi-Comp Inc.
Schwartz, M. D. (Ed.). (1984). *Using computers in clinical practice: Psychotherapy and mental health applications*. New York: Haworth.
Seligman, M. E. P., Steen, T. A., Park, N., & Peterson, C. (2005). Positive psychology progress: Empirical validity of approaches. *American Psychologist, 60*, 410-421.
Smith, J. C. (1985). *Relaxation dynamics*. Champaign, IL: Research Press.
Smyth, J., & L'Abate, L. (2001). A meta-analytic evaluation of workbook effectiveness in physical and mental health. In L. L'Abate (Ed.), *Distance writing and computer-assisted interventions in psychiatry and mental heath* (pp. 77-90). Westport, CT: Ablex.
Snowden, S. (2001). *Aging with grace: What the nun study teaches us about leading longer, healthier, and more meaningful lives*. New York: Bantam Books.
Snyder, C. R., & Ingram, R. E. (Eds.).(2000). *Handbook of psychological change: Psychotherapy processes & practices in the 2ist century*. New York: Wiley.
Sperry, L., Brill, P. L., Howard, K. I., & Grissom, G. R. (1996).*Treatment outcomes in psychotherapy and psychiatric interventions*. New York: Brunner/Mazel.
Sobell, M. B., & Sobell, L. C. (2000). Stepped help as a heuristic approach to the treatment of alcohol problems. *Journal of Consulting and Clinical Psychology, 68*, 573-589.

Strecher, V. (2007). Internet methods for delivering behavioral and health-related interventions (eHealth). *Annual Review of Clinical Psychology, 3*, 53-76.

Stricker, G. (2007). Psychodynamic therapy. In N. Kazantzis & L. L'Abate (Eds.), *Handbook of homework assignments in psychotherapy: Research, practice, and prevention* (pp. 101-111). New York: Springer Science

Thomas, J. L., & Cummings, J. L. (Eds.). (2000). *The collected papers of Nicholas A. Cummings: The value of psychological treatment.* Phoenix, AZ: Zeig, Tucker & Company.

Tompkins, M. A. (2004). *Using homework in psychotherapy: Strategies, guidelines, and forms.* New York: Guilford.

Torres, A., Mendez, L. F., Merino, H., & Moran, E. A. (2002). Rehab rounds: Improving social functioning in schizophrenia by playing The Train game. *Psychiatric Services, 53*, 799-801.

Twohig, M. P., Pierson, H. M., & Hayes, S. C. (2007). Acceptance and commitment therapy. In N. Kazantzis & L. L'Abate (Eds.), *Handbook of homework assignments in psychotherapy: Research, practice, and prevention* (pp. 113-130). New York: Springer Science

United States Public Health Service (1999). *Mental health: A report of the Surgeon General.* Rockville, MD: Department of Health and Human Services.

Van Hasselt, V. B., & Hersen, M. (Eds.).(1998). *Sourcebook of psychological treatement manuals for adult disorders.* New York: Lexington Books.

Wilson, G. T., Vitousek, K. M., & Loeb, K. L. (2000). Stepped care treatment for eating disorders. *Journal of Consulting and Clinical Psychology, 68*, 564-572.

Wilson, S. R., Shi, X., Tirmenstein, L., Norris, A., & Rack, J. J. (2006). Parental physical negative touch and child noncompliance in abusive, neglectful, and comparison families: A meta-analysis of observational studies. In L. H. Turner & R. West (Eds.), *The family communication sourcebook* (pp. 237-257). Thousand Oaks, CA: Sage.

Witty, M. C. (2007). Client-centered therapy. In N. Kazantzis & L. L'Abate (Eds.), *Handbook of homework assignments in psychotherapy: Research, practice, and prevention* (pp. 85-99). New York: Springer Science

Young, J. F., & Mufson, L. (2007). Interpersonal psychotherapy. In N. Kazantzis & L. L'Abate (Eds.), *Handbook of homework assignments in psychotherapy: Research, practice, and prevention* (pp. 51-63). New York: Springer Science

Zeig, J. K. (Ed.).(1997). *The evolution of psychotherapy: The third conference.* New York: Brunner/Mazel.

In: Toward a Science of Clinical Psychology
Editor: Luciano L'Abate, pp. 385-392
ISBN: 978-1-60456-062-6


*Appendix*

# PROPOSED CURRICULUM FOR A DIPLOMA OR GRADUATE DEGREE IN "STRUCTURED ONLINE MENTAL HEALTH INTERVENTIONS"

***Luciano L'Abate***

The purpose of this proposal is to present for discussion and elaboration a graduate curriculum based strictly on structured online mental health interventions administered through distance writing rather than face-to-face (F2f) talk.

## RATIONALE FOR PROPOSED CURRICULUM

The last 20 years have seen the proliferation of various types of writing that can be used to promote mental health and prevent mental illness through the Internet, discussed in Chapter 19 of this volume (Lange, Rietdijk, Hudcovicova, van de Ven, et al., 2003; Pulier et al., 2006; Ritterband, Cox, Walker, Kovatchev, et al., 2003; Ritterband, Gonder-Frederick, Cox, Clifton, et al., 2003). Most types of writing have not been used or have been mostly underused by the mental health professions. A recent survey with a sample of psychotherapists, for instance, indicated that that is indeed the case. Responses to how frequently these structured interventions are used in psychotherapy ranged from a complete rejections to their use by a strong representative of the existential psychotherapy school to a non-systematic, occasional, and sporadic use of writing interventions in cognitive-behavioral school.

Seemingly, the psychotherapeutic professions prefer talk to writing, in spite of the shortcomings of talk over writing (L'Abate, 1999; L'Abate, 2005). As far as this writer knows, there is no formal coursework in the area of "*Structured Distance Writing or Structured Mental Health Interventions Online*." Of course, it takes more than one course to learn what is and could, in the future, become a specialty area in its own rights. Hence, this proposal takes into consideration the possible structured types of distance writing that could be used to promote mental health and prevent mental illness online.

The term "Structured" means that instead of mimicking unstructured talk therapies online, which require a professional license and advanced expertise (Kraus, Zack, & Stricker, 2005), in this case "structured" means using distance writing approaches that involve a finite number of possibilities included in this proposed curriculum. This curriculum, therefore, would fall within the provinces of *health promotion* and of *primary prevention* to be administered to functional or semi-functional rather than only dysfunctional populations. This proposed curriculum is not intended to produce second class therapists. It is intended to train specialists in a specific type of online interventions, that is: structured. Furthermore, the vast impact that computers have had socially, economically, medically, and professionally (Pulier et al., 2007; Rosenberg, 2005), indicates that new specialties will be necessary to work with computers to deliver services in health promotion and disease prevention through the Internet.

Nonetheless, the enthusiasm possibly provoked by this proposal is tempered by objections that some psychotherapists may have about a curriculum and coursework advocated here. George Stricker, for instance, a well known psychotherapist in academic circles, made these comments (personal communication, November 7, 20005):

> "Very interesting. I have some concerns, as you might suspect, both about the curriculum and about the trainees. In terms of the curriculum, it seems fine, and between you and Pennebaker, there is some support for doing what you propose. However, I'm not sure how you can limit the extent of the services offered, and I'd be afraid that more pathological people could wander into chat rooms (or wherever) looking for help, and the trainees would be over their heads. I've seen message boards with suicidal threats and such, and I don't see how these trainees would be prepared to deal with that.
>
> As far as the trainees are concerned, if they can't be licensed, I don't know why they would choose this field, and there would be an enormous economic temptation to overstep the boundaries of their competence. I do like the internet as a medium of help, and have no problem with self-help activities. I do have some similar concerns about licensed professionals offering services that may be beyond their competence to who knows who is on the other end, and with unclear licensing requirements because of the lack of definition of how far a license extends. I'm sure I don't have to add anything about the need to maintain good data collection, because you would do that anyway. Good luck with a fascinating project."

The concerns expressed by Dr. Stricker are quite valid. This is why two courses address those concerns directly. One course covers ethical and professional issues that define responsibilities and limitations of what trainees can do, even though restrictions to their practice will come from state and federal laws. A second course covers evaluation, to screen out those very individuals, couples, or families that would not benefit by online interventions because of their disturbed or troubled state. A third precaution has been added to the courses on workbooks or protocols, and that is: trainees will experience only "normative" workbooks rather than workbooks dealing with clinical or pathological conditions. In spite of this precaution, however, nothing will prevent trainees to eventually use whatever workbooks are available to anyone on the market. Indeed, by the same token, anyone, including lay-persons can buy and use those workbooks without restrictions.

At least, the trainees in this curriculum will be informed about the possible dangers and costs of overstepping their functions. A fourth precaution consists of requiring a Signed Informed Consent Form from the trainees themselves, since all the coursework in this curriculum will involve a great deal of self-disclosure and revelation. Trainees, in turn will eventually learn to use the same Informed Consent Form from all their participants. A fifth precaution will be built in training trainees to operate within the ethical and professional bounds of their specialty, with their knowing full well that offering or providing unstructured interventions, that is, talk-based psychotherapy, would be not only unethical and unprofessional, but would also risk of being treated as criminals by going outside of their knowledge and training, that is: practicing psychology without a license. Sixth, trainees are required to take one course on personality theories and a second course on abnormal psychology to become acquainted with existing psychopathologies. Trainees will be trained on how to refer to relevant mental health services, potential participants (individuals, couples, or families) who are too deviant, distressed, or troubled to be treated with structured online interventions alone and who could not benefit by those interventions.

The staggering statistics about the large numbers of untreated but dysfunctional individuals, couples, and families, reported in L'Abate (2007), plus the reports of the Surgeon General (1999) and the President's New Freedom Commission on Mental Health (2003), indicate the need for the creation of specialists who will be able to deal with functional or semi-functional populations to decrease the burden put on existing mental health facilities by many overwhelming dysfunctionalities and ever increasing mental health needs. This proposal, therefore, indicates one way to deal with large populations of less troubled people. Between those who do need professional, face-to-face talk and/or medication and those who do not need professional help, there are those who might not need expensive interventions, but who could use interventions directed toward promoting healthier solutions to their problems decreasing the intensity of problems that, left unattended, may exacerbate into full-blown disorders.

According to both reports, promotion of physical and mental health as well as prevention of mental health illness have not even been attempted for a variety of issues. One issue includes the creation of specialties trained to deal effectively in both promotion and prevention, areas, either directly or indirectly by assisting existing mental health professions to deal with as many functional and semi-functional populations who avoid existing mental health facilities but who could profit by working on their problems in the privacy of their homes. The American Psychological Association (2005) developed three categories for the potential need of practice guidelines: (a) legal and regulatory, (b) public benefit, and (c) professional guidance. Relevant to this proposal is public benefit where an improved service delivery may reach emerging underserved or vulnerable client populations. Without denying the need for laws, court decisions and changes in regulatory and administrative systems, professional guidance includes the development of new technology, as included in this proposal.

If costs are an issue in the delivery of mental health services, as indicated above, any innovation that would reduce costs should be relevant. In this case, this curriculum would allow specialists from this program help deliver low-cost online interventions that could be added to existing, expensive, traditional face-to-face talk-based interventions, either on their own or in addition to those traditional practices.

## Goal

Therefore, the goal of this proposed curriculum is to create a new, ancillary, middle-level specialty of individuals who can add to the promotion of physical and mental health, by helping to prevent mental illness, and supplement additionally or alternatively the work of existing mental health professionals. By offering structured (rather than unstructured) distance writing online interventions, different from talk-based face-to-face psychotherapy, they would offer a larger spectrum of options already available. As far as this writer knows, most of the online procedures contained in the suggested coursework offered in this curriculum are not used by most mental health professionals.

Potential trainees for this curriculum could include college graduates who are looking for an innovative, challenging curriculum that will allow them to work in ancillary positions in the mental health field, either from home or in other mental health settings. Specialists graduating from this curriculum could work in group private practice settings as well as in mental health clinics, hospitals, and correctional institutions to aid existing mental health professions by adding structured online interventions. These interventions could be delivered either before participants have to move on to more expensive treatments, such as f2f talk-based psychotherapy, during other treatments, like medication, as well as follow-up to such treatments, either promotionally, preventively, or rehabilitatively. These specialists could also participate in helping populations that are underserved or not served by most private and public institutions, namely: shut-ins, handicapped, and less disturbed individuals, couples, and families who could accept less threatening and less expensive approaches that do not require face-to-face, unstructured talk (Hahm & Segal, 2005).

Proposing a completely new mental health specialty is fraught with many legal, conceptual, and professional dangers that can be barely addressed here. For instance, how are graduates from this program going to be hired by professions or professionals who may perceive distance learning as a threat to their livelihood and to the status quo in the mental health field? In spite of demonstrating the usefulness of gathering information that is crucial for reaching a diagnosis and a treatment plan, like autobiographies and diaries and journals, it will take more than this argument to change negative perceptions about distance learning when a perceived threat is involved. No matter how much research could be included to supports the use of the Internet in the actual promotion, prevention, therapy, and rehabilitation of many disorders (Lange, Rietdijk, Hudcovicova, van de Ven et al., 2003: Pullier et al., 2007), the issue is not a rational one. Threats to established practices are inherent in creating a completely novel specialty. Much more thought will need to be given about whether many of these issues are real or perceived based on fears rather than on reality. The issue, then, is whether change should be avoided because of fears or because of the reality facing us, as the information given by the Institutes of Drug Abuse about the incidence of mental illness in the USA (L'Abate, 2007). This proposal, therefore, is based on that reality, being aware of the very real possible and potential dangers that such innovation may provoke.

Two of the many hurdles that an innovative proposal of this kind has to confront is (1) recruiting competent faculty members willing to instruct trainees online, and (2) securing jobs for its graduates. This is the reason for submitting this proposal for publication, and that is: to receive feedback from knowledgeable colleagues in the field of cyber-communication, psychotherapy, and clinical psychology.

Consequently, on the basis of the foregoing statements and other considerations (L'Abate, 2007), the following online coursework is proposed:

## Requirements to Enter Graduate Coursework

1. A Bachelor Degree or its equivalent from an approved institution.
2. Knowledge of Internet technology necessary to conduct online structured interventions.
3. Passing an undergraduate or graduate introductory course on tests and measurements to understand and be familiar with test construction and basic statistical concepts of test validity and reliability.
4. Passing an undergraduate or graduate course on personality and personality theories.
5. Passing an undergraduate or graduate course on abnormal psychology or psychopathology.
6. (Optional). Passing an undergraduate or graduate course in developmental psychology.

## First Semester Coursework

901. *Online Evaluation of Possible Participants*: This course includes taking a structured self-information form, and a battery of self-report tests available online (L'Abate, 1996) as well as another self-report instrument of the student's choice. In addition to such tests showing a modicum of statistical validity and reliability requirements for such a test-battery would be: (1) easy to administer; (2) easy to score; (3) theory-driven or -related; (4) relational rather than intrapsychic; and (5) available at various chronological ages (L'Abate, 1996; L'Abate & Cusinato, 2007). A report on the validity and reliability of these instruments is required. This course will also serve as an introduction to issues of Informed Consent by trainees themselves signing an Informed Consent Form for self-disclosures, not only for use in this course but also for future courses included in this curriculum that require a certain amount of self-disclosure from trainees.

902. *Ethics and Professional Issues in Online Interventions*. Trainees will be required to write a paper based on a review of the literature about the ethical and professional issues facing structured online interventions as well as the differences between structured and unstructured only face-to-face and talk-based interventions, their advantages and disadvantages. Possible textbook: (Kazantzis & L'Abate, 2007).

903. *Introduction to Self-help Mental Health Workbooks or Protocols*: This course will familiarize the student with the plethora of self-help mental health workbooks

available in print and online. In addition to readings, reported in book reviews, each student will have to complete one workbook of their choice available commercially (L'Abate, 2007b). In addition, trainees will be required to write book reports and pass an objective test to prove passing knowledge of required readings. Possible Textbooks: L'Abate (2001, 2002, 2007b).

## Second Semester Coursework

904. *Autobiography* as a way to help people as well as trainees deal with their *pasts*. Trainees will be required to search the literature for works available in print and online and will have to write their own autobiography with references to relevant publications on autobiography.
905. *Journaling and Diaries* to help people deal with their *presents*. Trainees will be required to search the literature for research works available in print and online and write a paper on the subject. They will have to work on their own journal or diary for at least three months and show the work they have done. This part can be fulfilled by completing an online course on personal information.
906. *Advanced Course on Self-help Mental Health Workbooks*: This course will review in greater depth the vast field of self-help mental health workbooks available on the market and online. Trainees will be required to complete a workbook of their choice, write two book reports on the two textbooks, and pass an objective test to prove passing knowledge of required readings. Possible Textbooks: L'Abate (2004a, 2004b, 2007b).

## Third Semester Coursework

907. *Expressive writing, i.e., Pennebaker's paradigm.* This course requires completion of a test battery, as completed in course No. 1, book report on the textbook, completion of a course of expressive writing, and a paper with a review of the literature on expressive writing with references not contained in the textbook. Textbook: Lepore and Smyth (2002)
908. *Applications of Self-help Mental Health Workbooks to Children, Couples, and Families.* In this course, trainees will be required to evaluate on a pre-post-workbook administration basis, three children, three couples, and three families, administering to them appropriate workbooks.
909. *Seminar on Additional Structured Interventions*; Represented among the many by Seligman's et al., (2005).

## Fourth Semester

*Thesis*: Proof of a completed program of Structured Online Mental Health Interventions with a class of participants (middle school, high school, college trainees, groups of volunteer couples or families) complete with pre-and post-intervention testing.

# REFERENCES


American Psychological Association (2005). Determination and documentation of the need for practice guidelines. *American Psychologist, 60*, 976-978.

Hahm, H. C., & Segal, S. P. (2005). Failure to seek health care among the mentally ill. *American Journal of Orthopsychiatry, 75*, 54-62.

Kraus, R., Zack, J., & Stricker, G. (2005). *Online counseling: A handbook for mental health professionals*. Mahwah, NJ: Erlbaum.

L'Abate, L. (1996). Workbooks for Better Living <*www.mentalhealthhelp.*com>

L'Abate, L. (1999). Taking the bull by the horns: Beyond talk in psychological interventions. *The Family Journal: Therapy and Counseling for Couples and Families, 7*, 206-220.

L'Abate, L. (Ed.).(2001). Distance writing and computer-assisted interventions in psychiatry and mental heath. Westport, CT: Ablex.

L'Abate, L. (2002). Beyond psychotherapy: Programmed writing and structured computer-assisted interventions. Westport, CTî Ablex.

L'Abate, L. (2004a). A guide to self-help workbooks for clinicians and researchers. Binghamton, NY: Haworth.

L'Abate, L. Ed.).(2004b), Using workbooks in mental health: Resources in prevention, psycho-therapy,, and rehabilitation for clinicians and researchers . Binghamton, NY: Haworth.

L'Abate, L. (2007a). Low-cost approaches to promote physical and mental health. In L. L'Abate (Ed.). *Low-cost interventions to promote physical and mental health: Theory, research, and practice* (pp. 3-48). New York: Springer.

L'Abate, L. (2007b). Sourcebook of self-help protocols in mental health. New York: Springer.

L'Abate, L., & Cusinato, M. (2007). Linking theory with practice: Theory-derived interventions in prevention and family therapy. *The Family Journal:Counseling and Therapy for Couples and Families, 15,* 318-327.

Lange, A., Rietdijk, D., Hudcovicova, M., van de Ven, J., et al. (2003). Interapy: A controlled randomized trial of the standardized treatment of posttraumatic stress through the internet. *Journal of Consulting & Clinical Psychology, 71*, 901-909.

Lepore, S. J. & Smyth, J. M. (Eds,),(2002) *The writing cure: How expressive writing promotes health and well-being* Washington, DC: American Psychological Association.

New Freedom Commission on Mental Health (2003). *Achieving the promise: Transforming mental healthcare in America: Executive summary*. Rockville, MD: DHHS Publication No. SMA- 03-3831.

Pulier, M., Mount, T., McMenamin, & Maheu, M. (2006). Computers and the Internet. In L. L'Abate (Ed.), *Low-cost interventions to promote physical and mental health: Theory, research, and practice* (pp. 000-000). New York: Springer.

Ritterband, L. M., Cox, D. J., Walker, L. S., Kovatchev, B., et al. (2003). An Internet intervention as adjunctive therapy for pediatric encopresis. *Journal of Consulting & Clinical Psychology, 71*, 910- 917.

Ritterband, L. M., Gonder-Frederick, L. A., Cox, D. J., Cliftorn, A. D., et al. (2003). Internet interventions: In review, in use, and into the future. *Professional Psychology: Research & Practice*, *34*, 527-534.

Rosenberg, R. S. (2005). *The social impact of computers*. Third Edition. Mahwah, NJ: Erlbaum.

Seligman, M. E. P., Steen, T. A., Park, N., & Peterson, C. (2005). Positive psychology progress: Empirical validation of interventions. *American Psychologist*, *60*, 410-421.

United States Public Health Service Office of the Surgeon General (1999). *Mental health: A report of the Surgeon General*. Rockville, MD: Department of Health and Human Services.

# INDEX

## A

## B

## C

## D

## E

## F



## G

## H



## I

## J



## K



## L



## M

## N



## O

## Q



## R

## S

## T

## Y



## Z